Male and Sperm Factors that Maximize IVF Success

Male and Sperm Factors that Maximize IVF Success

Edited by

R. John Aitken
University of Newcastle, New South Wales

David Mortimer
Oozoa Biomedical Inc., Vancouver

Gabor T. Kovacs
Epworth HealthCare, Melbourne

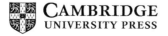

CAMBRIDGE UNIVERSITY PRESS

CAMBRIDGE
UNIVERSITY PRESS

University Printing House, Cambridge CB2 8BS, United Kingdom

One Liberty Plaza, 20th Floor, New York, NY 10006, USA

477 Williamstown Road, Port Melbourne, VIC 3207, Australia

314–321, 3rd Floor, Plot 3, Splendor Forum, Jasola District Centre, New Delhi – 110025, India

79 Anson Road, #06–04/06, Singapore 079906

Cambridge University Press is part of the University of Cambridge.

It furthers the University's mission by disseminating knowledge in the pursuit of education, learning, and research at the highest international levels of excellence.

www.cambridge.org
Information on this title: www.cambridge.org/9781108708319
DOI: 10.1017/9781108762571

First published 2020

Printed in the United Kingdom by TJ International Ltd, Padstow Cornwall

A catalogue record for this publication is available from the British Library.

ISBN 978-1-108-70831-9 Paperback

Cambridge University Press has no responsibility for the persistence or accuracy of URLs for external or third-party internet websites referred to in this publication and does not guarantee that any content on such websites is, or will remain, accurate or appropriate.

Every effort has been made in preparing this book to provide accurate and up-to-date information that is in accord with accepted standards and practice at the time of publication. Although case histories are drawn from actual cases, every effort has been made to disguise the identities of the individuals involved. Nevertheless, the authors, editors, and publishers can make no warranties that the information contained herein is totally free from error, not least because clinical standards are constantly changing through research and regulation. The authors, editors, and publishers therefore disclaim all liability for direct or consequential damages resulting from the use of material contained in this book. Readers are strongly advised to pay careful attention to information provided by the manufacturer of any drugs or equipment that they plan to use.

Contents

Contributors

Ahmad Aboukhshaba
Weill Cornell Medicine, Department of
Urology, New York, NY, USA

Rachel Agnew
Reproductive and Developmental
Biology, Division of Systems
Medicine, School of Medicine,
Ninewells Hospital and
Medical School, University of Dundee,
Dundee, UK

R. John Aitken
Priority Research Centre for
Reproductive Science, University of
Newcastle, Callaghan, NSW
Australia

Christopher L. R. Barratt
Reproductive and Developmental
Biology, Division of Systems Medicine,
School of Medicine, Ninewells Hospital
and Medical School, University of Dundee,
Dundee, UK

Elizabeth G. Bromfield
The University of Newcastle
Priority Research Centre for Reproductive
Science, School of Environmental
and Life Sciences, University of
Newcastle, Callaghan, NSW
Australia

Douglas T. Carrell
Surgery and Human Genetics, University
of Utah School of Medicine, Salt Lake City,
UT, USA

Gary N. Clarke
Andrology Unit, Royal Women's & Royal
Children's Hospitals, Melbourne, Victoria,
Australia

Michael Davies
Professor, The Robinson Research
Institute, University of Adelaide, South
Australia, Australia

Alberto Ferlin
Department of Clinical and Experimental
Sciences, Unit of Endocrinology and
Metabolism, University of Brescia, Brescia,
Italy

Javier González García
Urology Service University General
Hospital Gregorio Marañón, Madrid,
Spain

Russell P. Hayden
Weill Cornell Medicine, Department of
Urology, New York, NY, USA

Eleanor Heighton
Reproductive and Developmental
Biology, Division of Systems Medicine,
School of Medicine, Ninewells Hospital
and Medical School, University of Dundee,
Dundee, UK

Carlos Hernández-Fernández
Urology Service, University General
Hospital Gregorio Marañón and
Department of Surgery, Complutense
University of Madrid, Madrid, Spain

Emma R. James
Andrology and IVF Laboratories,
Department of Surgery, University of Utah
School of Medicine, Salt Lake City, UT, USA

José Jara-Rascón
Urology Service, University General
Hospital Gregorio Marañón and
Department of Surgery, Complutense
University of Madrid, Madrid, Spain

Shannon Hee Kyung Kim
University of New South Wales, Royal
Hospital for Women, Randwick, and IVF
Australia, Sydney, NSW, Australia

Gabor T. Kovacs
Monash University, Clayton, and Epworth
HealthCare, Richmond, Victoria, Australia

Csilla Krausz
Department of Biomedical,
Experimental and Clinical Sciences
"Mario Serio," University of Florence,
Florence, Italy

Enrique Lledó García
Department of Urology, University
General Hospital Gregorio Marañón,
Madrid, Spain and Complutense
University of Madrid, Madrid, Spain

Elena Martínez Holguín
Urology Service, University General
Hospital Gregorio Marañón, Madrid, Spain

Sarah Martins da Silva
Reproductive Medicine, Ninewells
Hospital and Medical School, University of
Dundee, Dundee, UK

David Mortimer
Oozoa Biomedical Inc., West
Vancouver, BC, Canada

Sharon T. Mortimer
Oozoa Biomedical Inc., West Vancouver
and Adjunct Professor, Division of
Endocrinology and Infertility,
Department of Obstetrics and
Gynaecology, Faculty of Medicine,
University of British Columbia,
Vancouver, BC, Canada

Victoria Nisenblat
Robinson Research Institute, School of
Medicine Department O&G, University of
Adelaide, Adelaide, Australia

Brett Nixon
Priority Research Centre for Reproductive
Science, School of Environmental and Life
Sciences, University of Newcastle,
Callaghan NSW, Australia, and Hunter
Medical Research Institute, New Lambton
Heights, NSW, Australia

Willem Ombelet
Genk Institute for Fertility Technology,
Department of Obstetrics and
Gynaecology, Genk and Hasselt
University, Department of Physiology,
Hasselt, Belgium

Allan Pacey
Department of Oncology and Metabolism,
University of Sheffield, Sheffield, UK

Ángel Rebollo Román
Unit of Clinical Management,
Endocrinology and Nutrition, Reina Sofía
University Hospital, Córdoba, Spain

Viktória Rosta
Department of Biomedical, Experimental
and Clinical Sciences "Mario Serio,"
University of Florence, Florence, Italy

Albert Salas-Huetos
Andrology and IVF Laboratories,
Department of Surgery, University of Utah
School of Medicine, Salt Lake City, UT,
USA

Viviane Santana
Andrology and IVF Laboratories,
Department of Surgery, University of
Utah School of Medicine, Salt Lake City,
UT, USA and Department of Gynecology
and Obstetrics, Ribeirao Preto Medical
School, University of Sao Paulo, Sao
Paulo, Brazil

Peter N. Schlegel
E. Darracott Vaughan Senior Associate
Dean for Clinical Affairs, Weill Cornell
Medicine, Urologist-in-Chief, New York
Presbyterian/Weill Cornell, New York,
NY, USA

Ciara Wright
Glenville Nutrition Ireland, Rathgar,
Dublin, Ireland

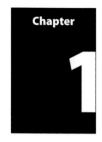

Chapter

Sperm Selection for ART Success

R. John Aitken

1.1 Introduction

One of the great challenges in assisted conception is to ensure that only the highest quality gametes are selected for fertilization. This is necessary not only to optimize the chances of successful conception but also to ensure the normality of any offspring generated as a consequence. In our species, around 200 million spermatozoa are normally released into the female reproductive tract at insemination and, in the journey that follows, all but a small minority of these cells will perish. The subpopulation of spermatozoa that reaches the surface of the oocyte in the ampullary region of the fallopian tubes *in vivo* is therefore highly selected. The selection process appears to be dependent on the intrinsic motility of the spermatozoa and their capacity to evade detection by the host's immune system. The outcome is to select spermatozoa that are highly motile, are morphologically normal and exhibit a clear ability to express all of the features of a capacitated cell, including hyper-activation and the ordered expression of receptors on the sperm surface for the zona pellucida. The selected spermatozoa are also characterized by high levels of DNA integrity, as befits a cell charged with the responsibility of transferring an intact paternal genome onto the next generation [1].

Sperm selection *in vivo* is an extremely sophisticated process involving changes in the pattern of motility, the creation of isthmic reservoirs, chemotaxis, thermotaxis, rheotaxis, complex interactions with the extracellular matrix and changes in the sperm surface expression of receptors and proteases. In the context of assisted reproductive technology (ART), an important aim is to replicate this complex sperm selection cascade, so that gametes selected *in vitro* for the purpose of fertilization will reflect those selected *in vivo*. This selection process is particularly important in the context of intracytoplasmic sperm injection (ICSI), which involves the physical injection of an individual spermatozoon into the ooplasm of the egg. This procedure is particularly forgiving of defects in sperm quality, with the result that even severely damaged spermatozoa possessing high levels of DNA damage can still achieve fertilization, if ICSI is used as the insemination protocol [2]. With IVF, the situation is less critical because the zona pellucida itself acts as a filter that will exclude any spermatozoon that does not possess the qualities of movement needed to achieve penetration of the zona matrix, has not successfully engineered the expression of zona receptors on the sperm surface or has not proven capable of acrosomal exocytosis once zona recognition has occurred [3]. However, even with IVF as the insemination procedure, the spermatozoa have not been subjected to the discrimination that normally occurs at the levels of the cervix and isthmic region of the fallopian tubes and, in mouse infertility models, this is frequently where sperm selection occurs [4].

1.2 Principles of Sperm Isolation: Preventing Leukocytic Attack

Human semen is an extremely complex cellular mixture containing live and dead spermatozoa, leukocytes (largely neutrophils), precursor germ cells, bacteria and cellular detritus originating from the secondary sexual glands. The clinical challenge is to extract the high-quality spermatozoa from this complex mélange, without inducing any iatrogenic damage. In this context, seminal plasma is our friend because it is richly endowed with antioxidants specifically designed to protect the spermatozoa during their short journey from the male reproductive tract into the female. These antioxidants include small molecular mass scavengers such as vitamin E, glutathione, uric acid and taurine as well as highly specialized antioxidant enzymes including catalase, glutathione peroxidase and superoxide dismutase [5]. This complex antioxidant mixture has evolved because the spermatozoa are very vulnerable to oxidative attack during the insemination process – and this attack may come from a variety of sources. In this context it is important to remember that spermatozoa have been matured and stored in the epididymal lumen, which is essentially free of phagocytic leukocytes capable of generating reactive oxygen species (ROS). Then, at the moment of ejaculation, the spermatozoa are suddenly exposed to macrophages and neutrophils that have infiltrated the ejaculate via the secondary sexual glands and urethra. These phagocytes are in an activated free-radical-generating state and would cause considerable damage to the sperm plasma membrane and other structures if it were not for the antioxidants in seminal plasma providing a high level of free radical scavenging protection (Figure 1.1) [6].

Very soon after insemination, the best quality spermatozoa with the highest levels of progressive motility leave the protection provided by seminal plasma and colonize the cervix. In this location the spermatozoa are safe – for a while. Within a few hours the presence of spermatozoa and semen in the cervix and vagina stimulates a leukocytic infiltration, largely neutrophils, designed to phagocytose any dead or moribund spermatozoa remaining at the site of insemination. The post-insemination phagocytosis of non-viable spermatozoa is generally "silent" in the sense that no ROS or pro-inflammatory cytokines are generated. The silent phagocytosis of senescent spermatozoa is thought to be a response to markers, such as phosphatidylserine (PS), which are expressed on the surface of spermatozoa as they engage in the intrinsic apoptotic cascade. This concept has arisen by analogy to silent phagocytosis in somatic systems, in which the expression of apoptotic markers such as PS on the surface of phagocytosed cells informs the phagocyte that engulfment must *not* be accompanied by an oxidative burst. Such silent phagocytosis is widespread in biology and can be seen, for example, when senescent neutrophils are being removed by macrophages from sites of tissue repair [7]. The silent nature of this phagocytic process ensures that under normal physiological circumstance, the spermatozoa do not have to contend with additional oxidative stress while they ascend the female reproductive tract. However, if surface expression of PS does not occur because the spermatozoa have died a necrotic death mediated by peroxynitrite [8] or attack by spermicidal detergents such as nonoxynol-9, then they may well be exposed to a post-insemination oxidative attack, only this time they will not be able to rely on the antioxidant properties of seminal plasma to protect them.

The protective role of seminal plasma is an important fundamental concept that has helped design optimized sperm isolation strategies. Whatever sperm preparation approach

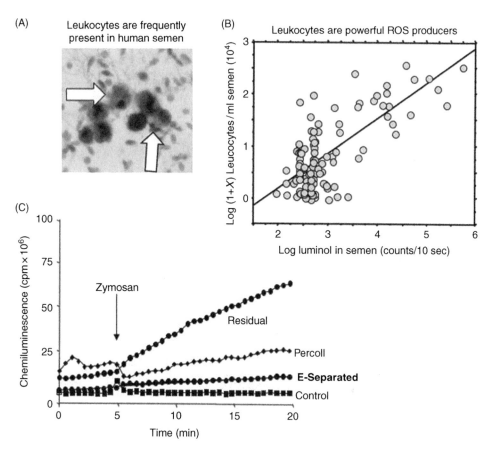

Figure 1.1 Human semen samples are invariably contaminated with leukocytes, particularly neutrophils, which are capable of generating reactive oxygen species (ROS) and damaging the spermatozoa. (**A**) Leukocytes in semen (arrowed) stained with an anti-CD45 antibody. (**B**) The concentration of leukocytes in human semen correlates very closely with ROS generation by the unfractionated ejaculate, indicating that a significant proportion of the seminal leukocyte population is in an activated state. (**C**) Using opsonized zymosan to investigate the presence of ROS-generating phagocytes in sperm samples prepared for IVF reveals that electrophoretically separated sperm suspensions (E-separated) possess lower levels of leukocyte contamination than those prepared by discontinuous gradient centrifugation (DGC) (Percoll). Following electrophoresis, most of the leukocytes remain trapped in the inoculation chamber (Residual) [6].

is used, it is important that seminal leukocytes and spermatozoa are not allowed to come into contact with each other in the absence of seminal plasma. When this is permitted to occur, as when spermatozoa are prepared by repeated cycles of washing and centrifugation or are swum up from a washed pellet, then sperm quality is invariably compromised [9]. This can occur inadvertently, if the sperm preparation procedure has not been successful in removing all of the contaminating leukocytes from the suspension used for IVF. Thus, in one study involving the use of discontinuous gradient centrifugation (DGC) to carefully purify spermatozoa for an IVF program, leukocyte contamination could still be demonstrated in 28.5% of the sperm preparations. Furthermore, the presence of these contaminating cells was associated with elevated levels of spontaneous ROS production, impaired

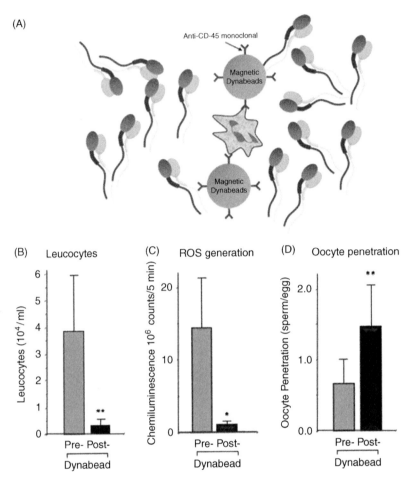

Figure 1.2 When leukocyte contamination is observed in human sperm suspensions, these cells can be removed, resulting in a reduction in oxidative stress and an increase in sperm function. (**A**) Principle behind the leukocyte separation procedure using magnetic beads coated with antibodies against the common leukocyte antigen (CD45). (**B**) The treatment is extremely effective in removing residual leukocytes from sperm suspensions. (**C**) The removal of contaminating leukocytes results in a massive reduction in oxidative stress as determined by the chemiluminescent measurement of ROS generation. (**D**) Leukocyte removal results in an increase in levels of sperm–oocyte fusion as observed with the hamster oocyte penetration assay [11].

movement, and a significantly reduced capacity for fertilization *in vitro* [10]. Treatment of such human sperm suspensions with magnetic beads or ferrofluids coated with antibodies against the common leukocyte antigen (CD45) has been found to successfully remove these cellular contaminants and, by so doing, significantly enhance the fertilizing capacity of the remaining spermatozoa (Figure 1.2) [11].

It follows from the above that any strategy for isolating spermatozoa for ART purposes should take its lead from nature and isolate the cells directly from semen rather than a washed sperm suspension. Given that this is the case, there are a limited number of strategies that can be pursued in order to achieve the effective isolation of high-quality spermatozoa from the ejaculate based on sperm motility, density, charge and other surface characteristics. In the sections that follow, we shall consider the effectiveness of these approaches and their potential for application in a clinical setting.

1.3 Intrinsic Motility

Because our species is a vaginal inseminator, we generate spermatozoa that are capable of progressive linear movement capable of penetrating the dense extracellular matrices that characterize the female reproductive tract, beginning with cervical mucus. If we wish to emulate nature in developing optimized methods for isolating high-quality spermatozoa, we could do worse than develop a medium resembling cervical mucus for the spermatozoa to colonize. In this context, cervical mucus itself, whether of human or bovine origin, is too logistically difficult to obtain and too difficult to standardize for routine sperm isolation purposes. Recognizing this, scientists in the early 1990s started to experiment with cervical mucus substitutes for the isolation of spermatozoa and discovered that hyaluronate polymers were extremely effective in this regard [12]. Furthermore, spermatozoa that have been isolated using hyaluronate solutions have been shown to be functionally normal as judged by their motility and ability to undergo both capacitation and the acrosome reaction [13]. Swim-up procedures involving the layering of a hyaluronate solution over human semen, followed by an incubation period of 50–60 minutes at 37°C in an atmosphere of 5% CO_2 in air, have been reported to generate sperm suspensions that are of significantly higher quality than those prepared by swim-up following centrifugation [14]. As a simple inexpensive technique for sperm isolation, the self-migration of spermatozoa directly from semen into medium that has been modified by the addition of sodium hyaluronate in order to increase its viscosity and limit contamination of the sample with seminal plasma constituents, has much to commend it. A variation on this theme has been a double-up technique in which spermatozoa are swum up from a pellet previously prepared by DGC [15]. Such a technique generates sperm suspensions of high purity and quality, although preparation time is prolonged and success ultimately depends on the intrinsic quality of the original semen sample in terms of motility and count.

1.4 Microfluidic Devices

The intrinsic motility of spermatozoa has also been exploited in the generation of microfluidic systems for sperm isolation that employ media based on hyaluronate or occasionally methylcellulose for the initial isolation of the spermatozoa [16]. A variety of such microfluidic systems have been developed that attempt to replicate the mechanisms by which spermatozoa are isolated *in vivo*. Most of these devices feature carefully engineered microchannels that spermatozoa colonize in the same way as they colonize cervical mucus by virtue of their own motility. Orientation of the spermatozoa in such channels has been achieved by a variety of different mechanisms, depending on such properties as rheotaxis, chemotaxis or thermotaxis, all of which spermatozoa display.

Rheotaxis, for example, refers to the orientation of spermatozoa in a fluid flow. In some respects, spermatozoa are like trout, in that faced with a mild flow in the extracellular environment, they will orientate upstream. Of course, unlike trout, spermatozoa do not possess a lateral line to detect the flow but rather depend on complex hydrodynamic interactions to achieve the upstream orientation [16]. The rate of flow is critical because if it becomes too strong the spermatozoa will simply be swept away. However, a carefully engineered flow of around 15–100 μm/s can facilitate the migration of spermatozoa through the device. Building on these fundamentals, an ingenious microfluidic corralling system has recently been developed for isolating subpopulations of highly motile human spermatozoa [17].

Chemotaxis is another potential mechanism for orientating spermatozoa, particularly for microfluidics systems that aim to not only isolate the spermatozoa but also fertilize the oocyte and culture the embryo. Some candidates for human sperm chemotaxis have already been identified, notably progesterone, and used as the basis for creating a sperm isolation system. In studies with this device, spermatozoa were initially separated on Percoll gradients and then inoculated into a system that mimicked the dimensions of the human female tract [18]. After a prolonged 150-min incubation at 37°C, spermatozoa attracted by the presence of a progesterone gradient were shown to have significantly better morphology and significantly reduced levels of DNA damage compared with spermatozoa isolated by virtue of their motility alone. Although the incubation time used in this study was protracted and the recovery efficiency low, the general principle of using chemotaxis as an aid to sperm isolation certainly has merit. Clearly, species exhibiting an internal mode of fertilization exhibit nothing like the strong chemotaxis evident in aquatic species where fertilization is external and conspecific gametes have to quickly find each other before becoming diluted to infinity in the water column. Nevertheless, there is strong evidence for the involvement of chemotaxis in human fertilization as suggested by the synthesis and insertion of olfactory receptors in the sperm plasma membrane [19]. Although progesterone is evidently a player in this context, there are other possibly more powerful chemotactic factors elaborated by the oocyte that still await definitive characterization [20]. Further resolution of such factors may greatly assist in the development of sperm isolation systems that reflect the *in vivo* situation.

Along similar lines, microfluidic devices have also been constructed based on the principle of thermotaxis and exploiting the fact that spermatozoa move along a temperature gradient as they ascend the female reproductive tract. Although the mechanisms that unpin this thermotaxis are currently unresolved, the capacity of these cells to discriminate changes in temperature has been analysed in detail with some astonishing results. According to Bahat and colleagues [21], human spermatozoa can sense and respond to a temperature difference of less than 0.0006°C! Using this principle, a novel microfluidics device has been constructed that appears to be effective in trapping spermatozoa that have migrated into regions of elevated temperature [22].

To date, there are no reports of how such microfluidic devices perform with pathological samples under real-life clinical laboratory conditions. The implementation of such studies will be important not just to determine whether microfluidics systems have any practical potential in a clinical context but also to determine whether such systems could be used as the initial component of a microfluidics system that will not only capture high-quality spermatozoa but also support fertilization and the early stages of embryo development – IVF on a chip. Using donated frozen-thawed human embryos, microfluidic devices have been assessed that appear to provide the same level of support for preimplantation embryonic development as conventional embryo culture methodologies [23]. This is clearly an extremely active area of research at the present time, which envisions development of a single microfluidics device that can achieve isolation of the highest quality spermatozoa, fertilization and the detailed monitoring of preimplantation development with a minimal degree of involvement on behalf of the embryologist overseeing the process. One could even imagine systems where the embryo culture fluid is automatically sampled and scanned for markers that will confirm their euploid status prior to being selected for transfer [24].

The difficulties with such a highly technical automated approach to IVF are cost, time and, ultimately, feasibility. The capacity to troubleshoot any unexpected problems that arise during the sperm isolation–fertilization–development continuum may be curtailed if the process becomes too automated and, at the end of the day, the embryo will still have to be recovered and manually transferred into the uterine cavity – and this comprises one of the most difficult risky phases of the entire ART process. Furthermore, the sperm selection component of such devices depends for its success on the intrinsic motility of the spermatozoa. In an IVF program where many of the semen samples that are being processed for treatment will be of poor quality and frequently suffering from low levels of motility, the ability of spermatozoa to self-select may be impaired. In order to compensate for the poor intrinsic motility of pathological sperm samples, alternative sperm separation strategies have been developed that actively recruit the spermatozoa rather than relying on their capacity to self-select. The two principle properties on which such selections have been based are sperm density and sperm charge.

1.5 Isolation According to Density

One of the features of mammalian spermatozoa is that they have a relatively high density by virtue of their lack of cytoplasmic space. Hence, if these cells are placed in a continuous density gradient and centrifuged, the highest quality cells with the greatest isopycnic densities will be carried to the densest region of the gradient [25]. Such DGC techniques have been progressively simplified with the passage of time and, in minimal two-step mode, have proven highly effective in isolating motile spermatozoa exhibiting high levels of fertilizing potential capable of establishing viable pregnancies following IVF [26].

The positioning of spermatozoa in such discontinuous gradients is a function of their density and thus, inversely, their volume. High-quality spermatozoa are the product of a highly efficient spermatogenic process that effectively removes most of the residual cytoplasm from the spermatozoa just prior to their release from the germinal epithelium. Any residual cytoplasm then snaps back into the midpiece of the cell to create a cytoplasmic remnant that, as far as we are aware, is not further processed by the cell. The retention of excess residual cytoplasm in this manner is in contrast to many other mammalian species where any cytoplasm remaining with the spermatozoon after spermiation is concentrated into a rounded cytoplasmic droplet which then slips down the shaft of the sperm tail to the annulus, where it is discarded or resorbed. Human spermatozoa do not behave in the same way. The retention of excess residual cytoplasm by human spermatozoa is a pathological change that inversely reflects the quality of the spermatogenic process involved in their creation and thus, ultimately, their functionality (Figure 1.3). The more cytoplasm is retained by the spermatozoa the worse their motility, the poorer their capacity for acrosomal exocytosis and sperm–oocyte fusion and the higher the levels of ROS generation [27].

Exactly why the retention of excess residual cytoplasm should be so detrimental to sperm function is still something of a mystery. For most cell types, cytoplasm is a virtuous possession that encapsulates most of the enzymes and all of the organelles needed to sustain life. The limited distribution and small volume of sperm cytoplasm actually creates vulnerabilities for this cell type, due to a lack of antioxidant protection and DNA-repair capacity which, in somatic cells, are orchestrated by enzymes that have their origins in the cytoplasm and the organelles housed within this space. Given the extreme vulnerability created by this

(A)

(B)

(C)

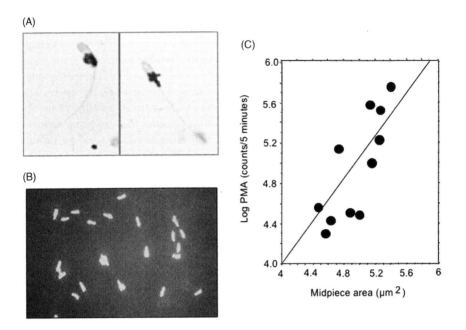

Figure 1.3 The behaviour of human spermatozoa in density centrifugation gradients depends on their density which, in turn, reflects the extent to which they have extruded their cytoplasm. (**A**) Any residual cytoplasm snaps back into the midpiece of the cells creating large cytoplasmic extensions, which can be readily imaged using an NADH-nitroblue tetrazolium reduction technique [27]. (**B**) The areas of nitroblue tetrazolium reduction can be readily imaged and quantified to generate an objective measure of how much residual cytoplasm a given sample might have retained. (**C**) The amount of residual cytoplasm correlates extremely well with the capacity of the purified spermatozoa to generate ROS, when all leukocytes have been removed [27].

strategy, there must be a very powerful set of reasons why spermatozoa go to such lengths to remove a majority of their cytoplasm and confine what remains to the midpiece of the cell.

Of course, for a highly motile cell, the presence of excess cytoplasm may simply represent a physical encumbrance that limits the capacity of these cells to move quickly though a viscous extracellular environment and, ultimately, to penetrate the zona pellucida. In addition, the drive to minimize the amount of cytoplasm retained by spermatozoa may be related to the need to protect the nucleus from endonuclease attack. Thus, the highly specialized architecture of human spermatozoa results in the cytoplasm and mitochondria being physically separated from the nucleus. This confers advantages upon the cell by limiting the vulnerability of their DNA to fragmentation during the early stages of apoptosis. The latter is usually accomplished by endonucleases activated in the cytoplasm or released from the mitochondria that then migrate into the cell nucleus in order to complete the apoptotic cascade. Because the sperm nucleus is physically separated from the mitochondria and a majority of the cytoplasm, such endonuclease-mediated DNA damage rarely features in these cells [28]. Another important reason to get rid of sperm cytoplasm is because its presence is associated with excess ROS generation, which not only damages the capacity of these cells for motility and sperm–egg interaction but also damages the DNA in the sperm nucleus and mitochondria [29]. Why excess cytoplasm should be responsible for generating excess ROS may be related to the capacity of spermatozoa to concentrate lipoxygenase in the cytoplasmic space and the fact that this enzyme is emerging as a possible candidate for the generation of ROS by defective human spermatozoa [30]. Alternative suggestions such as the involvement of cytoplasmic NADPH oxidase activity in ROS generation are currently unresolved [29].

Whatever the underlying mechanisms, there can be no doubt that DGC is an extremely effective means of isolating high-quality spermatozoa exhibiting low levels of ROS generation and high levels of functionality in terms of their motility and competence for fertilization. Moreover, because the energy required to effect the separation is achieved through the external imposition of a gravitational force, this technique should be more effective than self-migration swim-up protocols for isolating spermatozoa from poor-quality ejaculates. On the other hand, while DGC protocols are generally highly effective in getting rid of most of the leukocytes contaminating human semen samples, they are not perfect in this regard and sperm suspensions prepared in this manner can possess residual leukocytes in numbers sufficient to compromise the fertilizing capacity of the spermatozoa [10].

Another problem with DGC is that its application can be associated with an elevation in the levels of DNA damage seen in spermatozoa [31]. There is some inter-individual variation in the levels of DNA damage induced in this context that may be related to the specific vulnerability of individual samples to the oxidative stress created during centrifugation as a result of exposure to transition metals in the colloidal silicon solutions used to create the discontinuous gradients. Interestingly, cases where an increase in DNA fragmentation is observed following DGC exhibit lower pregnancy rates than samples where DNA damage is not elevated [32]. So, whatever vulnerability is being highlighted by this response to DGC has a bearing on the overall competence of the sample to establish a pregnancy. This makes DGC an interesting diagnostic procedure but does not necessarily commend it as an approach to sperm isolation.

1.6 Electrophoretic Isolation

An alternative to the use of sperm density as a criterion for isolating spermatozoa is to use sperm charge. Spermatozoa are negatively charged cells that have been known for several decades to migrate towards the anode in an electric field. This property has been exploited to generate a device for the isolation of human spermatozoa for assisted conception purposes (Figure 1.4) [33]. This system was found to be effective in generating suspensions of human spermatozoa exhibiting high levels of motility, good morphology and low levels of DNA damage that were essentially free from leukocyte contamination. The sperm preparations are generally similar in quality to those generated by DGC except that levels of sperm DNA damage are lower, possibly because this method does not involve exposure of the spermatozoa to any extraneous reagents capable of triggering ROS generation. Moreover, one of the major advantages of the electrophoretic technique is its great rapidity, generating suspensions containing more than 10 million spermatozoa/ml within 5 minutes (Figure 1.4). Subsequent studies confirmed that the electrophoretically isolated spermatozoa were competent to establish viable pregnancies in a clinical setting and were associated with measures of fertilization and embryo quality that were not significantly different from traditional methods [34]. In addition, it was established that the electrophoretic isolation of spermatozoa did not bias the genotype of the selected cells towards either an X- or Y-bearing genotype. Furthermore, the electrophoretic method was found to be effective with

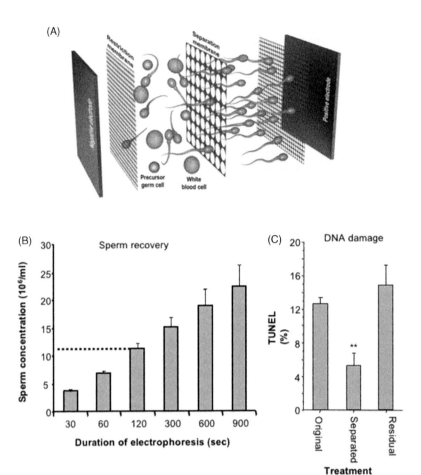

Figure 1.4 Electrophoresis represents a promising approach to sperm isolation. (**A**) The principle behind this approach is that high-quality spermatozoa are negatively charged and move towards the anode in an electric field. The creation of a cassette containing a separation membrane with pore sizes of around 5 μm allows spermatozoa to be pulled away from other cell types such as leukocytes or precursor germ cells that might also carry a net negative charge but are too large to pass through the pores. (**B**) The technique is extremely efficacious allowing the isolation of more than 10 million highly motile spermatozoa/ml within 5 minutes. (**C**) The separated cells possess significantly lower levels of DNA damage than the original sperm population [33].

severely compromised samples including testicular biopsy material, where the spermatozoa are immotile and deeply buried within an extremely complex cellular mixture. Electrophoretically isolated cells were also shown to capacitate normally when washed free from seminal decapacitation factors that co-migrate with the spermatozoa during their electrophoretic migration [35]. It was also established in these studies that the negative charge responsible for the migration of spermatozoa in an electric field is largely determined by surface sialic acid residues. This conclusion was based on the ability of neuraminidase to significantly suppress the electrophoretic isolation of spermatozoa, suggesting that this association between cell surface sialation and sperm behaviour in an electric field has a causative basis [35].

With this method, the application of current for sperm isolation purposes has to be carefully controlled because while field strength is positively correlated with sperm recovery rates it is negatively correlated with sperm movement, irrespective of whether the current or the voltage is held constant. Importantly, the loss of motility observed when the intensity of the electric field is high, or the duration of exposure is prolonged, is not associated with any increase in ROS generation or the induction of DNA damage. Indeed, the levels of oxidative stress and DNA damage observed following exposure of human spermatozoa to an electric field are so minimal that this may constitute an effective method for immobilizing sperma-tozoa for ICSI [36].

Exploiting the negative charge expressed by high-quality human spermatozoa, others have developed microelectrophoresis systems for the small-scale isolation of individual spermatozoa for ICSI [37]. In another variation on this theme, a zeta method has been developed which depends on the creation of a positively charged surface to which the negatively charged spermatozoa can adhere. This method has been reported to result in a doubling in the rates of hyperactivation and progressive motility and a halving in the levels of DNA damage observed in the isolated populations of spermatozoa [38]. Taken together, these results suggest that the isolation of human spermatozoa on the basis of their charge is as rapid as it is efficacious. Furthermore, this approach is safe because it does not carry with it the risk of inadvertent DNA damage as a consequence of enhanced ROS generation.

1.7 Consequences of Sperm Preparation Protocols

Does the method of sperm preparation make much of a difference to overall success rates? The answer to this question depends on how you measure success. If the latter is assessed in terms of pregnancy or live birth rate then the method of sperm preparation probably makes very little difference, except when semen quality is so poor that methods relying on the intrinsic motility of the spermatozoa or adequate sperm numbers (swim-up, for example) become ineffective. For poor-quality human semen samples of the type that might be commonly encountered in an infertility clinic, methods that are less dependent on sperm motility or number such as mini-DGC, glass wool columns or electrophoresis might be preferred [40]. Outside of the extremes of semen quality, when direct comparisons have been made between sperm suspensions prepared by repeated centrifugation, swim-up from a washed pellet, glass wool filtration or DGC, then little difference has been revealed in terms of the per-cycle pregnancy rate [39]. Similarly, when pregnancy rates have been compared between spermatozoa prepared DGC and electrophoresis, neither conception rates nor pregnancy rates were very different between the two methods [34].

However, pregnancy rate is an extremely crude method of determining whether sperm preparation methodologies have made a difference. Using a variety of methods for assessing sperm quality, it is clearly possible to detect highly significant differences in the quality of the gametes isolated as a function of the isolation procedure used in their preparation. Of particular importance is the impact of sperm preparation techniques on the levels of DNA damage seen in the spermatozoa [36]. Such differences in DNA integrity may not have a major impact on pregnancy rates, *per se*. However, they have every possibility of generat-ing differences in the genetic/epigenetic make-up of the offspring [40].

As a process, fertilization appears to be relatively forgiving of differences in DNA integrity, particularly when ICSI is used as the insemination strategy [4]. If spermatozoa are isolated using less-than-optimal techniques, such that they still contain such damage or have it iatrogenically induced as a consequence of the procedure, then there is a risk that these DNA lesions will become translated into genetic/epigenetic changes in the offspring, following inefficient or aberrant post-fertilization repair in the oocyte [29]. Such changes have the potential to significantly impact the progeny's long-term health trajectory and, if genetic changes are involved, to impact the wellbeing of progeny for many generations to come. What the field needs now are studies that examine the impact of sperm preparation strategy, not on rates of fertilization or implantation, but on the levels of DNA damage carried by the spermatozoa and the genetic/epigenetic mutational load subsequently imposed upon the offspring. Techniques that are simple, rapid and capable of effecting the isolation of spermatozoa with minimal DNA damage from a range of pathological samples, including those characterized by low sperm numbers and little intrinsic motility, will become the methods of the future. In an era dominated by ICSI, we require studies that focus less on the functional attributes of the spermatozoa and more on the mutational load carried by, and developmental normality of, the offspring. The techniques we are currently using are almost half a century old. Hopefully, some of the new insights discussed in this chapter on the behaviour of spermatozoa in fluid flows, gradients and electric fields will provide the basis for a new generation of safer, more effective sperm isolation methodologies in the future.

References

1. Hourcade, J. D., Pérez-Crespo, M., Fernández-González, R., Pintado, B. and Gutiérrez-Adán, A. (2010) Selection against spermatozoa with fragmented DNA after postovulatory mating depends on the type of damage. *Reprod Biol Endocrinol* 8:9.

2. Twigg, J. P., Irvine, D. S. and Aitken, R. J. (1998) Oxidative damage to DNA in human spermatozoa does not preclude pronucleus formation at intracytoplasmic sperm injection. *Hum Reprod* 13:1864–1871.

3. Liu, D. Y., Liu, M. L., Clarke, G. N. and Baker, H. W. (2007) Hyperactivation of capacitated human sperm correlates with the zona pellucida-induced acrosome reaction of zona pellucida-bound sperm. *Hum Reprod* 22:2632–2638.

4. Nishimura, H., Kim, E., Nakanishi, T. and Baba, T. (2004) Possible function of the ADAM1a/ADAM2 Fertilin complex in the appearance of ADAM3 on the sperm surface. *J Biol Chem* 279:34957–34962.

5. Aitken, R. J. and Roman, S. D. (2008) Antioxidant systems and oxidative stress in the testes. *Adv Exp Med Biol* 636:154–171.

6. Aitken, R. J. and Baker, M. A. (2013) Oxidative stress, spermatozoa and leukocytic infiltration: relationships forged by the opposing forces of microbial invasion and the search for perfection. *J Reprod Immunol* 100:11–19.

7. Leitch, A. E., Duffin, R., Haslett, C. and Rossi, A. G. (2008) Relevance of granulocyte apoptosis to resolution of inflammation at the respiratory mucosa. *Mucosal Immunol* 1:350–363.

8. Uribe, P., Cabrillana, M. E., Fornés, M. W., Treulen, F., Boguen, R., Isachenko, V., et al. (2018) Nitrosative stress in human spermatozoa causes cell death characterized by induction of mitochondrial permeability transition-driven necrosis. *Asian J Androl* 20:600–607.

9. Aitken, R. J. and Clarkson, J. S. (1988) Significance of reactive oxygen species and antioxidants in defining the efficacy of sperm preparation techniques. *J Androl* 9:367–376.

10. Krausz, C., Mills, C., Rogers, S., Tan, S. L. and Aitken, R. J. (1994) Stimulation of oxidant generation by human sperm suspensions using phorbol esters and formyl peptides: relationships with motility and fertilization *in vitro*. *Fertil Steril* 62:599–605.

11. Aitken, R. J., Buckingham, D. W., West, K. and Brindle, J. (1996) On the use of

paramagnetic beads and ferrofluids to assess and eliminate the leukocytic contribution to oxygen radical generation by human sperm suspensions. *Am J Reprod Immunol* 35:541–551.

12. Neuwinger, J., Cooper, T. G., Knuth, U. A. and Nieschlag, E. (1991) Hyaluronic acid as a medium for human sperm migration tests. *Hum Reprod* 6:396–400.

13. Perry, R. L., Barratt, C. L., Warren, M. A. and Cooke, I. D. (1996) Comparative study of the effect of human cervical mucus and a cervical mucus substitute, Healonid, on capacitation and the acrosome reaction of human spermatozoa *in vitro*. *Hum Reprod* 11:1055–1062.

14. Wikland, M., Wik, O., Steen, Y., Qvist, K., Söderlund, B. and Janson P. O. (1987) A self-migration method for preparation of sperm for *in-vitro* fertilization. *Hum Reprod* 2:191–195.

15. Yamanaka, M., Tomita, K., Hashimoto, S., Matsumoto, H., Satoh, M., Kato, H., et al. (2016) Combination of density gradient centrifugation and swim-up methods effectively decreases morphologically abnormal sperms. *J Reprod Dev* 62:599–606.

16. Suarez, S. S. and Wu, M. (2017) Microfluidic devices for the study of sperm migration. *Mol Hum Reprod* 23:227–234.

17. Zaferani, M., Cheong, S. H. and Abbaspourrad, A. (2018) Rheotaxis-based separation of sperm with progressive motility using a microfluidic corral system. *Proc Natl Acad Sci USA* 115:8272–8277.

18. Li, K., Li, R., Ni, Y., Sun, P., Liu, Y., Zhang, D. and Huang, H. (2018) Novel distance-progesterone-combined selection approach improves human sperm quality. *J Transl Med* 16:203.

19. Flegel, C., Vogel, F., Hofreuter, A., Schreiner, B. S., Osthold, S., Veitinger, S., et al. (2016) Characterization of the olfactory receptors expressed in human spermatozoa. *Front Mol Biosci* 2:73.

20. Armon, L., Ben-Ami, I., Ron-El, R. and Eisenbach, M. (2014) Human oocyte-derived sperm chemoattractant is a hydrophobic molecule associated with a carrier protein. *Fertil Steril* 102:885–890.

21. Bahat, A., Caplan, S. R. and Eisenbach, M. (2012) Thermotaxis of human sperm cells in extraordinarily shallow temperature gradients over a wide range. *PLoS One* 7: e41915.

22. Li, Z., Liu, W., Qiu, T., Xie, L., Chen, W., Liu, R., et al. (2014) The construction of an interfacial valve-based microfluidic chip for thermotaxis evaluation of human sperm. *Biomicrofluidics* 8:024102.

23. Kieslinger, D. C., Hao, Z., Vergouw, C. G., Kostelijk, E. H., Lambalk, C. B. and Le Gac, S. (2015) *In vitro* development of donated frozen-thawed human embryos in a prototype static microfluidic device: a randomized controlled trial. *Fertil Steril* 103:680–686.e2.

24. Xu, J., Fang, R., Chen, L., Chen, D., Xiao, J. P., Yang, W., et al. (2016). Noninvasive chromosome screening of human embryos by genome sequencing of embryo culture medium for *in vitro* fertilization. *Proc Natl Acad Sci USA* 113:11907–11912.

25. Gorus, F. K. and Pipeleers, D. G. (1981) A rapid method for the fractionation of human spermatozoa according to their progressive motility. *Fertil Steril* 35:662–665.

26. Hyne, R. V., Stojanoff, A., Clarke, G. N., Lopata, A. and Johnston, W. I. (1986) Pregnancy from *in vitro* fertilization of human eggs after separation of motile spermatozoa by density gradient centrifugation. *Fertil Steril* 45:93–96.

27. Gomez, E., Buckingham, D. W., Brindle, J., Lanzafame, F., Irvine, D. S. and Aitken, R. J. (1996) Development of an image analysis system to monitor the retention of residual cytoplasm by human spermatozoa: correlation with biochemical markers of the cytoplasmic space, oxidative stress, and sperm function. *J Androl* 17:276–287.

28. Koppers, A. J., Mitchell, L. A., Wang, P., Lin, M. and Aitken, R. J. (2011) Phosphoinositide 3-kinase signalling pathway involvement in a truncated

apoptotic cascade associated with motility loss and oxidative DNA damage in human spermatozoa. *Biochem J* **436**:687–698.

29. Aitken, R. J. (2018) Not every sperm is sacred: a perspective on male infertility. *Mol Hum Reprod* **24**:287–298.

30. Walters, J. L. H., De Iuliis, G. N., Dun, M. D., Aitken, R. J, McLaughlin, E. A., Nixon, B., et al. (2018) Pharmacological inhibition of arachidonate 15-lipoxygenase protects human spermatozoa against oxidative stress. *Biol Reprod* **98**:784–794.

31. Aitken, R. J., Finnie, J. M., Muscio, L., Whiting, S., Connaughton, H. S., Kuczera, L., et al. (2014) Potential importance of transition metals in the induction of DNA damage by sperm preparation media. *Hum Reprod* **29**:2136–2147.

32. Muratori, M., Tarozzi, N., Cambi, M., Boni, L., Iorio, A. L., Passaro, C., et al. (2016) Variation of DNA Fragmentation levels during density gradient sperm selection for assisted reproduction techniques: a possible new male predictive parameter of pregnancy? *Medicine (Baltimore)* **95**:e3624.

33. Ainsworth, C., Nixon, B. and Aitken, R. J. (2005) Development of a novel electrophoretic system for the isolation of human spermatozoa. *Hum Reprod* **20**:2261–2270.

34. Fleming, S. D., Ilad, R. S., Griffin, A. M., Wu, Y., Ong, K. J., Smith, H. C., et al. (2008) Prospective controlled trial of an electrophoretic method of sperm preparation for assisted reproduction: comparison with density gradient centrifugation. *Hum Reprod* **23**:2646–2651.

35. Ainsworth, C. J., Nixon, B. and Aitken, R. J. (2011) The electrophoretic separation of spermatozoa: an analysis of genotype, surface carbohydrate composition and potential for capacitation. *Int J Androl* **34**: e422–e434.

36. Aitken, R. J., Hanson, A. R. and Kuczera, L. (2011) Electrophoretic sperm isolation: optimization of electrophoresis conditions and impact on oxidative stress. *Hum Reprod* **26**:1955–1964.

37. Simon, L., Murphy, K., Aston, K. I., Emery, B. R., Hotaling, J. M. and Carrell, D. T. (2016) Optimization of microelectrophoresis to select highly negatively charged sperm. *J Assist Reprod Genet* **33**:679–688.

38. Chan, P. J., Jacobson, J. D., Corselli, J. U. and Patton, W. C. (2006) A simple zeta method for sperm selection based on membrane charge. *Fertil Steril* **85**:481–486.

39. Johnson, D. E., Confino, E. and Jeyendran, R. S. (1996) Glass wool column filtration versus mini-Percoll gradient for processing poor quality semen samples. *Fertil Steril* **66**:459–462.

40. Aitken, R. J., Bronson, R., Smith, T. B. and De Iuliis, G. N. (2013) The source and significance of DNA damage in human spermatozoa: a commentary on diagnostic strategies and straw man fallacies. *Mol Hum Reprod* **19**:475–485.

Chapter

2

New Horizons in Male Subfertility and Infertility

Brett Nixon and Elizabeth G. Bromfield

2.1 Introduction

Infertility is a distressingly common condition that afflicts up to 15% of couples of reproductive age. Male factor infertility is directly implicated in approximately 30% of couples experiencing problems with conception and is a contributory factor in as many as 50% of cases [1]. In the 40 years since the first description of successful human *in vitro* fertilisation (IVF), substantial improvements have been made in the efficacy of treatments for male subfertility. One such advance has been the introduction of gamete micromanipulation techniques such as intracytoplasmic sperm injection (ICSI), which have had a transformative impact on the treatment of individuals with compromised sperm parameters, effectively dispensing with the need for spermatozoa to display progressive motility or have the potential to recognise an oocyte and complete an acrosome reaction [2]. So profound has the impact on clinical andrology been, that ICSI has become the favoured choice for fertilisation irrespective of the male factor, now featuring in as many as two-thirds of IVF cycles undertaken in countries such as Australia [3]. However, despite technological advances, both worldwide clinical pregnancy and live birth rates remain relatively modest at approximately 26.8% and 20% per started cycle, respectively [2]. Notwithstanding confounders, recent epidemiological data has documented the potential for an elevated risk of birth defects and perpetuation of defective semen profiles in children conceived via ICSI [4,5]. Such data encourage caution in the utilisation of ICSI beyond its intended application for achieving pregnancy in couples with severely compromised semen parameters and highlight a pressing need to explore new horizons for diagnostic tools to assist with patient stratification, sperm selection and therapeutic treatment options for males suffering from subfertility and infertility. Here, we review the current state of the art and future directions in the field of male infertility with the goal of addressing the long-standing question of how best to approach the clinical management of these individuals. Out of necessity, we have also sought to direct the reader to a number of excellent reviews that critically appraise our current armoury of diagnostic and therapeutic strategies.

2.2 Diagnostic Andrology

Without question, there are many different pathologies captured under the umbrella of male infertility and each of these presents different implications for the clinical management of the patient. Until recently, our approach to diagnostic andrology has been based upon the tenet that fertility can be defined in terms of a routine descriptive semen profile that places emphasis on sperm count, morphology and motility. Regrettably, these conventional criteria reveal little about the underlying aetiology of the infertility or the functionality of the sperm, have proven to be relatively insensitive indicators of fertilisation success, and are therefore of limited utility in selecting the optimal clinical management regimen [6]. Indeed, we now appreciate that stalwarts of andrological assessment such as sperm number represent relatively weak criterion for the prediction of fertility. Likewise, despite progress towards automation of gross morphology assessments and the advent of ultra-high magnification (i.e. motile sperm organelle morphology examination [MSOME]) to standardise the detection of even very subtle morphological defects, limitations remain in terms of the ability to discriminate those morphological elements that define the functionality of a given sperm cell. Thus, whilst the combination of MSOME in tandem with ICSI (i.e. intracytoplasmic morphologically selected sperm injection [IMSI]) has a theoretical potential to improve reproductive outcomes, there is currently limited evidence supporting the positive effect of IMSI on live birth or miscarriage rates, and the veracity of evidence citing improved clinical pregnancy following IMSI remains questionable [7]. It has yet to be determined whether such deficiencies may be overcome through the application of selective stains to highlight particularly important attributes of sperm structure and quality, such as those reflecting sperm viability, acrosomal status, capacitation, mitochondrial membrane potential, reactive oxygen species (ROS) generation, lipid peroxidation, apoptotic markers and DNA damage.

As the final component of the routine descriptive semen profile, sperm motility holds promise, particularly when undertaken with the aid of objective computer-aided semen analysis (CASA) systems to accurately measure sperm trajectories [8]. Accordingly, positive correlations have been established between the motility and fertility of human spermatozoa [9]. Regrettably, owing to the fact that the motility profile of sperm is a constantly changing entity influenced by the differing physiological environments encountered by the cell, these correlations are often weak. Indeed, during their transport to the site of fertilisation, spermatozoa are variably characterised by forward progressive motility, complete quiescence associated with the formation of a storage reservoir in the isthmic region of the fallopian tubes, and the induction of hyperactivated motility characterised by high-frequency, high-amplitude, asymmetric flagellar waves. Whilst the measurement of these various forms of movement can be achieved by CASA [8], problems associated with the intermittent nature of these profiles render them difficult diagnostic criteria to apply in a clinical setting. Moreover, the selection of sperm on the basis of their motility using "swim-up" techniques has failed to deliver superior pregnancy rates to that of the most widely adopted sperm preparation procedures utilising colloidal silica density gradients [10].

2.3 Improvements in Diagnostic Andrology

In order to alleviate the limitations and variability inherent in current methodologies used for fertility diagnosis and selection of spermatozoa in assisted reproductive technology (ART), new modalities are urgently required. In terms of driving advances in this field, we have much to learn from the study of the mechanistic basis of sperm dysfunction and, conversely, the characteristics of those sperm cells that are able to participate in the cascade of events that underpin natural conception. In this setting, it is evident that only relatively

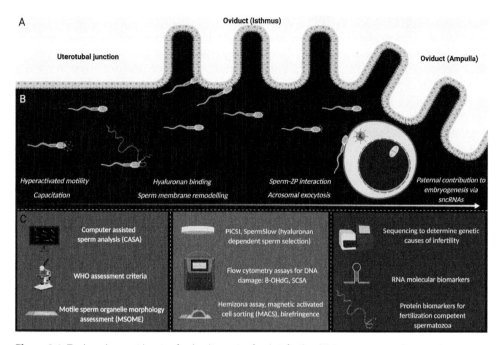

Figure 2.1 Tools under consideration for the diagnosis of male infertility. (A) As sperms enter the reproductive tract they transit through the uterus, navigate the uterotubal junction and progress through the isthmus and ampulla of the oviduct to contact the ovulated oocyte. (B) To achieve fertilisation, spermatozoa must first undergo an extensive period of membrane remodelling in the female reproductive tract, termed capacitation, where dynamic protein phosphorylation events give rise to important physiological changes in motility (hyperactivated motility). These dynamic protein changes also facilitate the presentation/unmasking of key receptors on the sperm surface that facilitate sequential cumulus matrix (hyaluronan) and sperm–zona pellucida binding and penetration. Spermatozoa are required to undergo exocytosis of their acrosomal contents and acrosomal membrane remodelling events prior to cell–cell membrane fusion and fertilisation. Post-fertilisation, there is mounting evidence that sperm-borne small non-coding RNAs (sncRNAs) influence pre-implantation embryogenesis. (C) Currently, routine protocols for the diagnosis of male infertility and subfertility include basic and advanced morphology, motility and sperm concentration assessments (including computer-assisted sperm analysis (CASA), World Health Organisation (WHO) assessment criteria and motile sperm organelle morphology assessment (MSOME). In addition, there are now several tools available to determine cell quality, DNA integrity and fertilisation capacity (including hyaluronan-based detection methods, high-throughput flow cytometry assays for the oxidised base 8-hydroxyl-2-deoxyguanosine (8-OHdG) and the sperm chromatin structure assay (SCSA). Finally, the advance of omics technology is permitting the development molecular biomarkers that can stratify infertile and fertile sperm populations and aid our understanding of the genetic causes of male infertility.

few sperm cells successfully navigate the female reproductive tract to reach the site of fertilisation in the oviduct. This highly selected population not only are endowed with the motility needed to penetrate through cervical mucus and gain entry into the uterus and the oviducts, but also complete the process of capacitation, which primes the cells for their interaction with the outer vestments of the oocyte [11], the cumulus oophorus and zona pellucida. Such interactions are coordinated by specialised sperm domains overlying the anterior region of the sperm head. These domains are formed during the latter phases of spermatogenesis before being dynamically modified upon passage through both the male and female reproductive tracts [12]. Accordingly, the development of bioassays that seek to impose the stringency of natural sperm selection barriers have been receiving increased attention (Figure 2.1).

2.3.1 Hyaluronic Acid Binding

Illustrative of strategies designed to mimic physiological sperm selection are protocols based on the hyaluronic acid (HA) binding properties of spermatozoa. Such techniques seek to exploit the principle that functionally mature spermatozoa express hyaluronic acid binding sites capable of adhering to, and digesting, the hyaluronic acid-rich matrix of the cumulus oophorus [13]. Two systems are currently marketed based on hyaluronic acid sperm selection, differing with respect to their use of either immobilised HA (i.e. physiological intracytoplasmic sperm injection (PICSI)) or HA suspended in a viscous medium (i.e. SpermSlow), which theoretically immobilises or retards mature sperm movement respectively, and is thus permissive of their selection away from immature counterparts in preparation for downstream ICSI [13]. Despite the promise of such interventions, meta-analyses have concluded that current evidence is insufficient to support their utility in terms of improved clinical pregnancy rates, miscarriage rates and, perhaps more importantly, in live birth rates from ART [14]. Available evidence is also insufficient to preclude adverse effects or establish differences in the efficacy of the PICSI versus SpermSlow HA binding systems [14]. By way of a biological explanation for the lack of a clear consensus regarding the efficacy of HA-based sperm selection, there is mounting evidence that human spermatozoa experience a dynamic, capacitation-associated remodelling of their surface architecture [11]. This process is characterised by an apparent reduction in the number of spermatozoa with hyaluronidase enzymes (i.e. sperm adhesion molecule 1, (SPAM1)) superficially exposed on their surface. Conversely, capacitated populations of human spermatozoa are characterised by an increase in the proportion of cells with zona pellucida (ZP) receptors presented on the outer leaflet of their plasma membrane [15]. One such receptor is arylsulphatase A (ARSA), an enzyme with affinity for the sulphated sugar ligands that decorate the ZP, and which is almost exclusively expressed on the surface of capacitated spermatozoa. Thus, HA adhesion may in fact be selecting the sub-population of spermatozoa that have failed to complete capacitation, but the extent to which this is reflective of underlying lesions in capacitation-associated signalling remains to be determined.

2.3.2 Zona Pellucida Binding

Downstream of HA binding, spermatozoa encounter the ZP, an acellular matrix that surrounds the ovulated oocyte and serves as a tenacious physiological barrier to fertilisation. Accordingly, a failure to bind and penetrate the ZP is a relatively common defect encountered in the spermatozoa of infertile patients. Indeed, approximately 10% of men with idiopathic infertility exhibit a failure of sperm–ZP recognition [16]. For most infertile males, however, failures of sperm–ZP recognition are a matter of degree and when carefully quantified using a hemizona assay (HZA) provide an accurate assessment of overall fertility, both *in vivo* and *in vitro* [17]. Thus, the HZA has historically been found to provide the highest discriminatory power for fertilisation success/failure of any sperm parameter assessed [17]. Such findings raise the prospect that the ZP may possess the ability to discriminate superior quality spermatozoa, a notion supported by demonstrations that the ZP selectively binds sperm with normal motility, morphology and high levels of nuclear chromatin DNA integrity [18]. This phenomenon may be attributed, at least in part, to the fact that each of these functional parameters are highly sensitive to physiological insults, such as those arising from elevated levels of ROS, which the sperm of infertile individuals commonly encounter [19].

As an extension of these observations, biological selection of sperm for ICSI on the basis of their ZP binding affinity has been shown to produce higher quality embryos and contribute to improved implantation and clinical pregnancy rate compared to sperm selected by conventional subjective approaches [18]. Despite the biological importance of ZP binding, the fact that this barrier can now be readily breached through ICSI has contributed to a situation whereby the molecular basis of sperm–ZP recognition remains poorly characterised [12]. What we do appreciate is that this interaction involves both lectin-like and protein–protein interactions, raising the prospect of utilising these ligands as unique molecular signatures with which to discriminate high-quality, fertilisation competent spermatozoa. Whilst resourcing and ethical limitations prohibit the use of native ZP for this purpose, it has long been known that complex carbohydrate substrates such as fucoidan or neoglycoproteins terminated with the sialyl-Lewisx (sLex) sequence can competitively inhibit human sperm–ZP binding [20,21]. These findings support the hypothesis that selective carbohydrate motifs could be employed for sperm selection. As an extension of this principle, the prospect of developing advanced sperm selection strategies based on surface properties that differentiate viable mature spermatozoa such as negative charge, exposure of apoptotic markers, or birefringence properties have also been trialled and are briefly discussed below. It is important to note, however, that while each of these sperm selection strategies has shown promise, more detailed randomised evaluation of their efficacy is needed to support their widespread adoption in clinical practice [14].

2.3.3 Sperm Surface Properties

As with all cell surfaces, the spermatozoon is adorned with a dense glycocalyx matrix comprising a heterogeneous array of complex carbohydrates. This extracellular coat is subjected to substantial temporal remodelling during the successive phases of sperm maturation, with an uptake of glycoproteins rich in terminal sialic acid residues being a key hallmark of those cells that have completed their epididymal maturation [22]. Thus, a gradient of increasing sialylation is associated with the attainment of full sperm fertilising ability and has also been linked to the masking of the allogeneic sperm cell from immune surveillance upon entering the female reproductive tract [22]. However, in addition to its protective role, the attendant increase in electronegativity associated with sialylation has been exploited as a means by which to electrophoretically separate mature sperm away from contaminating leucocytes, bacteria and immature germ cells, all of which can exert deleterious effects on sperm function, prior to their use in either IVF or ICSI. In recent developments, novel electrophoretic approaches have seen application for the rapid isolation of populations of motile, viable, morphologically normal spermatozoa exhibiting high levels of DNA integrity [23]. Clinical utility has also been demonstrated using a range of difficult starting materials (biopsies, cryostored semen and snap-frozen sperm suspensions), culminating in the first reported human pregnancy following electrophoretic sperm isolation [23]. In a similar context, electrokinetic properties such as the zeta potential (i.e. the charge that exists across the plasma membrane, which in mature spermatozoa is ~ −16 mV to −20 mV) has also been used to separate mature sperm cells via adherence to a positively charged solid support such as a glass slide or centrifuge tube [24]. Such methods have been reported to select for spermatozoa with enhanced levels of maturity, DNA integrity, normal morphology and kinematic parameters that are each associated with increased fertilisation and pregnancy success following ART [25].

One of the leading causative agents of male infertility is oxidative stress originating from elevated levels of ROS within the male germ line [19]. Spermatozoa are particularly susceptible to such stress, not only because they are enriched in vulnerable substrates (i.e. polyunsaturated fatty acids, proteins and DNA), but they also possess little capacity to protect themselves from oxidative attack or to effect any repair, should damage occur [19]. Upon the induction of oxidative stress, spermatozoa revert to an apoptotic cascade resulting in a loss of their fertilisation potential and the externalisation of phosphatidylserine, the latter being a late onset event that may facilitate the phagocytosis of senescent spermatozoa without the accompanying generation of an inflammatory response within the female reproductive tract [26]. Accordingly, the appearance of phosphatidylserine residues on the external surface of the apoptotic sperm membrane has been used for the development of negative selection protocols to effectively eliminate these moribund cells from within an ejaculate prior to ART interventions. Applications formulated on the basis of this strategy include magnetic activated cell sorting (MACS) and glass wool separation technologies [14]. However, whilst systematic review and meta-analyses of prospective randomised trials allude to improvements in pregnancy rates when MACS is used in tandem with standard sperm selection methods (i.e. density gradient centrifugation or swim-up techniques), at present no differences have been established in regard to implantation and miscarriage rates, and further studies of suitable quality are required before advocating for the use of this sperm selection technique in clinical practice [14].

Aside from physical changes in the sperm surface that correlate with their functional status, the maturing cells also experience changes in an optical property known as birefringence. Birefringence refers to a substrate having a refractive index, which is influenced by the polarisation and propagation direction of light. The anisotropic optical characteristics of the spermatozoon are attributed to a combination of longitudinally oriented protein filaments housed within the cell's nuclear, subacrosomal and axonemal domains. Accordingly, based on similar principles to the MSOME approach described in Section 2.2, the application of polarisation microscopy has been proposed as a novel diagnostic tool for structural evaluation of the maturity of a given sperm cell population, and as a promising method for selection of viable sperm cells with normal morphology and reduced levels of DNA fragmentation in preparation for ICSI [27].

2.3.4 Sperm Biomarkers

With the limitations inherent in existing strategies for defining male fertility, attention has increasingly been directed towards the identification of alternative non-invasive biomarkers with the sensitivity to discriminate signatures of the underlying pathophysiology giving rise to a particular infertility phenotype and/or to accurately diagnose the likelihood of fertilisation success. Indeed, the advent of advanced "omic" platforms has been the catalyst for a recent proliferation in studies seeking to differentiate the macromolecular composition (e.g. proteomic, metabolomic and epigenomic) of spermatozoa and seminal fluids from fertile individuals versus those produced by their subfertile/infertile counterparts [28].

In the absence of *de novo* protein synthesis, the maturation of spermatozoa is largely dependent on the acquisition of new proteins encountered during their transit of the male reproductive system and the post-translational modifications of their intrinsic protein complement during their post-ejaculatory capacitation [29]. These features highlight the utility of proteomic analyses in terms of characterising the changes that confer functionality on the male gamete. Accordingly, considerable effort has been devoted to defining the sperm proteome, as well as that of the acellular fraction of seminal fluid and the trillions of extracellular vesicles it contains [30]. In terms of the spermatozoon, this expanding resource has recently been consolidated into an inventory of some 6,198 unique proteins, a comprehensive reference library representing approximately 80% of the estimated 7,500 total proteins that constitute a human sperm cell [31]. Among the key challenges that remain in harnessing the transformative potential of this information, is to characterise the targets impacted by post-translational modifications, investigate the protein interactome, and define anomalies in protein expression associated with specific lesions in sperm function [29].

In this context, exciting advances have been made in sophisticated comparative and quantitative approaches that enable analysis of the proteomic signature of spermatozoa in different functional states (immature vs mature, non-capacitated vs capacitated, fertile vs infertile). These techniques are helping to define which specific elements of the proteome are of functional significance and to improve our understanding of the post-translational modifications (e.g. phosphorylation, glycosylation, acetylation, proteolytic cleavage) involved in generating a fertilisation competent spermatozoon [29]. Illustrative of the application of these technologies, mass spectrometry based proteomics has been used to map defects in human spermatozoa associated with failure to participate in ZP interaction. Among a small handful of significant alterations, the molecular chaperone heat shock protein A2 (HSPA2) was identified as being significantly under-represented in the spermatozoa of infertile patients [15]. Such findings accord with independent evidence that the overall levels of HSPA2 present in mature human spermatozoa provide a robust discriminative index of the success of the cumulus–oocyte interactions and reflect fertilising potential [13]. In accounting for these observations, HSPA2 has been implicated in the process of sperm plasma membrane remodelling associated with spermiogenesis and capacitation [15]. Thus, an under-representation of the protein likely comprises the formation of ZP binding domains on the surface of the mature spermatozoon. Moreover, the loss of HSPA2 from the sperm proteome has been causally linked to elevated levels of oxidative stress in various models [32], reinforcing the notion that the efficacy of sperm–oocyte interactions provide a highly sensitive readout of the legacy of this form of physiological insult.

Aside from sperm proteins, mounting interest has focused on alternative macromolecules such as the specific sperm RNAs and/or the overall integrity of the cell's DNA as predictive markers of fertilisation success [33,34]. Despite their transcriptionally and translationally inert status, it is now apparent that mature sperm cells are furnished with a complex cargo of RNA transcripts, including both mRNA and several species of small non-coding RNAs (sncRNA) [35]. Moreover, a subset of these transcripts has been implicated in regulating the initiation and/or trajectory of embryo development, as well as exerting influence over the lifetime health of the offspring [36]. Thus, far from being inconsequential remnants of the spermatogenic process, the sperm-borne RNA profile is gaining traction as a sensitive prognostic indicator for evaluating sperm quality and male infertility. There is also mounting interest in sperm-borne RNAs as a diagnostic readout of a male's exposure to reproductive toxicants as well as a surrogate to evaluate the fidelity of the spermatogenic and post-testicular development that gives rise to the mature spermatozoon [33,35]. In this context, compelling evidence now exists linking paternal exposure to a wide range of environmental stressors (e.g. dietary perturbations, corticosterone administration, psychological stress, cigarette smoke and environmental pollutants) to pronounced alterations in the sncRNA profile that the exposed spermatozoa carry. The clinical significance of these data rests with the fact that each of these changes represents a source of potential sperm dysfunction. Accordingly, a growing body of literature indicates that males with idiopathic infertility exhibit a specific sperm sncRNA expression profile that is clearly differentiated from that of fertile individuals [35]. The potential impact of such differences on the individuals' reproductive competence is highlighted by aberrant embryo miRNA expression detected in human blastocysts derived from patients with male factor infertility [37]. Notwithstanding the interest these studies have generated, the unique biology of a spermatozoon presents a number of challenges in seeking to characterise their RNA cargo for diagnostic purposes. Not least of these are the relatively low yield of RNA per spermatozoon and the absence of 18S and 28S ribosomal RNA subunits with which to rigorously assess the fidelity of sperm RNA isolation protocols. The continued refinement of isolation protocols that reliably yield high-quality sperm RNA will undoubtedly help to circumvent these limitations [38], aiding in the translation of data collected from animal models, as well as enhancing the reproducibility of clinical assessments of male factor fertility using RNA molecular biomarkers. In time, the assembly of a human sperm RNA inventory, equivalent to that already achieved for the proteome, may provide the opportunity to evaluate and monitor the effects of chemical, physical and environmental factors on semen quality.

2.4 Implications for Therapeutic Interventions

With ongoing limitations associated with the accurate diagnosis of male infertility, it is not surprising that a majority of the therapeutic interventions that have been clinically successful have been targeted to the treatment of pathologies with an obvious phenotype. Examples of these successful strategies lie in the treatment of varicocele through surgical means [39], the use of aromatase inhibitors in patients with abnormal testosterone-to-estradiol ratios [40], and extensive developments in ART procedures, such as ICSI [2], which have assisted patients with poor semen parameters, or those with an absence of sperm in the ejaculate through a combination of testicular sperm extraction (TESE) and ICSI.

In the case of varicocele, although the prevalence of the condition remains high at up to 20% of the male population, clinical varicocele now represents the most common correctable cause of male infertility [39]. Varicocele repair is aimed at the dilation of the pampiniform plexus, a venous network located in the spermatic cord, to relieve the causative retrograde blood flow through the internal spermatic vein. In current practice, surgical approaches to repair varicocele, including ligation and resection of the dilated vessels by open surgery or microsurgery, are preferred. Furthermore, the ability to tailor interventions to the grade and condition of each varicocele patient has led to a large array of treatment options [39]. These innovations have had a significant impact on the recovery of fertility in patients that have undergone varicocelectomy. However, complications due to the inflammation and testicular heating paradigms associated with this condition have led to the suggestion that varicocele may be a progressive, rather than a static pathological condition, with implications extending to both structural and functional damage within the testis [41]. Particularly concerning is that even in varicocele patients with normal semen parameters, or those with improved fertility post-surgery, the condition is commonly accompanied by an increased prevalence of sperm DNA fragmentation compared to that of fertile controls [42].

Thus, issues associated with reduced paternal DNA integrity may persist in embryos generated through either natural conception or through ART interventions after varicocelectomy.

Although the nature of the sperm DNA damage experienced in varicocele patients is not entirely understood, one hypothesis is that excessive production of ROS in varicocele testes may contribute oxidative DNA lesions in spermatozoa and/or damaged chromatin in developing germ cells [39]. One option for the management of these patients, pre- and post-surgery, is the administration of oral antioxidants to reduce the presence of ROS. While there is great theoretical merit in this strategy and strong evidence from recent animal models that report the efficacy of targeted antioxidant strategies to reduce DNA damage [43], the use of oral antioxidants in a clinical setting has been met with mixed success. Recent reviews have highlighted just five oral antioxidant supplements that have resulted in increases in clinical pregnancy rates and live birth rates [44,45], namely astaxanthin, L-carnitine + L-acetyl carnitine, Menevit, vitamin E and zinc sulphate. Despite the initial promise of these therapeutic candidates, there have been few reports regarding the longevity of this success or follow-up studies on the consistency of improved pregnancy outcomes following administration of these antioxidants. Moreover, throughout the analysis of 29 clinical studies of antioxidants targeted to individuals experiencing fertility problems, extensive variation in outcomes was observed, with some studies reporting profound improvement in several semen parameters and some reporting no effect using the same oral antioxidant [44].

A degree of this variability can certainly be attributed to disparities in the intrinsic design of clinical trials, with potential confounders including variations in dose regimens, methodology and the duration of treatment. However, recent reports have also highlighted a lack of selectivity in the patient populations that are recruited for each trial [44,46]. Regrettably, very few antioxidant trials have been performed with cohorts of patients specifically selected based on the presentation of oxidative defects in their spermatozoa or high levels of ROS in their ejaculate. Moreover, the measures of success for these trials, while encompassing important outcomes such as improved semen parameters and time-to-conception, do not commonly include assessments to ensure an initial reduction in ROS levels or DNA damage in the patient's spermatozoa [44]. This has led to a concerning inability to determine a rationale for why individual antioxidant trials have not been successful and compromises our ability to improve on formulations that may be beneficial in stratified patient cohorts.

The reasons for omitting crucial patient selection procedures are undoubtedly complex, though difficulties in the diagnosis of ROS-driven fertility issues and the accurate quantification of oxidative DNA damage remain major clinical roadblocks. Here, despite extensive validation of a number of reliable biomarkers for lipid peroxidation products, ROS and oxidative DNA damage [46], there are still major challenges associated with the cost-efficiency and accuracy of these tools. Consideration should be given to the development of these common laboratory tools to form clinically applicable markers that can be employed for the high throughput analysis of ROS and oxidative DNA damage in human spermatozoa. Towards this goal, validation has now been performed across several protocols to assess human DNA oxidation levels using an 8-hydroxy-2'-deoxyguanosine (8-OHdG) antibody and flow cytometry to discriminate patients with poor semen quality [47]. Indeed, this study has helped to establish a consensus for a clinically applicable protocol that allows for the stratification of patients based on 8-OHdG fluorescence. Moreover, great care has been taken to provide evidence of the repeatability and accuracy of the assay, and a rationale for its use as part of routine diagnostics in ART clinics [47]. It remains to be seen whether the clinical application of this technique will aid in the selection of patients for oral antioxidant trials. However, this approach is a step towards the development of better management strategies for patients with oxidative-stress derived infertility.

The examples provided here serve to highlight the necessity of a continuum between accurate diagnostics to stratify male reproductive pathologies and the successful development of appropriate treatment and management strategies. While there are many exceptions to this rule, such as the management of patients with non-obstructive azoospermia for which there are no current treatment options despite the clarity of the condition, gaining an advanced mechanistic understanding of male reproductive pathologies is essential to improve diagnostic and therapeutic strategies.

2.5 Conclusions

Despite a significant percentage of human infertility being attributed to the male partner, we currently lack the tools to accurately diagnose and treat this distressing condition. Traditional diagnostic approaches often overlook the subtleties associated with day-to-day variations in sperm production and have increasingly been found to be inadequate predictors of fertilisation outcome and live birth rates. These shortcomings underscore an urgent need for new diagnostic tools to assist with patient stratification, sperm selection and therapeutic treatment options for males suffering from subfertility and infertility. In terms of realising these ambitious goals, we have much to gain from continued research into the molecular mechanisms regulating normal sperm function and an understanding of how these facets of sperm cell biology become disrupted in cases of infertility. In particular, dissection of the highly specialised sequence of changes that accompany sperm production and their functional maturation during their transport through the male and female reproductive tracts promises to yield novel insights into how these cells behave during *in vitro* interventions (Figure 2.1). Moreover, with the growing realisation that poorer-quality sperm may impact offspring health, we have an obligation to define those contributions of the fertilising spermatozoon that limit the possibility of an adverse outcome after ART interventions. The development of specific sperm biomarkers for this purpose remains a significant goal as does seeking to define biological signatures indicative of the stress(ors) that the male may have experienced.

References

1. Kolettis, P. N. (2003) Evaluation of the subfertile man. *Am Fam Physician* 67:2165–2172.

2. O'Neill, C. L., Chow, S., Rosenwaks, Z. and Palermo, G. D. (2018) Development of ICSI. *Reproduction* 156:F51–F58.

3. Fitzgerald, O., Harris, K., Paul, R. C. and Chambers, C. G. (2017) *Assisted Reproductive Technology in Australia and New Zealand 2015.* Sydney: National Perinatal Epidemiology & Statistics Unit, University of New South Wales: 1–93.

4. Belva, F., Bonduelle, M., Roelants, M., Michielsen, D., Van Steirteghem, A., Verheyen, G., et al. (2016) Semen quality of young adult ICSI offspring: the first results. *Hum Reprod* 31:2811–2820.

5. Davies, M. J., Rumbold, A. R. and Moore, V. M. (2017) Assisted reproductive technologies: a hierarchy of risks for conception, pregnancy outcomes and treatment decisions. *Dev Orig Health Dis* 8:443–447.

6. Barratt, C. L. R., De Jonge, C. J. and Sharpe, R. M. (2018) "Man Up": the importance and strategy for placing male

reproductive health centre stage in the political and research agenda. *Hum Reprod* 33:541–545.

7. Teixeira, D. M., Barbosa, M. A., Ferriani, R. A., Navarro, P. A., Raine-Fenning, N., et al. (2013) Regular (ICSI) versus ultra-high magnification (IMSI) sperm selection for assisted reproduction. *Cochrane Database Syst Rev* CD010167.

8. Mortimer, D. and Mortimer, S. T. (2013) Computer-aided sperm analysis (CASA) of sperm motility and hyperactivation. *Methods Mol Biol* 927:77–87.

9. Hirano, Y., Shibahara, H., Obara, H., Suzuki, T., Takamizawa, S., et al. (2001) Relationships between sperm motility characteristics assessed by the computer-aided sperm analysis (CASA) and fertilization rates *in vitro*. *J Assist Reprod Genet* 18:213–218.

10. Boomsma, C. M., Heineman, M. J., Cohlen, B. J. and Farquhar, C. (2007) Semen preparation techniques for intrauterine insemination. *Cochrane Database Syst Rev* CD004507.

11. Aitken, R. J. and Nixon, B. (2013) Sperm capacitation: a distant landscape glimpsed but unexplored. *Mol Hum Reprod* 19:785–793.

12. Dun, M. D., Mitchell, L. A., Aitken, R. J. and Nixon, B. (2010) Sperm–zona pellucida interaction: molecular mechanisms and the potential for contraceptive intervention. *Handb Exp Pharmacol* 198:139–178.

13. Huszar, G., Jakab, A., Sakkas, D., Ozenci, C. C., Cayli, S., Delpiano, E., et al. (2007) Fertility testing and ICSI sperm selection by hyaluronic acid binding: clinical and genetic aspects. *Reprod Biomed Online* 14:650–663.

14. McDowell, S., Kroon, B., Ford, E., Hook, Y., Glujovsky, D. and Yazdani, A. (2014) Advanced sperm selection techniques for assisted reproduction. *Cochrane Database Syst Rev* 10: CD010461.

15. Nixon, B., Bromfield, E. G., Cui, J. and De Iuliis, G. N. (2017) Heat shock protein A2 (HSPA2): regulatory roles in germ cell

development and sperm function. *Adv Anat Embryol Cell Biol* 222:67–93.

16. Liu, D. Y. and Baker, H. W. (2000) Defective sperm–zona pellucida interaction: a major cause of failure of fertilization in clinical *in-vitro* fertilization. *Hum Reprod* 15:702–708.

17. Oehninger, S., Franken, D. R. and Ombelet, W. (2014) Sperm functional tests. *Fertil Steril* 102:1528–1533.

18. Liu, D. Y. (2011) Could using the zona pellucida bound sperm for intracytoplasmic sperm injection (ICSI) enhance the outcome of ICSI? *Asian J Androl* 13:197–198.

19. Aitken, R. J., Baker, M. A., De Iuliis, G. N. and Nixon, B. (2010) New insights into sperm physiology and pathology. *Handb Exp Pharmacol* 198:99–115.

20. Oehninger, S., Clark, G. F., Fulgham, D., Blackmore, P. F., Mahony, M. C. and Acosta, A. A., et al. (1992) Effect of fucoidin on human sperm-zona pellucida interactions. *J Androl* 13:519–525.

21. Pang, P. C., Chiu, P. C., Lee, C. L., Chang, L. Y., Panico, M., Morris, H. R., et al. (2011) Human sperm binding is mediated by the sialyl-Lewis(x) oligosaccharide on the zona pellucida. *Science* 333:1761–1764.

22. Tecle, E. and Gagneux, P. (2015) Sugar-coated sperm: unraveling the functions of the mammalian sperm glycocalyx. *Mol Reprod Dev* 82:635–650.

23. Ainsworth, C., Nixon, B., Jansen, R. P. and Aitken, R. J. (2007) First recorded pregnancy and normal birth after ICSI using electrophoretically isolated spermatozoa. *Hum Reprod* 22:197–200.

24. Said, T. M. and Land, J. A. (2011) Effects of advanced selection methods on sperm quality and ART outcome: a systematic review. *Hum Reprod Update* 17:719–733.

25. Simon, L., Ge, S. Q. and Carrell, D. T. (2013) Sperm selection based on electrostatic charge. *Methods Mol Biol* 927:269–278.

26. Aitken, R. J., De Iuliis, G. N., Gibb, Z. and Baker, M. A. (2012) The Simmet lecture:

new horizons on an old landscape-oxidative stress, DNA damage and apoptosis in the male germ line. *Reprod Domest Anim* **47** Suppl 4:7–14.

27. Vermey, B. G., Chapman, M. G., Cooke, S. and Kilanim, S. (2015) The relationship between sperm head retardance using polarized light microscopy and clinical outcomes. *Reprod Biomed Online* **30**:67–73.

28. Jodar, M., Sendler, E. and Krawetz, S. A. (2016) The protein and transcript profiles of human semen. *Cell Tissue Res* **363**:85–96.

29. Nixon, B., Dun, M. D. and Aitken, R. J. (2017) Proteomic analysis of human spermatozoa. In Krause, W. K. H. and Naz, R. K. (eds.), *Immune Infertility: The Impact of Immune Reactions on Human Infertility*, vol. **2**. Heidelberg, Germany: Springer Publishing Company: 3–22.

30. Jodar, M., Soler-Ventura, A. and Oliva, R. (2017) Semen proteomics and male infertility. *J Proteomics* **162**:125–134.

31. Amaral, A., Castillo, J., Ramalho-Santos, J. and Oliva, R. (2014) The combined human sperm proteome: cellular pathways and implications for basic and clinical science. *Hum Reprod Update* **20**:40–62.

32. Bromfield, E. G., Aitken, R. J., Anderson, A. L., McLaughlin, E. A. and Nixon, B. (2015) The impact of oxidative stress on chaperone-mediated human sperm-egg interaction. *Hum Reprod* **30**:2597–2613.

33. Jenkins, T. G., Aston, K. I., James, E. R. and Carrell, D. T. (2017) Sperm epigenetics in the study of male fertility, offspring health, and potential clinical applications. *Syst Biol Reprod Med* **63**:69–76.

34. Simon, L., Emery, B. R. and Carrell, D. T. (2017) Review: diagnosis and impact of sperm DNA alterations in assisted reproduction. *Best Pract Res Clin Obstet Gynaecol* **44**:38–56.

35. Jodar, M., Selvaraju, S., Sendler, E., Diamond, M. P. and Krawetz, S. A. (2013) Reproductive medicine: the presence, role and clinical use of spermatozoal RNAs. *Hum Reprod Update* **19**:604–624.

36. Burl, R. B., Clough, S., Sendler, E., Estill, M. and Krawetz, S. A. (2018) Sperm RNA elements as markers of health. *Syst Biol Reprod Med* **64**:25–38.

37. McCallie, B., Schoolcraft, W. B. and Katz-Jaffe, M. G. (2010) Aberration of blastocyst microRNA expression is associated with human infertility. *Fertil Steril* **93**:2374–2382.

38. Bianchi, E., Stermer, A., Boekelheide, K., Sigman, M., Hall, S. J., Reyes, G., et al. (2018) High-quality human and rat spermatozoal RNA isolation for functional genomic studies. *Andrology* **6**:374–383.

39. Zavattaro, M., Ceruti, C., Motta, G., Allasia, S., Marinelli, L., Di Bisceglie, C., et al. (2018) Treating varicocele in 2018: current knowledge and treatment options. *J Endocrinol Invest* **41**:1365–1375.

40. Khourdaji, I., Lee, H. and Smith, R. P. (2018) Frontiers in hormone therapy for male infertility. *Transl Androl Urol* **7**:S353–S366.

41. Jung, A. and Schuppe, H. C. (2007) Influence of genital heat stress on semen quality in humans. *Andrologia* **39**:203–215.

42. Moazzam, A., Sharma, R. and Agarwal, A. (2015) Relationship of spermatozoal DNA fragmentation with semen quality in varicocele-positive men. *Andrologia* **47**:935–944.

43. Gharagozloo, P., Gutierrez-Adan, A., Champroux, A., Noblanc, A., Kocer, A., Calle, A., et al. (2016) A novel antioxidant formulation designed to treat male infertility associated with oxidative stress: promising preclinical evidence from animal models. *Hum Reprod* **31**:252–262.

44. Majzoub, A. and Agarwal, A. (2018) Systematic review of antioxidant types and doses in male infertility: benefits on semen parameters, advanced sperm function, assisted reproduction and live-birth rate. *Arab J Urol* **16**:113–124.

45. Walters, J. L. H., De Iuliis, G. N., Nixon, B. and Bromfield, E. G. (2018) Oxidative stress in the male germ line: a review of novel strategies to reduce 4-hydroxynonenal production. *Antioxidants (Basel)* **7**:E132.

46. Aitken, R. J. (2018) Not every sperm is sacred: a perspective on male infertility. *Mol Hum Reprod* **24**:287–298.

47. Vorilhon, S., Brugnon, F., Kocer, A., Dollet, S., Bourgne, C., Berger, M., et al. (2018) Accuracy of human sperm DNA oxidation quantification and threshold determination using an 8-OHdG immuno-detection assay. *Hum Reprod* **33**:553–562.

Chromosome Abnormalities and the Infertile Male

Csilla Krausz and Viktória Rosta

3.1 Introduction

Male infertility is a highly heterogeneous, multifactorial, complex pathology of the reproductive system, affecting approximately 7% of the general male population. Genetic factors are estimated to contribute to nearly 20–25% of severe male infertility cases and inversely correlate with sperm production [1]. In fact, their frequency is 0.4% of the general population, while patients with a spermatozoa count of less than 5 million/ml already show a 10-fold higher incidence (4%) [2]. The aberrations include numerical defects, among them Klinefelter syndrome (47, XXY), which represents the most common karyotype abnormality in azoospermia. Structural chromosomal abnormalities, such as Robertsonian translocations (RobT), reciprocal translocations (RecT), or inversions are relatively frequent in severe male factor infertility. The most frequent molecular genetic causes of oligo/azoospermia are the submicroscopic deletions on the Y-chromosome (Yq), called AZF (azoospermia factor) deletions. The most widely accepted clinical indications for karyotype analysis are azoospermia and oligozoospermia below 10 million spermatozoa/ml and a family history of recurrent pregnancy loss (RPL), malformations, or mental retardation independent from the sperm count. AZF deletion screening is indicated in azoospermia and oligozoospermia below 5 million spermatozoa/ml [3]. In order to provide a better risk assessment for chromosomal abnormalities, besides sperm count, the integration of clinical characteristics (follicle stimulating hormone (FSH), luteinizing hormone (LH), and mean testicular volume) has been recently proposed [4]. Males with structural karyotype abnormalities are at an increased risk of producing aneuploid sperm or unbalanced chromosomal complements and uniparental disomies (in the case of RobTs), therefore genetic counseling in these couples is mandatory. Similarly, carriers of AZF deletions should be informed about the obligatory transmission of this genetic defect to the male offspring, who will be affected by spermatogenic disturbances.

The advent of high-resolution genomic platforms allowed the discovery of X chromosome linked genetic factors, such as copy number variations (CNVs) and *TEX11* intragenic deletion with potential clinical interest [5]. Genetic testing is an essential diagnostic tool, not only for personalized clinical decision making, but also for predicting the outcome of testicular sperm extraction (TESE) and indicates the risk of transmitting genetic disorders to the offspring through assisted reproductive technology (ART). This chapter aims to provide both an overview of the routine chromosomal testing and a description of clinically relevant novel data related to chromosomal anomalies involved in quantitative spermatogenetic disturbances (Table 3.1).

Table 3.1 Chromosomal abnormalities in quantitative disturbances of spermatogenesis

Chromosomal alterations		Semen phenotype	Testis volume/ histology	Genetic test	Biological parenthood (natural or ART)
Numerical chromosomal alterations	47, XXY	>90% men with azoospermia, rarely severe oligozoospermia or cryptozoospermia	hypotrophic, firm/ diffuse tubular hyalinization and fibrosis	Karyotype analysis	**ART:** (m)TESE + ICSI; **natural conception:** extremely rare
	Trisomy 21	from oligozoospermia to azoospermia	hypotrophic or normal/ hypospermatogenesis or meiotic arrest		**natural conception:** extremely rare #
Structural chromosomal alterations	RobT	most frequently oligozoospermia, but also normozoospermia	hypotrophic or normal/ hypospermatogenesis	Karyotype analysis	**ART:** ICSI or IVF with **PGT**; **natural conception:** possible
	RecT	most frequently azoospermia	hypotrophic/ SGA or SCOS or hypospermatogenesis		**ART:** TESE*+ ICSI with **PGT**
	idic Y	most frequently azoospermia *	hypotrophic or normal/ hypospermatogenesis* or SCOS* or SGA*, Leydig-cell hyperplasia		**ART:** TESE* + ICSI
	Yq (–) *AZFa* deletion	azoospermia* complete: azoospermia partial: oligozoospermia or normozoospermia	hypotrophic/SCOS hypotrophic/SCOS, Leydig-cell hyperplasia normal/ hypospermatogenesis	Microdeletion screening, based on ±PCR (according to the EAA-EMQN guidelines)	**Virtually impossible*** complete: mostly **unsuccessful** sperm retrieval by **TESE** ** partial: **ART:** TESE+ICSI; **natural conception:** rarely

Table 3.1 (cont.)

Chromosomal alterations		Semen phenotype	Testis volume/ histology	Genetic test	Biological parenthood (natural or ART)
	AZFb deletion	complete: azoospermia	normal/SGA		
		partial: oligozoospermia or normozoospermia	normal/ hypospermatogenesis		
	AZFc deletion	from severe oligozoospermia to azoospermia	hypotrophic or normal/ hypospermatogenesis, SCOS		ART: (m)TESE + ICSI; natural conception: rarely
	gr/gr deletion	from normozoospermia to oligozoospermia	hypotrophic or normal/ hypospermatogenesis		
	X chromosome linked CNV67	from oligozoospermia to azoospermia	hypotrophic or normal/ hypospermatogenesis or SCOS	Array-CGH	ART: TESE + ICSI; natural conception: rarely
	TEX11 hemizygous deletion	azoospermia	normal/meiotic arrest		ART: TESE likely to be unsuccessful
Sex reversal	XX male syndrome	azoospermia	hypotrophic, firm/ SCOS, Leydig-cell hyperplasia	Karyotype analysis and ±PCR or FISH for SRY detection	Virtually impossible

Abbreviations: AZF: azoospermia factor; ART: Assisted Reproduction Techniques; CGH: comparative genomic hybridization; EAA: European Academy of Andrology; EMQN: European Molecular Genetics Quality Network; ICSI: intracytoplasmic sperm injection; idic Y: isodicentric Y chromosome; IVF: in vitro fertilization; RecT: reciprocal translocation; RobT: Robertsonian translocation; SGA: Spermatogenic Arrest; SCOS: Sertoli-cell only syndrome; TESE: testicular sperm extraction; (m)TESE: micro-TESE; TGCT: testicular germ cell tumor; PCR: polymerase chain reaction; PGT: Pre-implantation Genetic Testing.

Three cases reported by Stefanidis et al. [11].

* Depends on the proportion of cells with the aberrant Y chromosome; whether the AZF subregions are intact or absent; and depends on the proportion of 45, X0 cells.

** Minimal chance in few cases, and depends on the proportion of 45, X0 cells.

3.2 Numerical Alterations of the Chromosomes

3.2.1 Klinefelter Syndrome

Klinefelter Syndrome (KS) represents the most common sex chromosome aneuploidy in humans, accounting for the main genetic cause of nonobstructive azoospermia (NOA). About 80–90% of KS patients carry the 47, XXY karyotype, while nearly 10% display various grades of mosaicism with the 46, XY/47, XXY karyotype or rarely present higher-grade sex chromosomal aneuploidy, such as 48, XXXY, 49, XXXXY, or structurally abnormal X chromosomes. Although the incidence of the syndrome is relatively high (1:660 in live births and 1:300 in spontaneous abortions), about two-thirds of KS patients are still misdiagnosed or remain undiagnosed [6]. The remaining 32% of KS patients are diagnosed in the following age groups: (i) in the fetus, during prenatal genetic diagnosis (10%); (ii) in childhood mainly for cognitive problems (3%); (iii) in adolescent age due to delayed puberty and gynecomastia (2%); and (iv) in adulthood due to infertility or sexual dysfunction (17%).

Heterogeneous clinical phenotypes of the disease, which may range from different grades of undervirilization, eunuchoid habitus, tall stature, long extremities, gynecomastia, hypergonadotropic hypogonadism, and azoospermia (90%), are likely related to the genotype. The overdosage of the *SHOX* (*short stature homeobox*) gene, located in the *pseudo-autosomal region 1 (PAR1)* on the short arm of Y and X chromosomes together with the delay of testosterone-induced closure of epiphyses have been proposed as possible explanations for the tall stature. In the majority of mosaic KS cases, few spermatozoa can be found in the ejaculate. A constant finding in KS patients is the small firm testis, due to testicular hyalinization and fibrosis, leading to testicular failure. Elevated LH and FSH levels are universal, whereas decline in the testosterone levels shows high interindividual variability. For most of the subjects, serum-testosterone concentrations after the age of 15 years remain in the low-normal adult range, and there is no absolute decline as they age. Testicular sperm extraction by conventional way (cTESE) and especially microsurgical TESE (micro-TESE) combined with intracytoplasmic sperm injection (ICSI) represent an opportunity for KS patients to father their own biological children. The average sperm retrieval rate (SRR) is about 40% [7] ranging from 28 to 62.5% [8], and it has been suggested that the success rates progressively decrease after the age of 30 [9]. Many different parameters have been studied with the aim to establish predictive factors for successful sperm retrieval, but available data have failed to identify clinically useful prognostic markers. Since apoptosis of spermatogonia and histological changes have been detected at onset of puberty, the question about the timing of testis biopsy has been the object of long debate. Preserving the fertility potential of young KS patients has been proposed in three different age groups: (i) pre-pubertal; (ii) peri-pubertal; and (iii) young adulthood. Some authors suggested that early pre-pubertal testicular sampling – before the complete germ cell loss occurs – might offer a greater chance of retrieving gametogenic cells. Although spermatogonia can be found in about 50% of a small number of adolescent KS boys by (m)TESE, testicular tissue freezing techniques as well as *in vitro* maturation strategies require further investigation. Data by Rohayem and colleagues in 2015 [9] suggest that the most promising predictive factors of finding spermatozoa in late adolescence and young adulthood are the patients' age (between 15 and 25 years at biopsy) and the near compensated Leydig cell function. The cut-off values for hormones have been found to be a combination of total serum testosterone above 7.5 nmol/l with an LH below 17.5 U/l; however, these findings need further validation. Still, overall data in the literature do not support the necessity of adolescent TESE, since various studies have not found higher retrieval rates of spermatozoa in post-pubertal boys versus young adult KS patients [9]. Regarding the data of 1,248 adult KS patients in the meta-analysis performed by Corona and colleagues [7], the SRR was on average 40% and the live birth rate was about 16% of subjects who underwent TESE approach. Sperm retrieval was independent of a number of clinical and biological parameters such as age, testis volume, hormonal status, and bilateral approach [7,9].

Another controversial topic is related to androgen replacement therapy, which was supposed to have a negative influence on the future fertility of KS patients. Recently published reports did not confirm the deleterious effect of testosterone supplementation [7,9]. Some authors found that using hormonal stimulation by aromatase inhibitors improved the chances of successful SRR.

In KS patients with successful sperm retrieval, the genetic constitution of spermatozoa has been questioned. Recent evidence suggests that non-mosaic KS patients who produce sperm have mosaicism confined to the testis, and only 46, XY spermatocytes can achieve meiosis. However, in the analysis of sperm from KS patients assessed by using cell fluorescence in situ hybridization (FISH), higher aneuploidy rates of sex chromosomes and autosomes (especially chromosomes 13, 18 and 21) have been revealed. It is highly likely that the elevated aneuploidy rate in spermatozoa from KS patients results from abnormal meiosis in 46, XY spermatocytes, rather than from 47, XXY spermatocyte cells, since the presence of a supernumerary X chromosome prevents meiosis. For the above reasons, Preimplantation Genetic Testing (PGT) is recommended, although with few exceptions, the nearly 200 babies born worldwide from KS fathers with ICSI without PGT were normal. According to a study on a large cohort undergoing prenatal genetic diagnosis, KS accounts for 0.17% (188 out of 106,000) of all cases, which was similar to the incidence detected at birth by various studies [10].

KS is not confined to infertility but includes a series of comorbidities leading to increased mortality and morbidity, such as metabolic syndrome, autoimmune diseases (i.e. systemic lupus erythematosus, rheumatoid arthritis, type 1 diabetes mellitus, etc.), venous thromboembolism, bone fractures due to osteoporosis, behavioral and socio-economic problems, etc. (Figure 3.1). They also present susceptibility to specific neoplasias, like breast cancer or extragonadal germ cell tumors and hematological malignancies [6]. The possible development of comorbidities implies that these patients need follow up (possibly by a multidisciplinary team) throughout their lifetime in order to actuate preventive strategies (life style change, diet, regular physical exercise, etc.) and therapies (i.e. testosterone replacement therapy, etc.).

3.2.2 Down Syndrome

Trisomy 21 occurs with an estimated frequency of 1:150 conceptions, 1:600 live births in the general population, and it correlates with advanced maternal age. The presence of an extra chromosome 21 has a detrimental direct and indirect effect on the reproductive capacity of the affected male subjects. The detailed pathophysiology of infertility in men with Down syndrome has not yet been elucidated. According to investigations addressing the causes of infertility, hormonal deficits, morphological alterations of the gonads, abnormal spermatogenesis, and psychological and social factors related to the mental retardations may play roles in this process. To date, three cases of parenting by fathers with Down syndrome have been described in the literature [11].

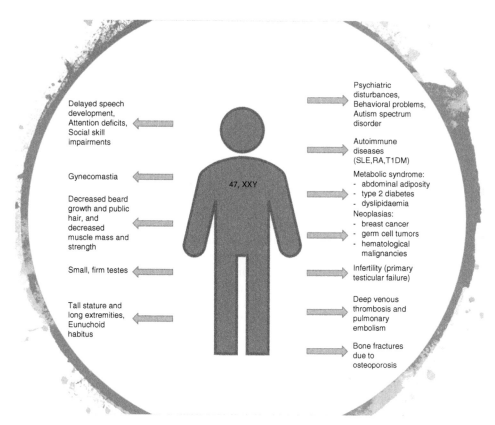

Figure 3.1 Phenotypic characteristics and co-morbidities in KS.

3.3 Structural Alterations of the Chromosomes

3.3.1 Detectable with Karyotyping

3.3.1.1 Structural Anomalies of the Autosomes

Couples with male carriers of structural abnormalities of the autosomes, such as Robertsonian translocations (RobT, inversions and reciprocal translocations (RecT) may experience reduced fertility, RPL and chromosomally unbalanced offspring. Most patients are likely to be fertile; however, structural chromosomal abnormalities occur in infertile patients 10 times more than in general populations. RobTs result from centromeric fusion of two acrocentric chromosomes (13,14,15,21,22) and more commonly occur between nonhomologous pairs. The short p-arms of the translocated chromosomes may be lost during early cell division, but it has relatively little impact, since the short arms of the acrocentric chromosomes consist largely of various classes of satellite DNA, as well as hundreds of copies of ribosomal RNA genes. Translocations can either be balanced or unbalanced, depending on the conservation of the genetic material. The vast majority of balanced translocations involve chromosomes 13 and 14 (13:14), which account for 75% of RobTs, and the most frequent unbalanced translocations involve chromosomes 21 (21:21). The prevalence of autosomal balanced translocations in infertile men ranges between 1.6 and 6.6%. RobT-s are considered the most common balanced chromosomal rearrangements, with an incidence of 1:1,000 in the general population and with normal sperm parameters in about 25.7% of patients. This type of rearrangement is more common in oligozoospermic versus azoospermic patients (1.6% vs 0.09%), while RecT-s – when two nonhomologous chromosomes exchange segments – are more commonly associated with azoospermia. Individuals with chromosomal translocations produce a very high rate of chromosomally abnormal embryos, such as a paternally derived trisomy 13 or 21 conceptus (Patau and Down syndrome). These abnormalities are often the cause of recurrent miscarriages or birth defects [12,13]. Several studies reported 54–72% of embryos to be unbalanced for RobT-s, while the even higher percentage of unbalanced embryos are RecT-s (75–82%) [13]. Furthermore, there is an increased risk of aneuploidy and uniparental disomy (UPD). Genomic imprinting – which refers to the differential expression of genes depending on its parental origin – among the acrocentric chromosomes have been observed in RobT cases. Chromosomes 14 and 15 have been documented as clinically relevant imprinted chromosomes; according to published reports, maternal UPD 15 is associated with Prader Willi Syndrome (PWS) in 30% of cases and paternal UPD 15 is associated with Angelman Syndrome (AS) in 2–5% of cases. The occurrence of UPD is estimated to be 1:3500 in newborn babies and 8–10% of all UDPs derive from parents with nonhomologous RobTs [14].

In vitro fertilization (IVF) with PGT represents a viable option for these couples to obtain chromosomally normal embryos. Comprehensive chromosome screening (CCS) with a variety of testing methods – including FISH, two main types of microarrays (comparative genomic hybridization (CGH) arrays and single nucleotide polymorphism (SNP) microarrays), or next generation sequencing (NGS), are available for embryo selection. Despite huge efforts that have been made enabling the selection of balanced and translocation-free embryos, so far PGT remains challenging and these new strategies need further validation [14].

3.3.1.2 Structural Anomalies of the Gonosomes

3.3.1.2.1 Isodicentric Y Chromosome (idic Y)

The structural abnormalities of the Y chromosome include dicentricism, truncation, or ring formation. Among these structural aberrations, dicentric Y chromosomes are the most commonly identified. If the dicentric chromosome has completely symmetric arms, it is considered an isodicentric chromosome. The site of breakage and fusions at Yp and Yq are highly variable, and whether spermatogenesis is present or not depends upon the proportion of cells with the aberrant Y chromosome, and whether the AZF subregions are intact or absent [15]. Patients may show mosaicism with a 45, X0 cell line, representing a poor prognosis for TESE [1,16].

3.3.1.2.2 Yq (−)

The absence of the long arm of the Y chromosome is inevitably associated with spermatogenic failure. The phenotype of these patients shows small testes, and their testicular histology is a picture of Sertoli-cell-only syndrome (SCOS), consistent with the loss of AZF regions.

3.3.2 Detectable with Molecular Genetic Tests

3.3.2.1 Submicroscopic Deletions of the Y-chromosome: AZF Deletions

The Y chromosome plays a critical role in the genetic regulation of the initiation and maintenance of spermatogenesis. The euchromatin long arm of the Y chromosome (Yq) contains a large set of testes expressed genes, most of them located in a specific region called the AZF region, which were discovered more than 40 years ago, in 1976 by Tiepolo and Zuffardi [17]. The peculiar feature of the AZF regions, characterized by highly homologous repeated sequences with the same orientations, represents a predisposing substrate for deletion/duplication formation through the mechanism called Non-Allelic Homologous Recombination (NAHR) [1]. Three different loci AZFs (*AZFa, AZFb*, and *AZFc*) have been mapped, in which the *AZFb* and *AZFc* regions overlap. Clinically relevant microdeletions partly or completely remove one or more AZF subregions. On the existing five Yq hotspots, disruption can result in the recurrent removal of large DNA sequences, leading to five different types of complete deletion patterns, and the likelihood of treatment success can be determined by the location of the deletion. The most fragile subregion is *AZFc* (~80%), followed by *AZFa* (~0.5–4%), *AZFb* (~1–5%), and *AZFb+c* (with two different breakpoints) (~1–3%) deletion. Deletions that are detected as *AZFabc* are often associated with abnormal karyotypes such as 46, XX male or iso(Y) [18].

The Y chromosome became the most important genetic target of male infertility, and AZF testing is part of routine clinical practice. AZF deletions are considered the most frequently known molecular genetic causes for oligo/azoospermia [19]. Based on global data, Yq microdeletions are estimated to occur in about 1:4,000 men in the general population, varying by geographic region or ethnicity (the lowest prevalence is in Europe and Australia), but its frequency rises to 5–10% of patients with idiopathic NOA, and 2–5% of severe oligozoospermic patients (mostly those with more than 2 million spermatozoa/ml) [16]. Most deletions occur *de novo* and are likely to arise during meiosis of the gametes from the patient's father, but some naturally transmitted cases of partial *AZFa* or *AZFb* and complete *AZFc* deletions have been described. According to the European Academy of Andrology (EAA) and European Molecular Genetics Quality Network (EMQN) guidelines, screening for Y chromosome microdeletions is indicated in men with less than 5 million spermatozoa/ml. In cases of partial *AZFa, AZFb*, and *AZFc* deletions, screening of other male members of the family is advised [3].

As a result of microdeletions, candidate genes within the AZF regions will be removed in the large majority en bloc, hence the role of a single AZF gene cannot be deduced from the AZF deletion phenotypes. Isolated gene-specific deletions are extremely rare, and they have been reported only in the *AZFa* region – which contains two protein-coding genes – for one gene (*USP9Y*), which acts as a fine tuner of spermatogenesis and is associated with variable semen phenotype. Hence the complete *AZFa* deletion phenotype SCOS is likely to be caused by the loss of the *DDX3Y* gene [20]. In fact, the deletion of the entire *AZFa* region invariably results in SCOS and involves both genes. The complete deletion of the *AZFb* region leads to spermatogenic arrest at different stages of germ cell maturation. The diagnosis of complete *AZFa* and *AZFb* deletions of the Y chromosome implies the virtual impossibility to retrieve testicular spermatozoa with (m)TESE [15,21]. It is worth noting that exceptionally the deletion only partially removes the *AZFa* or *AZFb* regions, which is related to residual sperm production and is compatible with natural pregnancy, or with a positive TESE result.

In the case of *AZFb* deletions, the determination of the extent of the deletion is essential, because the presence of the distal part of the *AZFb* deletion interval, of around 900 kb, is compatible with residual spermatogenesis [1]. Testicular size is generally smaller than normal in Y deletion carriers, unless caused by an *AZFb* deletion, which is typically associated with normal testis volume and normal FSH concentrations.

Largely variable semen phenotype can be identified with the deletions of the *AZFc* region. Up to 70% of men with *AZFc* deletion may have sperm in the ejaculate, typically less than 2 million/ml, and in rare cases natural fertilization may occur. In the case of azoospermia (ranging from SCOS to hypospermatogenesis), (m)TESE can be used to harvest sperm from the testicle in 50–60% [22]. As in a subset of *AZFc* microdeletion carriers, a progressive decline in sperm counts has been observed, and cryopreservation to prevent invasive techniques should be offered.

Since Y-microdeletions are obligatorily transmitted to the male offspring with consequent impaired spermatogenesis, genetic counselling is advised. However, the exact testicular phenotype cannot be predicted in the male offspring, as it depends on the various genetic backgrounds and the influencing environmental factors. So far, no significant differences in fertilization rates have been confirmed in different studies between men with or without Y deletion who have undergone ART. Besides the predicted reproductive consequences, concerns have been raised about the potential risk of Turner's syndrome (45, X0), other phenotypic anomalies associated with sex chromosome mosaicism (e.g. ambiguous genitalia), or other chromosomal anomalies in the offspring. Some authors suggest that there are associations between Yq-microdeletions and an overall Y-chromosomal instability, which might result in the formation of 45, X0 cell lines. Until now, the literature is scarce regarding the general health status of the descendants of AZF deletion carriers. Available data does not indicate a higher incidence of malformation rate/chromosomal anomalies. The two studies on PGT reported conflicting results about the risk of monosomy X in embryos. However, it must be noted that fetuses with 45, X0 karyotype have a very high risk of spontaneous abortion and there are no data about the abortion rate in these couples. Recently, additional alarming assumption was raised by the results of a study reporting 5.4% of men with AZF deletions and a normal karyotype also carried *SHOX* haploinsufficiency with consequent risk of short stature and skeletal anomalies. This observation has not been proved by a large multicenter study, implying that deletion carriers have no augmented risk of *SHOX*-related pathologies [1,3].

3.3.2.1.1 gr/gr Deletion

Partial deletion that removes half of the gene content of the *AZFc* subregion, known as "gr/gr deletion," represents a population-dependent risk factor for oligozoospermia. According to many investigations, all available meta-analyses and the largest multi-ethnic study [18], the gr/gr deletion shows a strong correlation – an average of 2–2.5-fold increased risk – with low sperm count. The phenotypic expression depends on the Y chromosome background and may vary in different ethnic groups. For instance, in the Caucasian population, the highest risk (OR 4.2, Cl 2.0–8.8, $p < 0.001$) has been reported in selected idiopathic oligozoospermic men of Italian and Spanish origin (with a frequency of 3.5%) when compared to normozoospermic controls of the same origin [18]. In specific Y haplogroups, which are common in Japan (D2b) and in a certain area of China (Q-M3), the deletion is fixed and does not have a negative impact on spermatogenesis [16]. The presence of gr/gr deletion has also been suggested to play a role in TGCT (testicular germ cell tumor) susceptibility; however, these data need further confirmation, considering that there was no ethnic and geographic matching of participants with or without malignancy [23]. Genetic counseling of the gr/gr carriers is recommended, because the deletion will obligatorily transmit to the male offspring and it might become a complete *AZFc* deletion (a clear-cut causative factor for spermatogenic impairment) [3].

3.3.3 Detectable with Array-CGH

3.3.3.1 X-linked Genetic Anomalies (CNVs and *TEX11* Intragenic Deletions)

CNVs are a class of structural variations that may involve complex gains or losses of homologous sequences at multiple sites in the genome. These variations cover about 12% of the human genome and represent the primary source of interindividual variability between genomes. Many CNVs generate alleles with a clear-cut impact on health status and human disease phenotypes [24]. So far, only a couple of studies have been conducted to ascertain the relationship between CNV load and male infertility, by performing array-CGH on the whole genome [25,26] or at high resolution on the X chromosome [5]. Although only a few partially overlapping CNVs have been observed, the conclusions of these investigations support a higher burden of CNVs in men with spermatogenic disturbances. The number of CNVs/person and the mean CNVs size/person were significantly increased in the oligo/azoospermic subject group compared to normozoospermic controls [5,26]. The observed CNV burden may reflect a high genomic instability in infertile patients, which may contribute to their higher morbidity and lower life expectancy in respect to the fertile male population [1].

The X chromosome accumulates a relevant number of testis specific genes involved in the regulation of spermatogenesis. Sex chromosomes harbor a notable number of segmental duplications, which favor the occurrence of the CNVs. Similar to the Y chromosome in males, no compensation is provided by another X-linked allele, so any deleterious *de novo* mutation or CNV have a potential direct pathogenic effect. CNVs on sex chromosomes are likely to play key roles in defective recombination leading to meiotic failure and the loss of germ cells. On the other hand, they may involve genes, which have regulatory effect in spermatogenesis, hence leading to fertility disturbances. Three recurrent X-linked microdeletions (CNV64, CNV67, CNV69) have been discovered, but only one of them has a potential clinical relevance (CNV67), since it is patient-specific. The Xq28 linked CNV67 has been reported with a frequency of 1.11% in a multicenter study in the Italian and Spanish populations [5,27] and 0.7% in the Han Chinese population [28]. The semen phenotype of deletion carriers ranges from azoospermia due to SCOS to oligozoospermia. The proposed biological mechanism for the observed phenotypes in the CNV67 carriers is the potential loss of the proximal copy of the testis specific *MAGEA9 (melanoma antigen family A,9B)* gene, belonging to the *CTA (cancer testis antigen)* gene family. This gene is one of those multi-copy X-linked genes, which have been acquired independently of the human X chromosome since the common ancestor of human and mice. These genes are expressed predominantly in testicular germ cells, and their independent acquisition indicates that they represent specialized portions of the X chromosome for sperm production [27,29].

Recently, with the use of high-resolution CGH micro-array, an intragenic, 99 kb loss – involving three exons – of the *TEX11 (testis expressed 11)* gene have been discovered in two patients affected by azoospermia due to meiotic arrest [30]. The role of *TEX11* mutations in

NOA was further corroborated by Yang and colleagues [31]. *TEX11* maps to chromosome Xq13.1 and encodes a protein crucial for male germ cell meiotic DNA recombination and chromosomal synapsis. Accordingly, *TEX11* linked mutations are considered a novel cause of pure meiotic arrest [1].

3.4 A Rare Sex Reversal: 46, XX Male Syndrome (46, XX Testicular Disorder of Sex Development)

According to the Chicago Consensus Statement by Lee and colleagues [32], disorders of sex development (DSD) are congenital conditions in which the development of chromosomal, gonadal, or anatomic sex is atypical. The 46, XX male syndrome or 46, XX testicular DSD – first reported by De la Chapelle and colleagues [33] – is a rare, heterogeneous clinical condition with an incidence of about 1:20,000 male neonates. The suggested genetic mechanisms leading to the 46, XX male DSD are: (i) translocation of part of the Y chromosome including the SRY gene, which is the master regulator of testis differentiation, to the X chromosome during paternal meiosis (up to 90% of cases); (ii) duplication of autosomal genes involved in testis determination, for instance *SRY box-related gene 9* (*SOX9*). *SOX9* is located on chromosome 17 and interacts with SRY during male sexual development. In around 10% of cases, the *SOX9* gene is duplicated or triplicated, but the SRY gene could not be detected hence leading to SRY-negative XX males; and (iii) Y chromosome mosaicism restricted to the gonads. Phenotypically, since genes harbored in the three AZF regions (AZFa, AZFb, AZFc) on the long arm of the Y chromosome are missing, patients are affected by SCOS and Leydig cell hyperplasia, appearing as small, firm testes. The majority of 46, XX SRY-positive DSD males have completely differentiated male external, internal genitalia and masculinization. 46, XX SRY-negative males usually have ambiguous genitalia because of the inadequate virilization. The hormonal status of 46, XX male patients features as hypergonadotropic hypogonadism. In contrast to KS, 46, XX male patients represent short stature, even shorter than healthy men in the population, with an average height of between 160 and 165 cm, suggesting a role for Y-linked gene(s) in height determination [34]. Micropenis, hypospadiasis, cryptorchidism, gynecomastia, and breast cancer may occur [35]. Seldomly, the diagnosis happens during childhood due to ambiguous genitalia or pubertal disorders, but the vast majority remain unidentified until adulthood, and diagnosed due to fertility disorders.

3.5 Conclusions

Karyotype and Y chromosome microdeletion analyses – which represent the most frequent genetic factors in severe oligo/azoospermia – allow diagnosis in about 25% of infertility cases. Genetic screening is not only important for diagnostic purposes; some of them have also predictive value for TESE. In addition, the diagnosis of chromosomal anomalies allows performing PGT in embryos derived from carriers of chromosomal anomalies to be advised in order to ensure the transfer of embryos with normal chromosomal constitution.

Monogenic forms of infertility are relatively rare and have been identified mainly in pre-testicular etiologies, post-testicular etiologies, and monomorphic teratozoospermia. In approximately half of patients with quantitative impairment of spermatogenesis (primary testicular forms), the etiology remains unknown and we refer to it as "idiopathic infertility." It is highly likely that not yet identified genetic/epigenetic factors are responsible for these pathological conditions [15,21]. Discovering the "hidden" genetic factors is essential both for clinical decision making regarding surgical or pharmacological treatment options, and for appropriate genetic counseling for the couples undergoing ART. An emerging clinical issue is related to the CNV burden (especially deletions) phenomenon, which may derive from a generalized genomic instability in some idiopathic infertile patients, with potential impact on general health. In addition to the CNV burden, mutations in genes involved in DNA repair have been reported as a common genetic link between NOA and different types of cancers. Molecular genetics, especially the diffusion of whole exome analysis, will likely lead to the implementation of the diagnostic armamentarium of male infertility. To this purpose, large international consortiums have been established with the aim of promoting fast progress in this field.

References

1. Krausz, C. and Riera-Escamilla, A. (2018) Genetics of male infertility. *Nat Rev Urol* **15**:369–384.

2. Jungwirth, A., et al. (2012) European Association of Urology Guidelines on Male Infertility: the 2012 update. *Eur Urol* **62**:324–332.

3. Krausz, C., Hoefsloot, L., Simoni, M. and Tüttelmann, F. (2014) EAA/EMQN best practice guidelines for molecular diagnosis of Y-chromosomal microdeletions: state-of-the-art 2013. *Andrology* **2**:5–19.

4. Dul, E. C., et al. (2012) The prevalence of chromosomal abnormalities in subgroups of infertile men. *Hum Reprod* **27**:36–43.

5. Krausz, C., et al. (2012) High resolution X chromosome-specific array-CGH detects new CNVs in infertile males. *PLoS ONE* **7**: e44887.

6. Kanakis, G. A. and Nieschlag, E. (2018) Klinefelter syndrome: more than hypogonadism. *Metab Clin Exp* DOI:10.1016/j.metabol.2017.09.017

7. Corona, G., et al. (2017) Sperm recovery and ICSI outcomes in Klinefelter syndrome: a systematic review and meta-analysis. *Hum Reprod Update* **23**:265–275.

8. Donker, R. B., et al. (2017) Chromosomal abnormalities in 1,663 infertile men with azoospermia: the clinical consequences. *Hum Reprod* **32**:2574–2580.

9. Rohaye, J., et al. (2015) Age and markers of Leydig cell function, but not of Sertoli cell function predict the success of sperm retrieval in adolescents and adults with Klinefelter's syndrome. *Andrology* **3**:868–875.

10. Gruchy, N., et al. (2011) Pregnancy outcomes in 188 French cases of prenatally diagnosed Klinefelter syndrome. *Hum Reprod* **26**:2570–2575.

11. Stefanidis, K., et al. (2011) Causes of infertility in men with Down syndrome. *Andrologia* **43**:353–357.

12. Xu, J., et al. (2017) Mapping allele with resolved carrier status of Robertsonian and reciprocal translocation in human preimplantation embryos. *PNAS* **114**: E8695–E8702.

13. Harton, G. L. and Tempest, H. G. (2012) Chromosomal disorders and male infertility. *Asian J Androl* **14**:32–39.

14. Zhang, W., et al. (2016) Clinical application of next-generation sequencing in preimplantation genetic diagnosis cycles for Robertsonian and reciprocal translocations. *J Assist Reprod Genet* **33**:899–906.

15. Tournaye, H., Krausz, C. and Oates, R. D. (2017) Novel concepts in the aetiology of male reproductive impairment. *Lancet Diab Endocrinol* **5**:544–553.

16. Krausz, C., Cioppi, F. and Riera-Escamilla, A. (2018) Testing for genetic contributions to infertility: potential clinical impact. *Exp Rev Mol Diag* **18**:331–346.

17. Tiepolo, L. and Zuffardi, O. (1976) Localization of factors controlling spermatogenesis in the nonfluorescent portion of the human Y chromosome long arm. *Hum Genet* **34**:119–124.

18. Krausz, C. and Casamonti, E. (2017) Spermatogenic failure and the Y chromosome. *Hum Genet* **136**:637–655.

19. Krausz, C. (2011) Male infertility: pathogenesis and clinical diagnosis. *Best Pract Res Clin Endocrinol Metab* **25**:271–285.

20. Tyler-Smith, C. and Krausz, C. (2009) The Will-o'-the-Wisp of genetics: hunting for the azoospermia factor gene. *N Engl J Med* **360**:925–927.

21. Tournaye, H., Krausz, C. and Oates, R. D. (2017) Concepts in diagnosis and therapy for male reproductive impairment. *Lancet Diab Endocrinol* **5**:554–564.

22. Flannigan, R. and Schlegel, P. N. (2017) Genetic diagnostics of male infertility in clinical practice. *Best Pract Res Clin Obstet Gynaecol* **44**:26–37.

23. Nathanson, K. L., et al. (2015) The Y deletion gr/gr and susceptibility to testicular germ cell tumor. *Am J Hum Genet* **77**:1034–1043.

24. Krausz, C., Escamilla, A. R. and Chianese, C. (2015) Genetics of male infertility: from research to clinic. *Reproduction* **150**(5):R159–R174.

25. Tüttelmann, F., et al. (2011) Copy number variants in patients with severe oligozoospermia and Sertoli-cell-only syndrome. *PLoS ONE* **6**:e19426.

26. Lopes, A. M., et al. (2013) Human spermatogenic failure purges deleterious mutation load from the autosomes and both sex chromosomes, including the gene DMRT1. *PLoS Genet* **9**(3):e1003349.

27. Giacco, D. L., et al. (2014) Recurrent X chromosome-linked deletions: discovery of new genetic factors in male infertility. *J Med Gen* **51**:340–344.

28. Shen, Y., Yang, X., Xu, J. and Liu, Y. (2017) Evidence for the involvement of the proximal copy of the MAGEA9 gene in Xq28-linked CNV67 specific to spermatogenic failure. *Biol Reprod* **96**(3):610–616.

29. Mueller, J. L., et al. (2013) Independent specialization of the human and mouse X chromosomes for the male germ line. *Nat Genet* **45**:1083–1087.

30. Yatsenko, A. N., et al. (2015) X-linked TEX11 mutations, meiotic arrest, and azoospermia in infertile men. *N Engl J Med* **372**:2097–2107.

31. Yang, F., et al. (2015) TEX11 is mutated in infertile men with azoospermia and regulates genome-wide recombination rates in mouse. *EMBO Mol Med* **7**:1198–1210.

32. Lee, A., et al. (2016) Global disorders of sex development update since 2006: perceptions, approach and care. *Horm Res Paediatr* **85**:158–180.

33. De la Chapelle, A., et al. (1964) XX sex chromosomes in a human male. *J Int Med* **175**:25–38.

34. Chakraborty, P. P., Bhattacharjee, R., Roy, A., Mukhopadhyay, S. and Chowdhury, S. (2016) Male factor infertility: clues to diagnose 46, XX Male. *J Obstet Gynaecol India* **66**:662–665.

35. Röpke, A. and Tüttelmann, F. (2017) Mechanisms in endocrinology: aberrations of the X chromosome as cause of male infertility. *Eur J Endocrinol* **177**:R249–R259.

4

The Effect of Endocrine Disruptors and Environmental and Lifestyle Factors on the Sperm Epigenome

Viviane Santana, Albert Salas-Huetos, Emma R. James, and Douglas T. Carrell

4.1 Introduction

Epigenetics is the field of study of heritable factors, other than DNA base pair coding, that regulate gene expression. It is important to emphasize the heritable component of epigenetics, both in terms of the definition and in terms of the scope of epigenetic effects, since by definition epigenetic alterations not only affect the health of the primary individual but also may have transgenerational effects on future progeny [1]. Hence, in a world in which individuals are increasingly exposed to industrial chemicals, environmental pollutants, and lifestyle changes such as increased obesity and advanced ages of paternity, epigenetic perturbations potentially induced by these types of environmental exposures are of prime importance in both individual and societal health concerns [2–5].

The male gamete is unique in its specialized structure and functions. The mature sperm cell is terminally differentiated to provide a mechanism by which the paternal genome can be transported through the female reproductive tract, undergo biochemical and morphological changes that facilitate fertilization of the oocyte, then undergo profound chromatin remodelling events during syngamy. One aspect of the sperm cell's uniqueness is its epigenome, both a historical record of the pathway of spermatogenesis, as well as a blueprint for early embryogenesis events [6–9]. Not only are key spermatogenesis genes marked in specific patterns that reflect spermatogenesis fidelity, but key developmental genes are bivalently marked to "poise" the genes for timely expression during embryogenesis. This pattern appears to be conserved in nature, and has been shown to be associated with poor embryo development and infertility.

In this chapter, we briefly review the basic aspects of the sperm epigenome, including DNA methylation, histone modifications, and non-coding RNAs (ncRNAs). We then highlight the known effects of some lifestyle and environmental influences on the sperm epigenome, highlighting the potential ramifications to the reproductive and general health of the male and his future progeny.

4.2 Overview of the Epigenome

The basic epigenetic factors that exist in spermatozoa are DNA methylation, histone and chromatin modifications, and ncRNAs (Figure 4.1). These epigenetic markers demonstrate extreme plasticity throughout sperm development as a consequence of cellular reprogramming and have also been shown to be modifiable by environmental

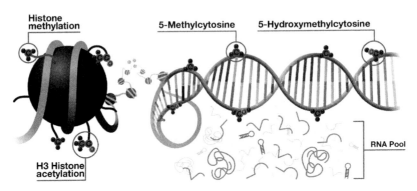

Figure 4.1 The major components of the sperm epigenome. This figure highlights the three major components of the sperm epigenome, which include DNA methylation and histone modifications. The epigenome also includes small ncRNAs, which include miRNAs and tRFs.

conditions, as will be discussed in Section 4.3. There are two main epigenetic repro-gramming events during mammalian development: the first one occurs in primordial germ cells (PGC) in the early stages of spermatogenesis, and the second reprogramming event occurs following fertilization, at the onset of embryogenesis [10,11]. These reprogramming periods are potential windows of susceptibility for the development of aberrant epigenetic programming. Aberrations in the sperm epigenome can lead to defects throughout spermatogenesis, thereby reducing fertilization capabilities and pregnancy rates. Evidence also suggests that alterations in the sperm epigenome may lead to defects or failures in embryonic development, miscarriage, or inheritance of paternal disease phenotypes in offspring [6,12].

4.2.1 Sperm DNA Methylation

DNA methylation exists throughout all stages of mammalian development. Methylation is a critical modification that provides regulation of tissue-specific gene expression patterns. In the male gamete, methylation is responsible for genomic imprinting, a mechanism for generating parent-of-origin specific gene expression in early embryos [13,14]. In mammals, DNA methylation consists of the covalent addition of a methyl group at position 5 of the cytosine ring, resulting in the formation of 5-methylcytosine (5meC). This epigenetic modification occurs mainly in cytosine-phosphate-guanine (CpG) dinucleotides and is initiated and maintained by DNA methyltransferases (DNMTs). CpG islands are usually found at gene promoters, and can prevent gene expression when hypermethylated by preventing access of transcriptional machinery to the DNA strand.

Sperm DNA is relatively hypermethylated in comparison to the hypomethylated pat-terns seen in oocytes, but is actively demethylated following fertilization prior to methyla-tion patterns being reset in the developing embryo [15]. Several studies have investigated associations between changes in sperm DNA methylation patterns and male fertility. Changes in sperm methylation markers may imply a number of changes in spermatogen-esis, leading to a decrease in sperm quality [16]. Moreover, DNA methylation patterns are involved in control of the functional capacity of germ cells and these alterations may affect fertilization and pregnancy rates [17]. It has also been shown that sperm methylation patterns can be predictive of male fertility and embryo quality during *in vitro* fertilization treatment, since methylation levels at specific regions were reduced significantly in the infertile men analyzed [18].

4.2.2 Sperm Histone Modifications

In order to protect sperm DNA from damage and deliver paternal nuclear content to the oocyte, sperm chromatin is organized in a very compact structure in which sperm DNA is wrapped around protamines as opposed to histones. During the late stages of spermatogenesis, sperm cells undergo dramatic chromatin structural rearrangements and approximately 85–90% of histones are replaced by protamines. In mammals, the protamination process occurs in two steps, first with a substitution of canonical histones by transition proteins, and then subsequent replacement by protamines 1 and 2 (P1 and P2) [19]. Protamines are capable of facilitating the very tight, toroid structure that sperm DNA forms by modulating interactions between themselves and the DNA sequence. In order to bind to DNA, protamines must be phosphorylated, and then, for DNA condensation, protamines are dephosphorylated, resulting in a chromatin structure 6 to 20 times more condensed than the classical somatic nucleosome [20]. In normal fertile men, the ratio of P1:P2 is tightly regulated and is approximately 1:1 [21]. Aberrant P1:P2 ratio is associated with abnormal semen parameters, DNA fragmentation, and reduced fertilization capabilities [22–24].

After the histone-to-protamine transition, the remaining 5–10% of histones were first considered remnants of an inefficient replacement process, but several studies have shown that histone retention does not occur randomly. Histones appear to be retained at specific genomic loci, such as developmental gene promoters, genes encoding microRNAs, and imprinted loci, which are regions related to fertilization and important to the developing embryo [25,26]. The modifications of histone proteins, via modification of lysine and serine residues on tail regions, promote activation or inactivation of gene transcription, a critical epigenetic regulator [17]. For example, modifications like acetylation of H3 and H4, ubiquitination of H2B, or trimethylation of H3K4, H3K36, and H3K79, create a more open chromatin structure, which can lead to gene activation [27]. On the other hand, deacetylation of H3 and H4, ubiquitination of H2A, and methylation of H3K9 and H3K27 can generate transcriptional inhibition [15].

4.2.3 Sperm Non-coding RNAs

It was thought that RNA transcripts present in sperm were just RNAs stored after meiosis or produced in the early stages of spermatogenesis. However, in recent years, different types of RNAs present in human spermatozoa have been described, as well as their activity in sperm development, fertilization, embryogenesis, and epigenetic inheritance [28–30]. Recent studies provide evidence that the spermatozoa RNA signature undergoes reprogramming during epididymal transit [31,32]. Sperm isolated from the caput epididymis show reduced abundance of RNA species that are found in the testes and cauda epididymis. These results indicate that sperm undergo either a random or programmed post-testicular loss of RNA species, and subsequent gain of ncRNAs during epididymal transit mediated by epididymosomes [31] (Figure 4.2).

Spermatozoal ncRNAs represent important epigenetic factors that may act as controllers for gene expression at the transcriptional and post-transcriptional level [29]. The most abundant RNAs found in sperm are the piwi-interacting RNAs (piRNAs) [28]. These are

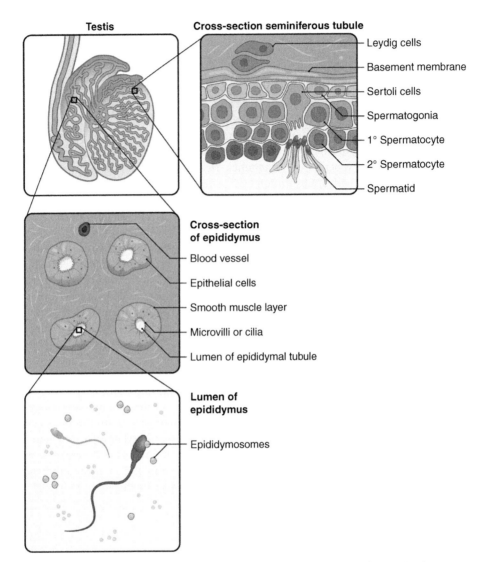

Figure 4.2 The sources of the sperm RNA pool. This figure demonstrates that species of RNA molecules originate in two diverse regions of the testis. First, mRNA fragments and small RNAs are added in the seminiferous tubule throughout spermatogenesis. During transport though the epididymis, removal of some RNAs appears to occur in the caput epididymis, with subsequent replacement as the sperm traverse the epididymis. This replacement occurs via epididymosomes, exosomes containing miRNAs, tRFs, and various proteins.

single stranded RNAs (24–30 nucleotides) that are associated with PIWI proteins and are responsible for transposon silencing. piRNAs predominantly contribute to spermatogenesis and embryogenesis in specific stages [33], and altered piRNA profiles could result in reduced male fertility, and may be related to testicular cancer [34,35]. miRNAs are also found in sperm and are transcripts that are 19–25 nucleotides long and promote gene silencing by binding to target mRNAs, leading to either mRNA degradation or translational repression. Sperm miRNAs have been associated with apoptosis, mitochondrial membrane integrity, failures in spermatogenesis and embryogenesis, and idiopathic male infertility [36–40]. Further studies are essential to confirm these hypotheses and to provide a better understanding of the role of these ncRNAs in embryo development and paternal inheritance.

4.3 Endocrine Disruptors, Male Fertility, and the Sperm Epigenome

A global trend in the reduction of male fertility has prompted research into potential environmental conditions that may play a role in male infertility [4,41]. Exposure to toxins in the form of pesticides, air pollution, and pharmaceutics has become increasingly common. Endocrine disruptors are a class of chemicals that exist in the environment due to many industrial and agricultural uses. Included in this class are agricultural and industrial chemicals such as DDT, dioxin, and plastics (i.e. bisphenol A, bis(2-ethylhexyl)phthalate, dibutyl phthalate). These chemicals are termed "endocrine disruptors" because of their ability to either mimic natural hormones in the body, inhibit the action of hormones, or alter normal functioning of the endocrine system [42].

4.3.1 Epidemiologic Evidence

Evidence from epidemiologic studies has suggested an association between males exposed to endocrine disruptors, either *in utero* or as adults, and reduced fertility [43,49]. Studies in mouse models have shown that embryonic exposure to certain endocrine disruptors such as vinclozolin result in male mice displaying increases in sperm cell apoptosis as well as other reproductive-related phenotypes [50–57]. Additionally, these mice produce sperm with alterations in DNA methylation patterns at promotors of multiple genes [52,55–57]. These observations prompt questions as to how exposure to these chemicals is capable of affecting fertility, and what consequences exist for offspring of exposed individuals.

Multiple reproductive phenotypes have been observed in men in association with endocrine and disruptor exposure. These include reduced sperm concentration, poor sperm motility and morphology, infertility, increased risk of testicular cancer, increased incidence of cryptorchidism, and others. Bibbo and colleagues reported reduced semen parameters such as sperm concentration in the sons of women treated with diethylstilbestrol, a synthetic estrogen previously prescribed to women to prevent miscarriage [43]. Polychlorinated biphenyl (PCB) metabolites and heavy PCB exposure in adult men has also been associated with poor semen parameters [44,45]. PCBs were once widely used in many applications as heat transfer fluids and coolants. Together, this evidence suggests that endocrine disruptor exposure, both *in utero* and in adulthood, has the potential to affect male fertility.

In addition to reduced fertility, individuals exposed to endocrine disruptors display increased risk of other reproductive-related disorders. Plastics workers can be exposed to multiple endocrine disruptors, such as bisphenol A (BPA) and bis(2-ethylhexyl)phthalate (DEHP). Increased incidence of testicular cancer has been observed in plastics workers, suggesting a role for endocrine disruptors as a risk factor for testicular cancer in adult men [46]. Additionally, based on a high prevalence of testicular cancer in specific populations and concurrent high dietary exposure to endocrine disruptor ochratoxin A in these populations, this chemical has been hypothesized as an additional risk factor for testicular cancer

[47]. Increased incidence of cryptorchidism has also been observed in the sons of women working with pesticides, many of which have previously contained endocrine disruptors [48]. This suggests again that both *in utero* and adult exposure to certain endocrine disruptors may increase risk for reproductive-related disorders in men.

4.3.2 Evidence in Model Systems

In addition to the epidemiologic evidence that exists regarding endocrine disruptors and male reproductive effects, studies in model systems have been conducted. These studies have allowed the characterization of both phenotypic and epigenetic modifications occurring in male offspring of endocrine disruptor exposed pregnant females. Interestingly, research in mice has shown reduced fertility in male progeny transgenerationally following embryonic exposure to endocrine disruptors [58].

Multiple studies in mice have shown a host of phenotypic changes such as reduction in sperm cell counts and cell viability, increases in male infertility, testis disease, prostate disease, obesity, and pubertal abnormalities in the male offspring of pregnant females treated with endocrine disruptors such as vinclozolin, methoxychlor, and plastics compounds [50–54,56–58]. Interestingly, many of these phenotypes are observed in males from F1, F2, F3, and, in some cases, F4 litters. These studies provide evidence that the detrimental effects of endocrine disruptor exposure are not limited to exposed animals, but that these effects may be inherited transgenerationally by an epigenetic mechanism. It is important to note that for this inheritance to be considered "transgenerational," the effects must be seen at least through the F3 generation. This is due to potential exposure of the *in utero* (F1) animal's germ cells to the endocrine disruptor treatment during development. These potentially exposed germ cells give rise to F2 animals, therefore, if effects are only shown through the F2 generation, it is possible that effects are due to germ cell exposure and not inheritance from the F1 animal [50].

An interesting study involving the transgenerational inheritance of endocrine-disruptor mediated effects recorded the incidence of adult-onset prostate abnormalities in male offspring of vinclozolin exposed females. Vinclozolin exposure during the period of F1 embryonic gonadal sex determination resulted in the development of adult-onset prostate disease in males from the F1 to F4 generation. These prostate abnormalities included prostatitis, hyperplasia of the ventral prostate, and epithelial cell atrophy. Analysis of the prostate and ventral prostate epithelial cell transcriptomes revealed significantly altered expression of 954 and 259 genes, respectively, in the F3 generation. Included in these genes are *MSP* and *FADD*, which have both previously been associated with prostate disease and cancer. Additionally, other affected genes are involved in pathways such as calcium and WNT signaling [52]. These data suggest that endocrine disruptor exposure, during specific periods of embryonic development, is capable of inducing epigenetic transgenerational abnormalities in the prostate transcriptome and male germ line.

In addition to transcriptome changes and infertility and disease phenotypes observed in offspring of exposed animals, alterations to the sperm epigenome of F1 and F3 animals have been recorded. Specifically, regions of differential DNA methylation have been observed at promotors of multiple genes [50,55,57,59,60]. Interestingly, some of the genes associated with the differentially methylated regions are involved in a functional connection network involved in cell signaling pathways [50,57]. Due to the ability of some regions of paternal DNA methylation to partially escape reprogramming events in the early embryo, it is possible that altered germ cell DNA methylation is at least partially responsible for the incidences of epigenetic inheritance observed. In fact, some of the differentially methylated regions identified overlap imprinted genes known to escape epigenetic reprogramming [59,60]. Additionally, it has been hypothesized that changes in the germ line epigenome of early generations may induce genetic or transcriptome changes, such as observed copy number variants and gene expression changes, respectively, in later generations [52,55].

With the knowledge that endocrine disruptor exposure is associated with alterations to the sperm epigenome, Manikkam and colleagues aimed to determine whether DNA methylation alterations were consistent between exposures to different types of endocrine disruptors. They exposed pregnant females to pesticides, dioxins, and plastics, separately, in order to characterize differences in F3 sperm DNA methylation. Differentially methylated regions were observed for dioxin, plastics, and pesticide groups. Interestingly, there was very limited overlap between the differentially methylated regions recorded for each group. These data suggest that individually each endocrine disruptor may have a unique effect on the sperm epigenome in F3 animals [56,58]. This observation is especially interesting considering the wide range of reproductive phenotypes that have been observed in the male offspring of exposed females, ranging from infertility to pubertal abnormalities to testicular or prostate disease.

Additional alterations to the epigenome have been recorded following embryonic exposure to endocrine disruptors in the mouse. Vinclozolin exposure to pregnant females resulted in an increase of germ cell apoptosis, as previously described, as well as a reduction in PGC numbers, resulting in reduced fertility. These abnormalities were present in F1 to F3 generation males. Analysis of PCG miRNA populations in all generations revealed altered expression of multiple miRNAs, including *miR-23b* and *miR-21*, which induced alterations in the *Lin28/let-7/Blimp1* pathway responsible for regulating PCG differentiation. These data suggest an epigenetic mechanism of transgenerational inheritance centered around the deregulation of miRNAs involved in cell differentiation [54].

The transgenerational phenotypic effects of embryonic endocrine disruption have been well characterized, and it is clear that an epigenetic mode of inheritance must be at least partially responsible for these observations. The recorded epigenome alterations, however, are often inconsistent between studies and between various endocrine disruptors. It is possible that different endocrine disruptors have unique effects on the epigenome and resultant unique phenotypes associated with their exposure, leading to the mosaic of reproductive phenotypes that have been observed. It is also likely that a combination of different epigenetic factors are responsible for the phenotypes observed [56,58]. Therefore, additional research on exposure is needed in other areas of the sperm epigenome, specifically in spermatozoal RNAs which have recently been strongly implicated as a mechanism for epigenetic inheritance. A more complete picture of sperm epigenome alterations as a result of embryonic endocrine disruptor exposure will also help to determine what cell types, tissues, and functions are acted upon following exposure.

4.3.3 Targets of Endocrine Disruptors in the Male Reproductive Tract

Many potential target sites exist for endocrine disruptors to act on male reproduction. Importantly, hormones produced in the testis are essential regulators of spermatogenesis. Therefore, endocrine disruptor action within the testis is a potential explanation for reduced fertility in exposed males. Leydig cells are found adjacent to seminiferous tubules within the connective tissue between tubules and are the primary endocrine cells within the testis. Production of testosterone by Leydig cells is under hormonal control by the pituitary. As the primary endocrine cells within the testis, these cells are potential targets for endocrine disruptor activity that may affect reproduction [42,61,62].

Sertoli cells form the inner lining of the seminiferous tubules and have important functions for sperm development. These cells function as endocrine cells, with the release of hormones inhibin and follicle stimulating hormone (FSH), which are important for the regulation of sperm development. Sertoli cells have additional functions, which may be perturbed by endocrine disruptor activity. These functions include the destruction of defective sperm cells, the provision of fluids important to sperm transport, and the provision of nutrients necessary for sperm development. Additionally, Sertoli cells are the basis for the blood–testis barrier, which is responsible for maintaining separation of the specialized tubule lumen environment from plasma components as well as preventing passage of agents, which may be toxic to sperm cells, into the tubule lumen. Disturbance of any of these regulatory or protective mechanisms, individually or in concert, by endocrine disruptors could be responsible for some of the epigenetic and phenotypic effects observed in exposed males [42,62].

As described, there are multiple cell types and structures within the testis which are potential targets for endocrine disruptor activity. In addition to these testicular structures, it is possible that endocrine disruptors have a direct effect on germ cells during development. During spermatogenesis, immature spermatogonia undergo mitotic divisions to become primary spermatocytes. These spermatocytes undergo meiosis to generate haploid spermatids, which condense and elongate and are eventually released as spermatozoa into the seminiferous tubule lumen. These cells then travel to the epididymis where final maturation and storage occurs prior to ejaculation. There are multiple stages during development, such as mitotic arrest, where developing germ cells are especially susceptible to toxic agents and damage. Additionally, the sperm epigenome undergoes significant remodeling during development and maturation, including changes to chromatin structure, development of DNA methylation patterns, and multiple waves of spermatozoal RNA payload remodeling [6,19,25,31,42]. These periods of susceptibility provide potential windows for endocrine disruptors to act directly on germ cells, leading to the phenotypic alterations observed as well as epigenetic alterations, which are likely involved in inheritance of these traits.

4.4 Age, Environmental Factors, Lifestyle Factors, and the Sperm Epigenome

4.4.1 Age and the Sperm Epigenome

Aging is associated with changes in dynamic biological, physiological, environmental, psychological, behavioral, and social processes that result in a decline in function of the senses and an increase of the susceptibility to diseases [63]. It is well known that aging is related to a decline in the male reproductive system, sperm quality, and fertility [64]. Also, recent evidences demonstrate a role for paternal aging on offspring disease susceptibility [65]. Notwithstanding these robust epidemiological evidences, in most cases the mechanisms that drive these processes are unclear, although it is thought that the sperm epigenome is possibly the key [66].

In that sense, one study analyzed sperm DNA methylation from fertile sperm donors in which semen was collected in the 1990s and again in 2008, and identified 139 regions that are significantly hypomethylated and 8 significantly hypermethylated regions associated with aging. Analyzing these regions, the authors found that the affected regions were associated with genes linked with schizophrenia and bipolar disorder, establishing the first non-causative relationship between paternal aging and the incidence of neuropsychiatric and other disorders in the offspring [67]. Moreover, Atsem and colleagues in a cohort study with 162 sperm DNA donors described two genes (*FOXK1* and *KCNA7* genes) with negative correlation between sperm methylation and paternal age. Also, the study suggested that the levels of methylation of the *FOXK1* gene were transmitted into the next generation [68].

Both studies suggest that age-related DNA methylation changes in sperm may contribute to increased disease risk in offspring because changes can be transmitted to the next generation, and found that changes accumulate gradually with aging, not in a sudden precipice at a given age. These changes are particularly relevant with the known societal changes in regards to advancing paternal age generally.

4.4.2 Environmental Factors, Lifestyle Factors, and Sperm Epigenome

Male reproductive health is declining year by year, raising serious concerns and implications about human fertility [69]. There are multiple possible causes of this decline; however, the most plausible seems to be related to environmental and lifestyle factors such as psychological stress, air quality and pollution, unhealthy diets, overweight or obesity, and smoking and alcohol consumption.

4.4.2.1 Psychological Stress

Physiological stress can be defined as an organism's response (e.g. biochemical, physiological, or/and behavioral changes) to a stressor such as an environmental condition. Some clinical studies reveal an inverse relationship between psychological stress and some quality semen parameters [70,74]. However, the relationship between male infertility and psychological stress is still controversial.

The hypothalamic–pituitary–gonadal (HPG) axis is one of the major systems that respond to stress disrupting endocrine homeostasis, mainly increasing or decreasing testosterone levels in the testes, affecting Sertoli cells that leads arrest of the spermatogenesis process and alters sperm quality [75]. However, it seems that this physiological stress also can affect the sperm epigenetic signatures, not only through DNA methylation changes, but also at the miRNA level.

There is only one longitudinal non-clinical study conducted to date that examined the association of psychological stress with DNA methylation in gametes [76]. In that study, combined physical, emotional, and sexual abuse in childhood was characterized in 34 men. The authors identified 12 DNA methylation regions differentially methylated by childhood abuse that contains genes associated with neuronal function (*MAPT, CLU*), fat cell regulation (*PRDM16*), and immune function (*SDK1*). These results confirmed that childhood abuse is associated with sperm DNA methylation changes and suggested that this may have implications for offspring development. However, further human and animal studies will need to be undertaken to prove this transgenerational inheritance hypothesis.

In that sense, some recent mouse studies suggest a mechanistic role for sperm miRNAs in the transgenerational transmission of paternal traumatic experiences [77,79]. Gapp and colleagues found that early traumatic stress induced remodeling of sperm miRNA expression in F0 but not F1 sperm. Notwithstanding, the behavioral and metabolic phenotypes were detected into the second (F2) generation [78]. On the other hand, Rodgers and colleagues discovered nine miRNAs (miR-29c, miR-30a, miR-30c, miR-32, miR-193-5p, miR-204, miR-375, miR-532-3p, and miR-698) that were altered in paternal sperm after exposure to chronic stress. Additionally, these miRNAs promoted and altered stress responses of the offspring [79]. Finally, in a very recent study, multiple miRNAs of the miR-449/34 family were differentially expressed in mice and men exposed to adolescent chronic social instability stress [77].

Taken together, these studies provide some evidence for the idea that miRNAs and DNA methylation markers contribute to the transmission of traumatic experiences, and therefore psychological stress, in mammals.

4.4.2.2 Air Quality and Pollution

The evidence that semen quality has been decreasing during the last 50 years is today very strong. It is also a fact that this decrease is stronger in certain geographic regions of the world, specifically in the developed and industrialized countries [41,80].

Currently there is some evidence that indicates that air quality and pollution could alter sperm parameters and result in male infertility [81,83]. However, to the best of our knowledge, only one study examined the relationship between air pollution and sperm epigenetics. In that study, the sperm DNA methylation was globally analyzed in 607 male partners of pregnant women from a large cohort and the authors found a significant association between exposure to persistent organic pollutants and a global decrease in sperm methylation [84]. With only this study it seems evident that further research needs to examine more closely the links between air quality and pollution and sperm epigenome.

4.4.2.3 Diet

Several observational studies suggest that adhering to a healthy diet (e.g. the Mediterranean diet) may improve male sperm quality parameters [85,86]. Also, a recent meta-analysis of randomized clinical trials (RCTs) proposes that some dietary supplements (e.g. omega-3, CoQ10, selenium, zinc, and carnitines) could beneficially modulate sperm quality parameters and affect male fertility [87]. However, results must be cautiously interpreted due to the limited sample size of the meta-analyzed studies and the considerable observed inter-study heterogeneity.

Presently only a few studies assessing the impact of diet on the sperm epigenetic signature have been published, therefore limited clinical conclusions or recommendations can be drawn. The effect of some nutrients, like folic acid and vitamin D, were analyzed in four different studies in mammals. First, Lambrot and colleagues identified multiple regions of the mouse sperm epigenome that are environmentally programmed. They discovered that, compared with folate sufficient males, mice receiving a folate deficient diet displayed alteration of sperm DNA methylation at genes implicated in development and some metabolic processes. Moreover, they have also demonstrated that a folate deficient diet is associated with negative pregnancy outcomes [88]. In humans, to the contrary of the aforementioned study, the administration of a high dose of folic acid (up to 10 times the daily recommended dose) daily, for 6 months, has been shown to also alter the sperm methylome. The general loss of methylation detected in this study was influenced by the presence of the *MTHFR* C677T polymorphism [89,90]. However, other authors have observed no effect on human sperm DNA methylation with the use of short-term (400 µg/day for 90 days) and long-term exposures to low-dose folic acid supplementation [91]. The only study testing the effect of vitamin D on the sperm epigenome revealed that depletion of vitamin D in mice resulted in more than 15,000 differentially methylated loci, and that most of these showed a loss of methylation. These differentially methylated CpGs were mainly localized in regions enriched for developmental and metabolic genes and pathways [92].

To the best of our knowledge, the only foods that have been tested in an RCT were nuts (walnuts, hazelnuts, and almonds). Healthy individuals consuming 60 g/d of raw nuts in the context of a Western-style diet during a period of 14 weeks improved various sperm quality parameters, but nut supplementation did not demonstrate any effect on global sperm DNA methylation. However, a significant reduction in hsa-miR-34b-3p expression levels in the group of individuals supplemented with nuts compared to the control group has been reported [93]. These data suggest that the sperm epigenome can be modulated by diet supplementation with certain nutrients and food. Nevertheless, due to the small number of studies published to date, further research may lead to a better understanding of the relationship between diet and the sperm epigenome.

4.4.2.4 Overweight and Obesity

Beyond diet, overweight and obesity are other possible factors to consider. The immediate effects of obesity on sperm quality are well documented [94]. However, the effects of this condition on the sperm epigenome are still debated [95,96]. In mice, Fullston and colleagues demonstrated that paternal obesity affected the next generation's risk of obesity and associated diseases through sperm miRNAs and DNA methylation disturbances. This experimental mouse study (control diet vs high-fat diet) reveals that expression of 11 miRNAs were affected in the F0 generation mice, initiating metabolic disturbances in two generations of mice (F1 and F2) that altered the transcriptional profile of testis and sperm [97].

In humans, there is also evidence that male overweight/obesity status is traceable in the sperm epigenome through multiple generations. In a study of sperm from overweight or obese men (n = 23), lower DNA methylation percentages at the *MEG3, NDN, SNRPN, and SGCE/PEG10* associated differentially methylated regions have been reported compared with men of a healthy weight (n = 46) [98]. These results suggest that paternal obesity promotes the transgenerational transmission of obesity status and associated metabolic alterations like type 2 diabetes via epigenetic changes of germ cell DNA. However, future studies investigating sperm epigenetic aberrations due to paternal adiposity status are warranted.

4.4.2.5 Smoking

Cigarettes are smoked by nearly 20% of the world's population and about 800 million of these smokers are men. Even though cigarette consumption has gradually declined it represents a worldwide health problem because it harms nearly every organ of the body and causes many diseases (e.g. cardiovascular and respiratory diseases, cancer, and infertility).

The most recent systematic review and meta-analysis to determine whether cigarette smoking affects human semen parameters suggests that smoking has an overall negative effect on conventional semen parameters like sperm count, motility, and morphology [99]. Also, in many cases, smoking can cause chromatin and DNA damage during spermatogenesis [100]. Similarly, there are some recent studies on the effect of smoking in sperm miRNAs and DNA methylation. Regarding the miRNAs, as far as we know, there is only one small case-control study (6 smokers and 7 non-smokers participants). In total, 28 miRNAs were differentially expressed in smokers compared with non-smokers and the validated targets are involved in cellular proliferation, differentiation, and cell death pathways [101].

In the last two years, three different groups published their work about smoking in men and sperm DNA methylation. While Hamad and colleagues, with a population of 55 smokers and 54 non-smokers, discovered a significantly lower global sperm DNA methylation in non-smokers compared with smokers individuals [102], the other two groups found some CpG-specific alterations. Jenkins and colleagues analyzed the sperm DNA methylation patterns in 78 men who smoke and 78 non-smokers and identified 141 significantly differentially methylated CpGs; however, the differentially methylated CpGs were not associated with a specific biologic pathway [103]. On the other hand, Alkhaled and colleagues did a similar analysis with a smaller population (14 smokers and 14 proven non-smokers) and found that only 11 CpGs were differentially methylated [104]. Taken together, these results suggest that smoking exposure could have negative reproductive epigenetic health consequences, not only for the exposed individual, but also for the descendants of those who are exposed.

4.4.2.6 Alcohol Consumption

Although alcohol intake has been associated with a wide range of diseases (e.g. cirrhosis, different cancers, immune system dysfunctions, etc.), the most extensive study in humans found that occasional alcohol intake is not adversely associated with semen quality [67]. However, a recent meta-analysis has shown a detrimental effect of alcohol consumption on semen volume and sperm morphology in daily consumers [105].

In the same way, very little evidence was published investigating the relationship between alcohol consumption and the sperm epigenome. On the one hand, Ouko and colleagues found a correlation between chronic alcohol use and demethylation of *H19* and *IG-DMR* imprinted regions in human sperm DNA and hypothesized that this epigenetic change in imprinted genes could be transmitted to the offspring and alter normal prenatal development, resulting in fetal alcohol spectrum disorders [106]. In mice, likewise to the aforementioned human study, a significant reduction in methylation not only at *H19* but also in *CTCF 1* and *CTCF 2* binding sites, was observed in the offspring of ethanol-treated males, but not in sperm DNA methylation of alcohol-exposed males [107]. Lee and colleagues treated male mice with 0.5, 1, 2, and 4 g/kg alcohol and mated them with untreated females and observed different skull malformations in some fetuses. This group suggested that the abnormalities were due to changes in methylation signatures in sperm [108]. To conclude, these studies agree that sperm DNA could be a potential medium to transmit alcohol induced epigenetic mutations; however, there is not a study that shows a direct link.

4.5 Conclusions

Clearly, the sperm cell has developed a complex complement of epigenetic signals that are both a historical record of spermatogenesis and a programmatic set of signals to the future development of the embryo. Given the well-known link between environmental exposures and alterations to epigenetic markers generally, it is an obvious concern to evaluate environmental factors and the sperm epigenome. It is a unique trait of reproductive epigenetics that environmentally induced perturbations of the epigenome not only affect the reproductive health of the affected individual but also may affect the health of that individual's progeny.

In this chapter, we have discussed the effects of various classes of environmental exposure to the sperm epigenome. We have focused on the effects of endocrine disruptors, but also touched on other factors, such as obesity, smoking, and aging. The over riding conclusion of these studies is that it is clear that sperm epigenetic changes are possible and present following certain exposures, and that the changes may have profound implications for the reproductive health of the individual and of future offspring. These studies imply that future clinical evaluations should include a careful screening for exposures to the agents known to affect the sperm epigenome, and that future screening of the sperm epigenome is likely to become a standard of care for individuals at risk. Future studies must expand the scope of environmental and lifestyle toxicants studied, as well as improving the translation to the clinic.

References

1. Waddington, C. H. (1942) The epigenotype. *Endeavour*, 18–20.

2. Skinner, M. K., Manikkam, M. and Guerrero-Bosagna, C. (2010) Epigenetic transgenerational actions of environmental factors in disease etiology. *Trends Endocrinol Metab* 21:214–222.

3. Meldrum, D. R., et al. (2016) Aging and the environment affect gamete and embryo potential: can we intervene? *Fertil Steril* 105:548–559.

4. Skakkebaek, N. E., et al. (2016) Male reproductive disorders and fertility trends: influences of environment and genetic susceptibility. *Physiol Rev* 96:55–97.

5. Stuppia, L., Franzago, M., Ballerini, P., Gatta, V. and Antonucci, I. (2015) Epigenetics and male reproduction: the consequences of paternal lifestyle on fertility, embryo development, and children lifetime health. *Clin Epigenetics* 7:120.

6. Carrell, D. T. (2012) Epigenetics of the male gamete. *Fertil Steril* 97:267–274.

7. Castillo, J., Jodar, M. and Oliva, R. (2018) The contribution of human sperm proteins to the development and epigenome of the preimplantation embryo. *Hum Reprod Update* 24:535–555.

8. Denomme, M. M., McCallie, B. R., Parks, J. C., Schoolcraft, W. B. and Katz-Jaffe, M. G. (2017) Alterations in the sperm histone-retained epigenome are associated with unexplained male factor infertility and poor blastocyst development in donor oocyte IVF cycles. *Hum Reprod* 32:2443–2455.

9. Aston, K. I., Uren, P. J., Jenkins, T. G., Horsager, A., Cairns, B. R., Smith, A. D., et al. (2015) Aberrant sperm DNA methylation predicts male fertility status and embryo quality. *Fertil Steril* 104:1388–1397.

10. Ge, S. Q., Lin, S. L., Zhao, Z. H. and Sun, Q. Y. (2017) Epigenetic dynamics and interplay during spermatogenesis and embryogenesis: implications for male fertility and offspring health. *Oncotarget* 8:53804–53818.

11. McSwiggin, H. M. and O'Doherty, A. M. (2018) Epigenetic reprogramming during spermatogenesis and male factor infertility. *Reproduction* 156:R9–R21.

12. Schagdarsurengin, U., Paradowska, A. and Steger, K. (2012) Analysing the sperm

epigenome: roles in early embryogenesis and assisted reproduction. *Nat Rev Urol* 9:609–619.

13. Urdinguio, R. G., et al. (2015) Aberrant DNA methylation patterns of spermatozoa in men with unexplained infertility. *Hum Reprod* 30:1014–1028.

14. Jones, P. A. (2012) Functions of DNA methylation: islands, start sites, gene bodies and beyond. *Nat Rev Genet* 13:484–492.

15. Jenkins, T. G., Aston, K. I., James, E. R. and Carrell, D. T. (2017) Sperm epigenetics in the study of male fertility, offspring health, and potential clinical applications. *Syst Biol Reprod Med* 63:69–76.

16. Rajender, S., Avery, K. and Agarwal, A. (2011) Epigenetics, spermatogenesis and male infertility. *Mutat Res* 727:62–71.

17. Jenkins, T. G. and Carrell, D. T. (2011) The paternal epigenome and embryogenesis: poising mechanisms for development. *Asian J Androl* 13:76–80.

18. Ankolkar, M., et al. (2012) Methylation analysis of idiopathic recurrent spontaneous miscarriage cases reveals aberrant imprinting at H19 ICR in normozoospermic individuals. *Fertil Steril* 98:1186–1192.

19. Wykes, S. M. and Krawetz, S. A. (2003) The structural organization of sperm chromatin. *J Biol Chem* 278:29471–29477.

20. Carrell, D. T., Emery, B. R. and Hammoud, S. (2007) Altered protamine expression and diminished spermatogenesis: what is the link? *Hum Reprod Update* 13:313–327.

21. Carrell, D. T. and Liu, L. (2001) Altered protamine 2 expression is uncommon in donors of known fertility, but common among men with poor fertilizing capacity, and may reflect other abnormalities of spermiogenesis. *J Androl* 22:604–610.

22. Aoki, V. W., et al. (2005) DNA integrity is compromised in protamine-deficient human sperm. *J Androl* 26:741–748.

23. Aoki, V. W., Liu, L. and Carrell, D. T. (2005) Identification and evaluation of a novel sperm protamine abnormality in a population of infertile males. *Hum Reprod* 20:1298–1306.

24. Torregrosa, N., et al. (2006) Protamine 2 precursors, protamine 1/protamine 2 ratio, DNA integrity and other sperm parameters in infertile patients. *Hum Reprod* 21:2084–2089.

25. Hammoud, S. S., et al. (2009) Distinctive chromatin in human sperm packages genes for embryo development. *Nature* 460:473–478.

26. Brykczynska, U., et al. (2010) Repressive and active histone methylation mark distinct promoters in human and mouse spermatozoa. *Nat Struct Mol Biol* 17:679–687.

27. Kouzarides, T. (2007) Chromatin modifications and their function. *Cell* 128:693–705.

28. Krawetz, S. A., et al. (2011) A survey of small RNAs in human sperm. *Hum Reprod* 26:3401–3412.

29. Jodar, M., et al. (2013) The presence, role and clinical use of spermatozoal RNAs. *Hum Reprod Update* 19:604–624.

30. (2015) Absence of sperm RNA elements correlates with idiopathic male infertility. *Sci Transl Med* 7:295re296.

31. Sharma, U., et al. (2018) Small RNAs are trafficked from the epididymis to developing mammalian sperm. *Dev Cell* 46:481–494. e486.

32. Conine, C. C., Sun, F., Song, L., Rivera-Pérez, J. A. and Rando, O. J. (2018) Small RNAs gained during epididymal transit of sperm are essential for embryonic development in mice. *Dev Cell* 46:470–480. e473.

33. de Mateo, S. and Sassone-Corsi, P. (2014) Regulation of spermatogenesis by small non-coding RNAs: role of the germ granule. *Semin Cell Dev Biol* 29:84–92.

34. Zheng, K. and Wang, P. J. (2012) Blockade of pachytene piRNA biogenesis reveals a novel requirement for maintaining post-meiotic germ line genome integrity. *PLoS Genet* 8:e1003038.

35. Ferreira, H. J., et al. (2014) Epigenetic loss of the PIWI/piRNA machinery in human

testicular tumorigenesis. *Epigenetics* 9:113–118.

36. Capra, E., et al. (2017) Small RNA sequencing of cryopreserved semen from single bull revealed altered miRNAs and piRNAs expression between high- and low-motile sperm populations. *BMC Genomics* 18:14.

37. Abu-Halima, M., et al. (2014) Panel of five microRNAs as potential biomarkers for the diagnosis and assessment of male infertility. *Fertil Steril* 102:989–997. e981.

38. Bansal, S. K., Gupta, N., Sankhwar, S. N. and Rajender, S. (2015) Differential genes expression between fertile and infertile spermatozoa revealed by transcriptome analysis. *PLoS One* 10:e0127007.

39. Salas-Huetos, A., et al. (2015) Spermatozoa from patients with seminal alterations exhibit a differential micro-ribonucleic acid profile. *Fertil Steril* 104:591–601.

40. (2016) Spermatozoa from normozoospermic fertile and infertile individuals convey a distinct miRNA cargo. *Andrology* 4:1028–1036.

41. Carlsen, E., Giwercman, A., Keiding, N. and Skakkebaek, N. E. (1992) Evidence for decreasing quality of semen during past 50 years. *BMJ* 305:609–613.

42. Sikka, S. C. and Wang, R. (2008) Endocrine disruptors and estrogenic effects on male reproductive axis. *Asian J Androl* 10:134–145.

43. Bibbo, M., Haenszel, W. M., Wied, G. L., Hubby, M. and Herbst, A. L. (1978) A twenty-five-year follow-up study of women exposed to diethylstilbestrol during pregnancy. *N Engl J Med* 298:763–767.

44. Dallinga, J. W., et al. (2002) Decreased human semen quality and organochlorine compounds in blood. *Hum Reprod* 17:1973–1979.

45. Guo, Y. L., Hsu, P. C., Hsu, C. C. and Lambert, G. H. (2000) Semen quality after prenatal exposure to polychlorinated biphenyls and dibenzofurans. *Lancet* 356:1240–1241.

46. Ohlson, C. G. and Hardell, L. (2000) Testicular cancer and occupational exposures with a focus on xenoestrogens in polyvinyl chloride plastics. *Chemosphere* 40:1277–1282.

47. Schwartz, G. G. (2002) Hypothesis: does ochratoxin A cause testicular cancer? *Cancer Causes Control* 13:91–100.

48. Weidner, I. S., Moller, H., Jensen, T. K. and Skakkebaek, N. E. (1998) Cryptorchidism and hypospadias in sons of gardeners and farmers. *Environ Health Perspect* 106:793–796.

49. Eertmans, F., Dhooge, W., Stuyvaert, S. and Comhaire, F. (2003) Endocrine disruptors: effects on male fertility and screening tools for their assessment. *Toxicol in Vitro* 17:515–524.

50. Anway, M. D., Cupp, A. S., Uzumcu, M. and Skinner, M. K. (2005) Epigenetic transgenerational actions of endocrine disruptors and male fertility. *Science* 308:1466–1469.

51. Anway, M. D., Memon, M. A., Uzumcu, M. and Skinner, M. K. (2006) Transgenerational effect of the endocrine disruptor vinclozolin on male spermatogenesis. *J Androl* 27:868–879.

52. Anway, M. D. and Skinner, M. K. (2008) Transgenerational effects of the endocrine disruptor vinclozolin on the prostate transcriptome and adult onset disease. *Prostate* 68:517–529.

53. (2008) Epigenetic programming of the germ line: effects of endocrine disruptors on the development of transgenerational disease. *Reprod Biomed Online* 16:23–25.

54. Brieno-Enriquez, M. A., et al. (2015) Exposure to endocrine disruptor induces transgenerational epigenetic deregulation of microRNAs in primordial germ cells. *PLoS One* 10:e0124296.

55. Guerrero-Bosagna, C., Settle, M., Lucker, B. and Skinner, M. K. (2010) Epigenetic transgenerational actions of vinclozolin on promoter regions of the sperm epigenome. *PLoS One* 5(9).

56. Manikkam, M., Guerrero-Bosagna, C., Tracey, R., Haque, M. M. and Skinner, M. K. (2012) Transgenerational actions of environmental compounds on

reproductive disease and identification of epigenetic biomarkers of ancestral exposures. *PLoS One* 7:e31901.

57. Manikkam, M., Tracey, R., Guerrero-Bosagna, C. and Skinner, M. K. (2013) Plastics derived endocrine disruptors (BPA, DEHP and DBP) induce epigenetic transgenerational inheritance of obesity, reproductive disease and sperm epimutations. *PLoS One* 8:e55387.

58. Nilsson, E. E. and Skinner, M. K. (2015) Environmentally induced epigenetic transgenerational inheritance of reproductive disease. *Biol Reprod* 93:145.

59. Stouder, C. and Paoloni-Giacobino, A. (2010) Transgenerational effects of the endocrine disruptor vinclozolin on the methylation pattern of imprinted genes in the mouse sperm. *Reproduction* **139**:373–379.

60. (2011) Specific transgenerational imprinting effects of the endocrine disruptor methoxychlor on male gametes. *Reproduction* **141**:207–216.

61. Svechnikov, K., Izzo, G., Landreh, L., Weisser, J. and Söder, O. (2010) Endocrine disruptors and Leydig cell function. *J Biomed Biotechnol* 2010:684504.

62. Sharpe, R. M. (2006) Pathways of endocrine disruption during male sexual differentiation and masculinization. *Best Pract Res Clin Endocrinol Metab* 20:91–110.

63. Masoro, E. J. (2011) A. S. Handbook of the biology of aging. *J Psychosom Res* **23**.

64. Paul, C. and Robaire, B. (2013) Ageing of the male germ line. *Nat Rev Urol* **10**:227–234.

65. Miller, B., et al. (2011) Meta-analysis of paternal age and schizophrenia risk in male versus female offspring. *Schizophr Bull* **37**:1039–1047.

66. Jenkins, T. G., Aston, K. I. and Carrell, D. T. (2018) Sperm epigenetics and aging. *Transl Androl Urol* 7:S328–S335.

67. Jenkins, T. G., Aston, K. I., Pflueger, C., Cairns, B. R. and Carrell, D. T. (2014) Age-associated sperm DNA methylation alterations: possible implications in

offspring disease susceptibility. *PLoS Genet* 10:e1004458.

68. Atse, S., et al. (2016) Paternal age effects on sperm FOXK1 and KCNA7 methylation and transmission into the next generation. *Hum Mol Genet* 25:4996–5005.

69. Levine, H., et al. (2017) Temporal trends in sperm count: a systematic review and meta-regression analysis. *Hum Reprod Update* 23:646–659.

70. Abu-Musa, A. A., Nassar, A. H., Hannoun, A. B. and Usta, I. M. (2007) Effect of the Lebanese civil war on sperm parameters. *Fertil Steril* 88:1579–1582.

71. Clarke, R. N., Klock, S. C., Geoghegan, A. and Travassos, D. E. (1999) Relationship between psychological stress and semen quality among *in-vitro* fertilization patients. *Hum Reprod* 14:753–758.

72. DeStefano, F., Annest, J. L., Kresnow, M. J., Schrader, S. M. and Katz, D. F. (1989) Semen characteristics of Vietnam veterans. *Reprod Toxicol* 3:165–173.

73. Fenster, L., et al. (1997) Effects of psychological stress on human semen quality. *J Androl* 18:194–202.

74. Lampiao, F. (2009) Variation of semen parameters in healthy medical students due to exam stress. *Malawi Med J* 21:166–167.

75. Nargund, V. H. (2015) Effects of psychological stress on male fertility. *Nat Rev Urol* 12:373–382.

76. Roberts, A. L., et al. (2018) Exposure to childhood abuse is associated with human sperm DNA methylation. *Transl Psychiatry* 8:194.

77. Dickson, D. A., et al. (2018) Reduced levels of miRNAs 449 and 34 in sperm of mice and men exposed to early life stress. *Transl Psychiatry* 8:101.

78. Gapp, K., et al. (2014) Implication of sperm RNAs in transgenerational inheritance of the effects of early trauma in mice. *Nat Neurosci* 17:667–669.

79. Rodgers, A. B., Morgan, C. P., Leu, N. A. and Bale, T. L. (2015) Transgenerational epigenetic programming via sperm microRNA recapitulates effects of paternal

stress. *Proc Natl Acad Sci USA* **112**:13699–13704.

80. Swan, S. H., Elkin, E. P. and Fenster, L. (2000) The question of declining sperm density revisited: an analysis of 101 studies published 1934–1996. *Environ Health Perspect* **108**:961–966.

81. Deng Z., et al. (2016) Association between air pollution and sperm quality: A systematic review and meta-analysis. *Environ Pollut* **208**:663–669.

82. Lafuentem, R., Garcia-Blaquez, N., Jacquemin, B. and Checa, M. A. (2016) Outdoor air pollution and sperm quality. *Fertil Steril* **106**:880–896.

83. Leiser, C. L., Hanson, H. A., Sawyer, K., Steenblik, J., Al-Dulaimi, R., et al. (2019) Acute effects of air pollutants on spontaneous pregnancy loss: a case-crossover study. *Fertil Steril* **111** (2):341–347.

84. Consales, C., et al. (2016) Exposure to persistent organic pollutants and sperm DNA methylation changes in Arctic and European populations. *Environ Mol Mutagen* **57**:200–209.

85. Giahi, L., Mohammadmoradi, S., Javidan, A. and Sadeghi, M. R. (2016) Nutritional modifications in male infertility: a systematic review covering 2 decades. *Nutr Rev* **74**:118–130.

86. Salas-Huetos, A., Bullo, M. and Salas-Salvado, J. (2017) Dietary patterns, foods and nutrients in male fertility parameters and fecundability: a systematic review of observational studies. *Hum Reprod Update* **23**:371–389.

87. Salas-Huetos, A., et al. (2018) The effect of nutrients and dietary supplements on sperm quality parameters: a systematic review and meta-analysis of randomized clinical trials. *Adv Nutr* **9**:833–848.

88. Lambrot, R., et al. (2013) Low paternal dietary folate alters the mouse sperm epigenome and is associated with negative pregnancy outcomes. *Nat Commun* **4**: 2889.

89. Aarabi, M., et al. (2018) Testicular MTHFR deficiency may explain sperm DNA hypomethylation associated with high dose folic acid supplementation. *Hum Mol Genet* **27**:1123–1135.

90. (2015) High-dose folic acid supplementation alters the human sperm methylome and is influenced by the MTHFR C677T polymorphism. *Hum Mol Genet* **24**:6301–6313.

91. Chan, D., et al. (2017) Stability of the human sperm DNA methylome to folic acid fortification and short-term supplementation. *Hum Reprod* **32**:272–283.

92. Xue, J., et al. (2018) Impact of vitamin D depletion during development on mouse sperm DNA methylation. *Epigenetics* **13**:959–974.

93. Salas-Huetos, A., et al. (2018) Effect of nut consumption on semen quality and functionality in healthy men consuming a Western-style diet: a randomized controlled trial. *Am J Clin Nutr* **108**:953–962.

94. Ramaraju, G. A., Teppale, S., Prathigudupu, K., Kalagara, K., Thota, S., Kota, M. et al. (2018) Association between obesity and sperm quality. *Andrologia* **50**(3).

95. Craig, J. R., Jenkins, T. G., Carrell, D. T. and Hotaling, J. M. (2017) Obesity, male infertility, and the sperm epigenome. *Fertil Steril* **107**:848–859.

96. Raad, G., et al. (2017) Paternal obesity: how bad is it for sperm quality and progeny health? *Basic Clin Androl* **27**:20.

97. Fullston, T., et al. (2013) Paternal obesity initiates metabolic disturbances in two generations of mice with incomplete penetrance to the F2 generation and alters the transcriptional profile of testis and sperm microRNA content. *FASEB J* **27**:4226–4243.

98. Soubry, A., et al. (2016) Obesity-related DNA methylation at imprinted genes in human sperm: results from the TIEGER study. *Clin Epigenetics* **8**:51.

99. Sharma, R., Harlev, A., Agarwal, A. and Esteves, S. C. (2016) Cigarette smoking and semen quality: a new meta-analysis

examining the effect of the 2010 World Health Organization laboratory methods for the examination of human semen. *Eur Urol* **70**:635–645.

100. Polyzos, A., Schmid, T. E., Pina-Guzman, B., Quintanilla-Vega, B. and Marchetti, F. (2009) Differential sensitivity of male germ cells to mainstream and sidestream tobacco smoke in the mouse. *Toxicol Appl Pharmacol* **237**:298–305.

101. Marczylo, E. L., Amoako, A. A., Konje, J. C., Gant, T. W. and Marczylo, T. H. (2012) Smoking induces differential miRNA expression in human spermatozoa: a potential transgenerational epigenetic concern? *Epigenetics* **7**:432–439.

102. Hamad, M. F., et al. (2018) The status of global DNA methylation in the spermatozoa of smokers and non-smokers. *Reprod Biomed Online* **37**:581–589.

103. Jenkins, T. G., et al. (2017) Cigarette smoking significantly alters sperm DNA methylation patterns. *Andrology* **5**:1089–1099.

104. Alkhaled, Y., Laqqan, M., Tierling, S., Lo Porto, C., Amor, H. and Hammadeh, M.E. (2018) Impact of cigarette-smoking on sperm DNA methylation and its effect on sperm parameters. *Andrologia*, **January**.

105. Ricci, E., et al. (2017) Semen quality and alcohol intake: a systematic review and meta-analysis. *Reprod Biomed Online* **34**:38–47.

106. Ouko, L. A., et al. (2009) Effect of alcohol consumption on CpG methylation in the differentially methylated regions of H19 and IG-DMR in male gametes: implications for fetal alcohol spectrum disorders. *Alcohol Clin Exp Res* **33**:1615–1627.

107. Knezovich, J. G. and Ramsay, M. (2012) The effect of preconception paternal alcohol exposure on epigenetic remodeling of the h19 and rasgrf1 imprinting control regions in mouse offspring. *Front Genet* **3**:10.

108. Lee, H. J., et al. (2013) Transgenerational effects of paternal alcohol exposure in mouse offspring. *Animal Cells and Systems* **17**:429–434.

Lifestyle Factors and Sperm Quality

Ciara Wright

5.1 Introduction

Sperm counts have decreased by 50–60% between 1973 and 2011 across North America, Europe, Australia and New Zealand [1]. This decline has been predominantly attributed to lifestyle factors, which include poor-quality diets, increased rates of obesity and sedentary lifestyles. This chapter will examine the role of these factors in sperm quality and subfertility, making recommendations based on the available evidence (see Table 5.1 and Table 5.2).

Table 5.1 Food sources of nutrients which support sperm quality

Nutrient	Sources
Zinc	Oysters, beef*, lamb*, cashew nuts, almonds, pumpkin seeds, oats, chickpeas, kidney beans, peas, shiitake mushrooms
Selenium	Brazil nuts, tuna, salmon, white fish, shellfish, beef*, lamb*, chicken, eggs, sunflower seeds
Iron	Oysters, organ meats*, red meat*, tofu, oats, pumpkin seeds, lentils, beans, chickpeas
Copper	Oysters, kale, shiitake mushroom, sesame seeds, chickpeas, cashew nuts, soybeans or tofu, spinach
Vitamin C	Red and yellow peppers, guava, papaya, kiwi, oranges, strawberries, pineapple, broccoli, red cabbage
Vitamin E	Almonds, almond butter, sunflower seeds, hazelnuts, peanut butter, egg, avocado, spinach, chard
Omega-3	Anchovies, sardines, salmon, mackerel, trout, halibut
Folic Acid	Edamame beans, spinach, artichoke, asparagus, lentils, beans, chickpeas, liver*, fortified cereals
Vitamin D	Sunshine, salmon, mackerel, albacore tuna, trout, fortified dairy, fortified bread, eggs

*Limit sources of red meat

Table 5.2 Lifestyle factors affecting sperm quality

Include and increase		Decrease	Avoid
Fruits and vegetables	• Include brightly coloured fruits and vegetables high in antioxidants and fibre • Include Brassica vegetables to support reduction in oestrogen	Red meat, processed meats	• Source of pro-inflammatory omega-6 source of saturated fat. Choose fish or vegetarian meals
Fish	• Low in saturated fat for weight control • Choose oily fish such as salmon, mackerel, anchovies, sardines rich in anti-inflammatory omega-3	Biscuits, cakes, pastries, some fried foods and ready meals	• Possible source of highly inflammatory and damaging trans fats
Pulses: lentils, beans, peas	• Low in fat, high in fibre • Good source of zinc, iron	High sugar foods, sugar sweetened beverages	• Linked to weight gain and reduced sperm quality
Nuts and seeds	• High in selenium, zinc, vitamin E	Excess heat	• Bicycling, heated seats, laptop on lap, phone in pocket, saunas, hot baths may cause reduced sperm quality, DNA fragmentation or inflammation
Exercise	• Reduce weight	Smoking	• Causes direct damage to sperm, DNA damage, reduced antioxidants
Sleep	• Good-quality sleep and routine		

5.2 Nutrition and Male Fertility: Limitations of Research

The research on the effects of nutrition on sperm is growing, although there are a number of limitations. First, observational studies can give us information on dietary patterns that are associated with better semen parameters or increased pregnancy rates but causality cannot be proven. However, with repeated confirmation of these associations through several different studies, it is prudent to take valuable information from this.

The second limitation is that many studies focus on improvement of parameters of a semen analysis but may not include follow-up data regarding increased pregnancy rates or live birth rates. While this information would be useful, there are many variables that contribute to a healthy and viable pregnancy, not least the female's reproductive health. In cohorts undergoing assisted reproduction, there are additional variables and often con-comitant conditions. The WHO methodology of semen analysis has a proven association with fecundity. It is therefore logical to extrapolate and suggest that improving semen analyses will increase fecundity.

A significant limitation to almost all dietary and nutrition research is control and measurement of food intake. The development of new apps and tracking monitors may improve recall and accuracy but there is currently no ideal solution. The inability to accurately measure dietary intake makes it difficult to control for confounding factors.

Estimating dietary intake also does not account for absorption of nutrients. Digestive complaints are extremely common, some associated with poor diet and lifestyle factors themselves, such as gastro-intestinal reflux disease (GERD), hyper- or hypochloridria and irritable bowel syndrome (IBS), which can lead to malabsorption. Measuring blood levels of nutrients is often a better way of monitoring recent nutrient intake and absorption but is not frequently performed.

When looking at specific nutrients or supplements, the major limitation in many studies is that the background diet or indeed starting measurements of the nutrient is not taken into account. If a cohort takes zinc supplements for example, and 60% of this cohort is already replete, then the effects of case versus control will be diluted significantly, and more importantly the true effect will be unknown.

Looking at whole dietary patterns and whole foods or meals as we eat them in the real world lends to better overall recommendations that can be used on a large scale. Individual requirements may be more accurately assessed by using blood testing and then tailoring dietary or supplement recommendations accordingly. This could be conserved for more severe cases where general dietary improvements could be recommended for anyone considering conception.

5.3 Dietary Patterns Associated with Improved Sperm Quality and Quantity

There are now a number of studies, which taken together, can define a "healthy diet" for men, which is associated with normal semen parameters and increased fecundity. This is a diet high in fish, fruits, vegetables, nuts and pulses and low in red meat, saturated fat, trans fats, processed foods and sugary snacks or sugar sweetened beverages [2]. Despite differences across study design, food intake measurement tools and dietary classifications, the association is clear. Improving the general diet of men, either before conception or when attending fertility clinics, is a simple recommendation to make and carries no risk.

5.3.1 Dietary Food Groups

5.3.1.1 Fruits and Vegetables

Brightly coloured fruits and vegetables are particularly high in antioxidant vitamins including vitamin C, vitamin E and beta-carotene and a wide range of polyphenols. Antioxidants neutralise reactive oxygen species (ROS) and thus may prevent damage to sperm from high levels of oxidative stress which may cause reduced concentration, motility, morphology and higher levels of DNA fragmentation [3].

Fruits and vegetables are excellent sources of fibre. High fibre diets are associated with reduction in weight which will be discussed later in (see Section 5.5, Overweight and Obesity). Fibre also binds to oestrogen in the digestive tract, which may support a healthy testosterone/oestrogen ratio necessary for spermatogenesis. Brassica vegetables in particular (cabbage, kale, cauliflower, broccoli, bok choi) are high in indole-3-carbinol, a phytochemical that may inhibit aromatase.

5.3.1.2 Fish

Fish is very low in saturated fat which may contribute to a reduction in weight and risk factors associated with the metabolic syndrome. This includes insulin resistance which is a risk for sperm abnormalities, high DNA fragmentation and infertility [4]. A diet high in fish is also by default likely to be lower in meat so there is a reduction in overall saturated fat intake.

Oily fish, such as salmon, mackerel, herring, sardines and anchovies, are an excellent source of omega-3 polyunsaturated fats (see Section 5.4.5, Omega-3).

5.3.1.3 Meat, Processed Meats and Saturated Fats

Red meat is high in saturated fat and omega-6 arachidonic acid. A dose–response association between increased intake of saturated fat and a lower total sperm count and sperm concentration has been observed [5]. Arachidonic acid can be metabolised to pro-inflammatory prostaglandins and leukotrienes, promoting the inflammatory cascade and ultimately oxidative stress. A balanced diet that includes more fish and less meat will have greater overall anti-inflammatory potential.

Beyond the above mechanisms, it is not well understood why processed meats in particular are detrimental to male fertility, though higher intakes have been shown to correlate with significantly reduced fertilisation rates in IVF [6]. It may be that soy-containing additives have oestrogenic activity and there may be other unknown effects of artificial preservatives, colourings or flavourings.

5.3.1.4 Pulses

Pulses or legumes such as beans, lentils and peas are high fibre, low fat foods. They are often part of vegetarian meals as a source of protein and replace higher fat, pro-inflammatory foods such as meat or processed meats. Again, by default, a diet higher in pulses and fish is likely to be low in meat, but also may be high in vegetables due to their incorporation into vegetable-based meals.

5.3.1.5 Trans Fats

Trans fats are known to be pro-inflammatory and may increase markers of oxidation. In an intervention study, increased intake of trans fats in young men caused a marked decrease in sperm concentration [5]. Trans fats are also found in foods high in saturated fat, omega-6 oils and sugar such as confectionary, pastries, biscuits, cakes and processed foods. Therefore trans fat intake could also be seen as a marker for a high-fat, high-sugar, high processed food diet.

5.3.1.6 High Sugar Foods and Sugar Sweetened Beverages

High sugar diets contribute to weight gain, obesity, insulin resistance, inflammation and other hallmarks of the metabolic syndrome (see Section 5.5, Overweight and Obesity). Sugar sweetened beverages (SSB) in particular have been highlighted as a source of additional calories that has largely been blamed for the over-consumption of sugar by the consumer. Many European countries have singled out SSB by adding additional taxation or by promoting their exclusion from schools.

Studies directly linking the intake of SSB with male fertility are limited. Analysis of the Rochester Young Men's Study showed that a higher intake of SSB was related to significantly decreased motility in lean men only but not in those overweight or obese, where other factors may be involved [7]. Intakes of cola of over one litre per day also showed association with significantly lower sperm count and concentration [8]. In terms of pregnancy outcome, the Pregnancy Study Online (PRESTO) in North America including 1,045 men showed that higher SSB intake was related to a decreased fecundability ratio of 0.67 with daily consumption of one SSB [9]. This ratio declined further to 0.42 for energy drinks regardless of caffeine content. It is known that lifestyle habits often co-exist and PRESTO participants who drank more SSBs were more likely to smoke, have a higher BMI, lower physical activity, lower Healthy Eating Index scores and higher caloric intake; all factors contributing to inflammation and ROS which can affect sperm health.

5.4 Individual Nutrients

As mentioned previously, it is important to note that studies investigating individual nutrients rarely take into account the baseline status or even the likely dietary intake of the cohort. In the case of antioxidants, a negative effect may be seen with over-supplementation. Pro-oxidant reactions play an essential role in the body and sperm produce small amounts of ROS in order to fuel reactions involved in capacitation, binding to the zona pellucida and the acrosome reaction and thus, ultimately, fertilisation. The balance of pro-oxidant reactions is closely regulated by antioxidants. Over-supplementation is not advised, which may inhibit essential reactions or even cause chromatin instability [10].

5.4.1 Zinc

Zinc plays a number of diverse roles in the body, acting as a co-factor for hundreds of enzymatic reactions. Zinc fingers represent an abundant binding motif of DNA-binding proteins, protamines involved in chromatin remodelling and transcription factors to name a few. Zinc is found in high concentrations in the male reproductive tissues and seminal fluid has a zinc concentration of approximately 100 times higher than that of plasma. Infertile men have significantly lower seminal zinc than normal controls [11].

Zinc is involved in regulating lipid flexibility and thus motility, and membrane integrity during capacitation and the acrosome reaction [12]. Zinc is also critical to chromatin unpacking in the sperm head after fertilisation within the oocyte and deficiency may inhibit this, even in the cases of intracytoplasmic sperm injection (ICSI) [13]. Zinc is also an essential component of the abundant antioxidant compound copper/zinc superoxide dismutase (Cu/Zn SOD or SOD1), found at high concentration in seminal fluid. Zinc prevents lipid peroxidation by copper and iron. Lastly, zinc is essential for the production of thyroid hormones which in turn regulate sex hormone production and balance. Zinc deficiency correlates with testosterone deficiency.

Good sources of zinc include lamb, beef and dark chicken meat, although red meat should be limited in a "healthy diet" for male fertility. Good plant sources of zinc include cashew nuts, almonds, pumpkin seeds, oats, chickpeas, kidney beans, peas and some mushrooms. Oysters contain 10 times more zinc than the next highest food but are unlikely to be consumed regularly.

Zinc deficiency is common worldwide. Zinc absorption is negatively affected by hypo-chloridria which may be a pre-existing condition or induced by medications such as proton pump inhibitors (PPI) or H2 blockers. PPIs are among the most commonly used medications in the world and are easily available over the counter. Zinc absorption is also decreased in a high phytate diet such as a vegetarian or vegan diet high in pulses or wholegrains. Thus the advantages of an anti-inflammatory diet versus possible inhibition of mineral absorption should be considered. Some efforts can be made to reduce the phytate content of a meal such as pre-soaking foods such as pulses, brown rice or oats.

Analysing seminal zinc is uncommon in routine testing but testing blood serum zinc is economic and relatively accessible. Though zinc is higher in seminal plasma, blood levels may indicate overall deficiency. Blood levels also do not reflect long-term stores but may be a good indicator for recent dietary intake and absorption. Blood samples for assaying should be collected after fasting, as high protein intake before sampling will falsely reduce serum zinc.

Zinc is commonly found in supplement formulations targeted at men and male fertility. A number of studies include zinc as a component of a multivitamin and mineral, which may improve semen parameters and DNA fragmentation. A Cochrane review identified a marked increase in pregnancy rates in males using these formulations (OR 4.5) but rated the evidence as low due to poor design and heterogeneity of studies [14]. As a single supplement, meta-analysis has shown a positive role in improving morphology, motility and semen volume [11]. Supplement dosage varies in studies, with some giving high doses, for example 440 mg zinc sulphate daily; however, bioavailability of zinc from zinc sulphate may be as low as 10%. Zinc glycinate or zinc citrate have markedly higher bioavailability (as high as 60%) where zinc oxide may be poorly absorbed in hypochloridria or conditions of elevated gastric pH. The WHO/FAO assigned a Daily Recommended Value (DRV) of zinc for men with low bioavailability diets (e.g. high in phytates) at 14 mg per day. On a low meat, high fibre diet as described herein, a supplement of zinc glycinate or zinc citrate containing approximately 23 mg of zinc glycinate/citrate would provide the DRV for a male.

5.4.2 Selenium

Selenium is also found in high concentrations in the male reproductive tract, mostly as part of the selenoproteins glutathione peroxidases [10]. Glutathione peroxidases (GPX) are a family of antioxidant proteins which are abundant in the testes, specifically GPX5 and GPX4, which is found in higher concentrations in the testis than any other tissue. GPX4 proteins are critical to the regulation of pro-oxidant and antioxidant reactions involved in chromatid compaction during sperm maturation. Later in development, inactive GPX4 is a structural protein of the mitochondria in mature spermatozoa.

Selenium status in a population can be related to the selenium in the soil with notable exceptions. Selenium accumulates in plants which are then consumed by people or by animals which enter the food chain. Selenium content is higher for example in the west of the UK than the east but can vary. This may also depend on intensive farming techniques which may deplete minerals more rapidly, or whether food is imported from other areas. Animals that are not grass-fed and are fed a formulated feed will have standardised levels of selenium. Another exception is where high quantities of Brazil nuts are consumed. There is much advice in the public domain to consume Brazil nuts to support male fertility and it is recommended to question patients on this. Brazil nuts are markedly higher than other foods in selenium and just one Brazil nut could provide up to 80 μg of selenium, where the recommended daily intake set by the WHO/FAO is just 34 μg for men. Due to risk of excess selenium, Brazil nuts should not be consumed daily but could be part of a well-balanced diet. Other good sources of selenium include meat, chicken, fish, shellfish and eggs. Selenium status varies widely, with the measurement in a number of EU countries finding suboptimal levels to support sufficient activity of GPX proteins [15].

Selenium is often found in supplement formulations targeted at male fertility and may be present as the organic form selenomethionine or selenium derived from yeast, or the more poorly absorbed selenite. There are only a small number of studies examining selenium supplementation as a single nutrient and no meta-analyses [16]. One small Scottish study measured the effect of supplementation on men with sub-optimal selenium status and showed an improvement in motility but no significant increase in sperm count. Another well-designed larger randomised controlled trial in Iran included an infertile population with sub-optimal selenium status. Selenium status was optimal post-treatment and lead to a significant improvement in sperm count, concentration, motility and normal morphology. Notably, a study of selenium supplementation in North America which was carried out on participants that were not only selenium replete, but at the upper end of the normal range, showed no effect. Studies also varied in types of supplement used and whether the cohorts were healthy men or infertile men. As with other nutrients, we propose that the effect is more likely to be seen in males with suboptimal status and serum selenium should be measured before supplementation.

5.4.3 Iron and Copper

Iron deficiency or excess may have implications for male fertility. Ferritin in Sertoli and Leydig cells represents a source of iron for maturing spermatids and may play a number of functions in sperm development [17]. Iron deficiency can reduce oxygen availability in the testes and may correlate with suboptimal semen parameters. Copper is also critical for iron transport as the ferroxidase enzyme ceruloplasmin and thus copper deficiency could manifest as decreased iron availability in the testes also.

Iron overload or haemochromatosis is a common genetic condition, particularly in Northern Europe and highest in Ireland. Iron toxicity along with hypogonadism may lead to atrophied testes, reduced sperm quality and quantity and increased DNA fragmentation.

Copper and iron both have antioxidant roles. Copper is a component of Cu/Zn SOD. SOD converts reactive O_2^- to form oxygen (O_2) and hydrogen peroxide. Catalase (CAT), with four iron-containing haem groups, converts hydrogen peroxide into harmless O_2 and water.

Given that iron deficiency is simple to restore and iron overload is relatively common, measuring iron studies including ferritin, transferrin saturation and TIBC (Total Iron Binding Capacity) is recommended in an initial assessment of the male patient. Foods rich in haem iron include red meat. Plant sources on a low-meat diet include lentils, beans and leafy green vegetables. It is important to note that non-haem iron is poorly absorbed but this can be improved by consuming vitamin C-rich fruits or vegetables with a meal. Hypochloridria may also affect this, including use of PPIs, as the reaction to convert ferric acid to the absorbable ferrous state involves HCl and is facilitated by ascorbic acid.

5.4.4 Antioxidant Vitamins: Vitamins C and E

Vitamin C is a water-soluble antioxidant found at a concentration 10 times higher in seminal plasma than blood, while vitamin E is a fat soluble antioxidant [18]. Seminal fluid analyses from infertile men were found to contain lower vitamin C and vitamin E levels and higher ROS levels than those obtained from fertile controls. There are few studies examining the administration of either vitamin C or vitamin E as a single supplement, although vitamin C may be particularly beneficial in smokers (see Section 5.8, Smoking). With regard to protective effects on sperm DNA, there are some small but convincing studies with regard to DNA fragmentation. The most commonly cited studies are an RCT using 1 g Vitamin C and 1 g Vitamin E to reduce DNA fragmentation and a follow-up study showing increased pregnancy rates in couples undergoing ICSI [19,20].

Antioxidants have gained a good deal of attention with regard to protecting sperm, which will be discussed later in Chapter 9 in greater detail. As with any other nutrient, the effects of antioxidant supplementation are likely to be greater under conditions of depletion or increased ROS. Baseline measurements are rarely taken, nor measurements of seminal ROS, which could greatly confound outcomes of RCTs. A diet rich in fruits, vegetables, nuts, seeds and healthy fats such as avocado, salmon and olives should provide sufficient vitamin C and E for general health. However, it is worth noting that most intervention studies using vitamin C use amounts of 1 g. This would be extremely difficult to reach with diet alone, where fruits high in vitamin C such as kiwi contain approximately 90 mg.

5.4.5 Omega-3

Omega-3 fatty acids, eicosapentaenoic acid (EPA) and more specifically docosahexaenoic acid (DHA) are a major component of sperm membranes which support the flexibility of sperm cells, sperm motility and allow membrane changes that are associated with the acrosome reaction. A systematic review showed that omega-3 supplementation increased motility in all participants where patients were selected for asthenozoospermia [21]. In the one trial that included patients with oligoasthenozoopermia, sperm concentration also increased. Dosages ranged from 400 mg DHA to 1,840 mg omega-3 including DHA and EPA.

The lipid membrane of sperm is highly susceptible to lipid peroxidation, a major source of damage by ROS. Poly-unsaturated fats (PUFA) are anti-inflammatory in nature, where inflammation is a major source of ROS. Omega-3:omega-6 ratios or PUFA:saturated ratios may reflect overall anti-inflammatory potential and these ratios are seen to be higher in fertile men [5].

Replacing dietary saturated or trans fats with omega-3 fats may be most beneficial and may also result in weight reduction. A systematic review showed that increasing PUFA reduced waist circumference [22]. Abdominal obesity is associated with increased levels of ROS and insulin resistance which in turn can affect sperm quality, but the evidence in this analysis was of low quality.

Dietary intake of omega-3 is typically low across many cultures, particularly in the "Western Diet." At least two portions of oily fish per week are recommended to obtain just 500 mg of omega-3 per day. Many recommendations based on the anti-inflammatory action of omega-3 are higher than this. It is recommended to include two to three portions of salmon, mackerel, herring, sardines and anchovies per week. Wild salmon is preferable where available as farmed salmon should be limited to less than one portion per week due to high levels of dioxins, pesticides and persistent polychlorinated biphenyls (PCBs) which may also negatively affect male fertility [23]. If the male fertility patient consumes no fish or less than one portion of oily fish per week, it could be recommended to supplement with a moderate amount of omega-3 to achieve at least 500 mg of omega-3 daily.

5.4.6 Folic Acid

Folate deficiency is proposed to induce DNA damage by promoting the incorporation of uracil instead of thymine into DNA, ultimately causing DNA strand breaks. Limited studies have suggested a correlation with sperm DNA fragmentation, but study design has been a major factor.

The folate cycle also fuels the methylation cycle and low folate could deplete S-adenosylmethionine (SAM), the universal methyl donor. This may lead to aberrant DNA synthesis, alterations in methylation patterns and accumulation of homocysteine. The role of the MTHFR enzyme in the folate cycle has gathered a good deal of attention. The most common mutation is C667T, where heterozygotes account for approximately 40–50% of the European population and homozygotes account for approximately 15%. It is debated as to whether heterozygotes have reduced function of the enzyme. Homozygotes appear to have reduced function mainly in the state of low folate or other cofactors such as B_6, B_{12} and specifically riboflavin B_2 [24]. Where folate deficiency or hyperhomocysteinemia is identified in the male patient, a B complex which includes 400 µg folic acid and riboflavin could be safely recommended. These are commonly found in multi-nutrient complexes targeted at male fertility and are particularly beneficial in people under stress or with demanding lifestyles due to increased demands for B vitamins. It has been suggested that high dose folic acid (5 mg) might actually deplete MTHFR in the testes and cause hypomethylation of the sperm genome [25]. Further studies are needed to determine the role of folic acid in sperm health and the effects of supplementation.

5.4.7 Vitamin D

Cellular response to vitamin D requires expression of the vitamin D receptor (VDR) and/or cellular expression of enzymes involved in vitamin D metabolism such as CYP2R1, CYP27B1 (both activating) and CYP24A1 (inactivating). CYP2R1 and CYP27B1 are both found in high concentrations in the testes [26]. CYP24A1 and concomitant VDR expression has been shown as a good predictive marker for fertility and correlate with semen parameters. Importantly, men with reduced expression of CYP24A1 and VDR who may be infertile may not respond to vitamin D supplementation.

While VDR can promote transcription via VDR-response elements, the mature sperm is almost transcriptionally silent. Non-genomic effects of the VDR may include inducing rapid calcium influx that triggers motility and the acrosome reaction. A number of observational studies have shown correlation between motility and serum vitamin D in young healthy males and infertile and fertile males [26]. Some studies have also shown a correlation with normal morphology but no influence on sperm count or concentration.

Epidemiological studies show a seasonal variation in conception rate in northern countries of the northern hemisphere which could corroborate a role for vitamin D in fertility [27]. Vitamin D deficiency is common in these countries with an estimated 50% of adults in the UK being deficient during winter months. Cross-sectional studies have used a range of 50–125 nmol/L to assume sufficiency in relation to male fertility. With regards to other effects of vitamin D, it has been postulated that levels to the upper end of this scale may be more beneficial, for example the effect of vitamin D on the immune system. The Endocrine Society recommends a level of more than 75 nmol/L for sufficiency.

Serum vitamin D should be measured in the male patient and adequate supplementation recommended. Vitamin D in high doses can cause toxicity as it is fat soluble so should not be supplemented at high doses without testing. Currently, no international consensus is available on the optimal level for vitamin D supplementation, in particular at the safe upper level. While the tolerable upper daily limit given by the Endocrine Society is 10,000 IU, the European Food and Safety Authority currently recommends to stay below 4,000 IU/day.

5.5 Overweight and Obesity

Given that the best available evidence indicates that a healthy diet lower in saturated fats, trans fats, sugar and meat is best for supporting male fertility and fecundity, it would be expected that diets high in fat and sugar and with the associated weight gain must correlate with reduced fertility. A recent systematic review showed that males with a BMI of more than 30 had reduced clinical pregnancy rates and live birth rates with assisted reproduction [28]. With regard to semen parameters, conclusions from meta-analyses have been mixed. Eligible studies are limited, and in some cases only two studies were pooled to produce the analysis. No reliable correlation currently exists between BMI and sperm parameters, although there is a strong correlation with reduced testosterone, likely due to aromatase activity and reduced SHBG [29]. Obesity and low testosterone are also strong risk factors for erectile dysfunction [30].

BMI is a crude measurement and more research is warranted to examine any association of male fertility or sperm parameters with accurate markers of body fat such as impedance, waist circumference or biomarkers of inflammation as these could be directly related to the pathology of male subfertility. Localised inflammation, is a major source of ROS and damage to sperm including lipid peroxidation and DNA fragmentation. Systemic inflammation in the case of the Metabolic Syndrome and insulin resistance may also increase seminal pro-inflammatory cytokines resulting in abnormal semen parameters and increased DNA fragmentation [31].

Weight loss intervention studies in men are rare. A small but convincing intervention was carried out with six men with excessive abdominal fat and DNA fragmentation of more than 25%. All men achieved pregnancy resulting in a live birth and reduced DNA fragmentation [32]. Men who are overweight or obese should be counselled on weight loss. Dietary recommendations should stay in line with those that support male fertility in general.

5.6 Exercise and Hobbies

There are very few studies that examine exercise alone without relation to weight. Given its impact on health, weight and the immune system, exercise is expected to be beneficial and analysis of the EARTH (Environment and Reproductive Health Study) cohort demonstrated positive correlations with exercise and sperm count with the notable exception of bicycling [33]. Bicycling has been identified as a particular risk due to increased testicular heat or friction which may cause DNA fragmentation. Bicycling can also increase seminal pro-inflammatory cytokines and a reduction in sperm parameters [34]. Exercise should be encouraged as part of a healthy lifestyle and to promote weight reduction, but bicycling either as a leisure or competitive activity should be avoided.

Other activities that cause an increase in scrotal heat should also be avoided due to the negative effect on sperm quality, local inflammation and increased DNA fragmentation [35]. This might include saunas, hot baths, heated car seats or using a laptop on the lap. Carrying a mobile phone in the pocket may reduce motility and viability of sperm and should also be avoided where possible [36].

5.7 Caffeine

Studies on the effects of caffeine on sperm quality are limited. A 2011 meta-analysis did not identify a significant risk from caffeine intake [37] and more recent studies have shown similar or inconclusive results. An analysis of the PRESTO cohort in North America included 662 male pregnancy planners which showed a non-significant trend over two or more cups of coffee per day (Fecundity Ratio of 0.88) but no marked effect with black tea and increased fecundity with green tea (FR 1.33) [38]. There is no current evidence to suggest the men trying to conceive should avoid coffee. General recommendations based on other health outcomes might suggest that two cups per day is a moderate and safe intake. Coffee and tea, particularly green tea, also contain antioxidants which may be beneficial.

5.8 Smoking

Over one-third of men of reproductive age smoke cigarettes, and Europe has the highest number of smokers of any WHO region. Cigarette smoke contains over 4,000 toxins, carcinogens and mutagens which may impact sperm health [39]. It is well known that DNA damage can be caused by smoking, and smoking has a clear association with high DNA fragmentation [10]. Cigarette smoke is also a significant source of ROS itself and smokers have lower serum ascorbic acid. This may lead to lower levels of seminal antioxidants and thus less protection for sperm. Smokers also have higher incidence of leukocytospermia, where seminal leukocytes are the greatest source of ROS.

Epigenetic modifications in sperm including methylation aberrations, and altered chromatin structures may also be involved in the aetiology of smoking-related sub-fertility, but the mechanisms need further exploration.

Surprisingly, studies on smoking have yielded inconclusive results, although perhaps further data on genetic susceptibility might shed light on the differing effects on individuals. However, a robust meta-analysis has shown that smoking is significantly correlated with a marked reduction in sperm count and motility with a lesser effect on morphology [40]. Any male smoker should be counselled to stop smoking and relevant support provided.

5.9 Sleep

Very few studies examine the relationship of sleep and sperm quality. It is possible that men with a high degree of sleep disturbance have lower sperm count [41], but further research is warranted in this area. Shift work has been associated with reduced semen parameters and fertility, in particular where associated with disordered sleep [42].

5.10 Conclusions

Dietary and lifestyle modifications can be recommended in males to improve sperm quality and pregnancy rates without any risks. Most are simple to implement given the correct supports such as a nutrition or lifestyle coach. Nutritional supplementation is most beneficial when the individual requirements are taken into account.

References

1. Levine, H., Jorgensen, N., Martino-Andrade, A., Mendiola, J., Weksler-Derri, D., et al. (2017) Temporal trends in sperm count: a systematic review and meta-regression analysis. *Hum Repro Update* 23:646–659.

2. Salas-Huetos, A., Bullo, M. and Salas-Salvado, J. (2017) Dietary patterns, foods and nutrients in male fertility parameters and fecundability: a systematic review of observational studies. *Hum Reprod Update* 23:371–389.

3. Aitken, R. J., Gibb, Z., Baker, M. A., Drevet, J. and Gharagozloo, P. (2016) Causes and consequences of oxidative stress in spermatozoa. *Reprod Fert Dev* 28:1–10.

4. La Vignera, S., Condorelli, R., Vicari, E., D'Agata, R. and Calogero, A. E. (2012) Diabetes mellitus and sperm parameters. *J Androl* 33:145–153.

5. Esmaeili, V., Shahverdi, A. H., Moghadasian, M. H. and Alizadeh, A. R. (2015) Dietary fatty acids affect semen quality: a review. *Andrology* 3:450–461.

6. Xia, W., Chiu, Y. H., Williams, P. L., Gaskins, A. J., Toth, T. L., et al. (2015) Men's meat intake and treatment outcomes among couples undergoing assisted reproduction. *Fert Steril* 104:972–979.

7. Chiu, Y. H., Afeiche, M. C., Gaskins, A. J., Williams, P. L., Mendiola, J., et al. (2014) Sugar-sweetened beverage intake in relation to semen quality and reproductive hormone levels in young men. *Hum Reprod* 29:1575–1584.

8. Jensen, T. K., Swan, S. H., Skakkebaek, N. E., Rasmussen, S. and Jorgensen, N. (2010) Caffeine intake and semen quality in a population of 2,554 young Danish men. *Am J Epidem* 171:883–891.

9. Hatch, E. E., Wesselink, A. K., Hahn, K. A., Michiel, J. J., Mikkelsen, E. M., et al. (2018) Intake of sugar-sweetened beverages and fecundability in a North American preconception cohort. *Epidemiology* 29:369–378.

10. Wright, C., Milne, S. and Leeson, H. (2014) Sperm DNA damage caused by oxidative stress: modifiable clinical, lifestyle and nutritional factors in male infertility. *Reprod Biomed Online* 28:684–703.

11. Zhao, J., Dong, X., Hu, X., Long, Z., Wang, L., et al. (2016) Zinc levels in seminal plasma and their correlation with male infertility: a systematic review and meta-analysis. *Sci Reports* 6:22386.

12. Fallah, A., Mohammad-Hasani, A. and Colagar, A. H. (2018) Zinc is an essential element for male fertility: a review of Zn roles in men's health, germination, sperm quality, and fertilization. *J Reprod Infert* 19:69–81.

13. Mortimer, D. (2018) The functional anatomy of the human spermatozoon: relating ultrastructure and function. *Mol Hum Reprod* DOI 10.1093/molehr/gay040

14. Showell, M. G., Mackenzie-Proctor, R., Brown, J., Yazdani, A., Stankiewicz, M. T. and Hart, R. J. (2014) Antioxidants for male subfertility. *Cochrane database of systematic reviews (Online)* CD007411.

15. Stoffaneller, R. and Morse, N. L. (2015) A review of dietary selenium intake and selenium status in Europe and the Middle East. *Nutrients* 7:1494–1537.

16. Mistry, H. D., Broughton Pipkin, F., Redman, C. W. and Poston, L. (2012) Selenium in reproductive health. *Am J Obst & Gyn* 206:21–30.

17. Tvrda, E., Peer, R., Sikka, S. C. and Agarwal, A. (2015) Iron and copper in male reproduction: a double-edged sword. *J Assist Reprod Gen* 32:3–16.

18. Majzoub, A. and Agarwal, A. (2018) Systematic review of antioxidant types and doses in male infertility: benefits on semen parameters, advanced sperm function, assisted reproduction and live-birth rate. *Arab J Urol* **16**:113–124.

19. Greco, E., Iacobelli, M., Rienzi, L., Ubaldi, F., Ferrero, S. and Tesarik, J. (2005) Reduction of the incidence of sperm DNA fragmentation by oral antioxidant treatment. *J Androl* **26**:349–353.

20. Greco, E., Romano, S., Iacobelli, M., Ferrero, S., Baroni, E., et al. (2005) CSI in cases of sperm DNA damage: beneficial effect of oral antioxidant treatment. *Hum Reprod* **20**:2590–2594.

21. Hosseini, B., Nourmohamadi, M., Hajipour, S., Taghizadeh, M., Asemi, Z., et al. (2018) The effect of omega-3 fatty acids, EPA, and/or DHA on male infertility: a systematic review and meta-analysis. *J Diet Supp* **1–12**.

22. Zhang, Y. Y., Liu, W., Zhao, T. Y. and Tian, H. M. (2017) Efficacy of omega-3 polyunsaturated fatty acids supplementation in managing overweight and obesity: a meta-analysis of randomized clinical trials. *J Nut Health Age* **21**:187–192.

23. Foran, J. A., Carpenter, D. O., Hamilton, M. C., Knuth, B. A. and Schwager, S. J. (2005) Risk-based consumption advice for farmed Atlantic and wild Pacific salmon contaminated with dioxins and dioxin-like compounds. *Environ Health Pers* **113**:552–556.

24. Reilly, R., McNulty, H., Pentieva, K., Strain, J. J. and Ward, M. (2014) MTHFR 677TT genotype and disease risk: is there a modulating role for B-vitamins? *Proc Nut Soc* **73**:47–56.

25. Aarabi, M., San Gabriel, M. C., Chan, D., Behan, N. A., Caron, M., et al. (2015) High-dose folic acid supplementation alters the human sperm methylome and is influenced by the MTHFR C677T polymorphism. *Hum Mol Gen* **24**:6301–6313.

26. Blomberg Jensen, M. (2014) Vitamin D and male reproduction. *Nature Rev Endocrin* **10**:175–186.

27. Martinez-Bakker, M., Bakker, K. M., King, A. A. and Rohani, P. (2014) Human birth seasonality: latitudinal gradient and interplay with childhood disease dynamics. *Proc Biol Sci* **281**:20132438.

28. Mushtaq, R., Pundir, J., Achilli, C., Naji, O., Khalaf, Y. and El-Toukhy, T. (2018) Effect of male body mass index on assisted reproduction treatment outcome: an updated systematic review and meta-analysis. *Reprod Biomed Online* **36**:459–471.

29. MacDonald, A. A., Herbison, G. P., Showell, M. and Farquhar, C. M. (2010) The impact of body mass index on semen parameters and reproductive hormones in human males: a systematic review with meta-analysis. *Hum Reprod Update* **16**:293–311.

30. Shamloul, R. and Ghanem, H. (2013) Erectile dysfunction. *Lancet* **381**:153–165.

31. Leisegang, K., Bouic, P. J. and Henkel, R. R. (1989) Metabolic syndrome is associated with increased seminal inflammatory cytokines and reproductive dysfunction in a case-controlled male cohort. *Am J Reprod Immun (New York)* **76**:155–163.

32. Faure, C., Dupont, C., Baraibar, M. A., Ladouce, R., Cedrin-Durnerin, I., et al. (2104) In subfertile couples, abdominal fat loss in men is associated with improvement of sperm quality and pregnancy: a case-series. *PloS one* **9**:e86300.

33. Gaskins, A. J., Afeiche, M. C., Hauser, R., Williams, P. L., Gillman, M. W., et al. (2014) Paternal physical and sedentary activities in relation to semen quality and reproductive outcomes among couples from a fertility center. *Hum Reprod* **29**:2575–2582.

34. Hajizadeh Maleki, B. and Tartibian, B. (2015) Long-term low-to-intensive cycling training: impact on semen parameters and seminal cytokines. *Clin J Sport Med: Official J Can Acad Sport Med* **25**:535–540.

35. Zhang, M. H., Zhang, A. D., Shi, Z. D., Wang, L. G. and Qiu, Y. (2015) Changes in levels of seminal nitric oxide synthase, macrophage migration inhibitory factor, sperm DNA Integrity and Caspase-3 in

fertile men after scrotal heat stress. *PloS one* **10**:e0141320.

36. Adams, J. A., Galloway, T. S., Mondal, D., Esteves, S. C. and Mathews, F. (2014) Effect of mobile telephones on sperm quality: a systematic review and meta-analysis. *Environ Int* **70**:106–112.

37. Li, Y., Lin, H., Li, Y. and Cao, J. (2011) Association between socio-psycho-behavioral factors and male semen quality: systematic review and meta-analyses. *Fertil Steril* **95**:116–123.

38. Wesselink, A. K., Wise, L. A., Rothman, K. J., Hahn, K. A., Mikkelsen, E. M., et al. (2016) Caffeine and caffeinated beverage consumption and fecundability in a preconception cohort. *Reprod Tox (Elmsford, NY)* **62**:39–45.

39. Harlev, A., Agarwal, A., Gunes, S. O., Shetty, A. and du Plessis, S. S. (2015) Smoking and male infertility: an evidence-based review. *World J Men's Health* **33**:143–160.

40. Sharma, R., Harlev, A., Agarwal, A. and Esteves, S. C. (2016) Cigarette smoking and semen quality: a new meta-analysis examining the effect of the 2010 World Health Organization laboratory methods for the examination of human semen. *Eur Urol* **70**:635–645.

41. Jensen, T. K., Andersson, A. M., Skakkebaek, N. E., Joensen, U. N., Blomberg Jensen, M., et al. (2013) Association of sleep disturbances with reduced semen quality: a cross-sectional study among 953 healthy young Danish men. *Am J Epidem* **177**:1027–1037.

42. Deng, N., Haney, N. M., Kohn, T. P., Pastuszak, A. W. and Lipshultz, L. I. (2018) The effect of shift work on urogenital disease: a systematic review. *Current Urol Rep* **19**:57.

Chapter 6

The Effect of Age on Male Fertility and the Health of Offspring

Allan Pacey and Sarah Martins da Silva

6.1 Introduction

Over the past few decades, the average age of both mothers and fathers has risen noticeably in many post-industrial countries. In the United Kingdom (UK), for example, the average age of fathers in 1976 was 29.6 years, whereas by 2016 it had risen to 33.3 years (Figure 6.1). Notably, in the past two decades, the percentage of fathers aged 30 and over in the UK has increased from 59% in 1996 to 66% in 2006 [1]. Similar increases have been reported in the United States (US) [2]. Whilst there are obvious social and demographic reasons for these shifts, such as young men (and their partners) focusing on educational opportunities and career development in their teens and twenties, these trends also present challenges for those working in reproductive medicine. The average age of men and women presenting for infertility and assisted reproduction is also increasing, and management of the "older couple" is therefore becoming increasingly common. This chapter will review the available evidence of the effect of male age on: (i) semen quality, sperm function and sperm DNA damage; (ii) conception and pregnancy outcomes; (iii) outcomes of assisted reproduction; and (iv) the health of offspring.

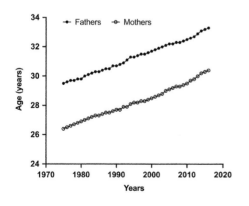

Figure 6.1 The age of fathers (solid circles) and mothers (open circles) in the UK from 1975 to 2016. Redrawn from data published in [1].

6.2 Effect of Male Age on Semen Quality, Sperm Function, and Sperm DNA Damage

Much has been previously written about the impact of male age on semen quality and/or aspects of sperm function. This section will summarise the relevant literature on how male age may impact on macroscopic measures of sperm quality as observed at semen analysis, functional aspects of sperm, and the quality of sperm nuclear DNA.

With regard to macroscopic and microscopic measures of semen quality, perhaps the largest meta-analysis undertaken to date included semen quality data from 93,839 men taken from a total of 90 studies [3]. Critically, the analysis controlled for a number of important confounding factors that can directly impact on semen analysis parameters, including duration of sexual abstinence (i.e. ejaculates produced after a long abstinence will likely contain fewer motile sperm). The conclusions of the meta-analysis were that there was a statistically significant age-associated decline in many of the macroscopic and microscopic measures of semen quality, including semen volume, total motility, progressive motility, and percentage of sperm with normal morphology. However, no age-related decline in sperm concentration was observed, which suggests that age does not impact on the speed of spermatogenesis, but more upon the "quality" of sperm produced.

Unfortunately, almost no studies have examined the influence of male age on the functional aspects of sperm, such as their ability to undergo acrosome reaction, or bind to the oocyte. This is probably a reflection on how difficult it is to perform such studies as well as poor availability, lack of standardisation, and therefore the lack of use of sperm function tests by diagnostic laboratories. However, it is plausible that the sperm of older men may function less well *in vivo* or *in vitro* during assisted reproduction. For example, age-related changes to subtle aspects of sperm movement can be measured by Computer Aided Sperm Analysis (CASA) [4]. Furthermore, a broad spectrum of alterations at the transcriptional and translational level have been described to occur in sperm of older men, which may impact on molecular mechanisms and function [5]. It is recognised that the acrosome reaction is impaired in the spermatozoa from obese men [6]. Since male obesity generally increases as men age, there is some validity in concluding that the sperm of older men may be similarly compromised. But whether this is independent from, or a consequence of, the ageing process is currently unknown.

In comparison to sperm function, much more has been written about the quality of sperm nuclear DNA in older men. For example, a meta-analysis including data from 10,220 men where information about sperm DNA fragmentation was available concluded that the number of sperms with unfragmented DNA (i.e. undamaged) generally decreases as men age [3]. However, given the controversy about sperm DNA fragmentation testing, and the array of tests that can be used to examine this [7], little could be concluded about the type of damage. This is discussed in detail in Chapter 4. It is also uncertain whether male age contributes to the risk of sperm aneuploidy, although age-related alterations in sperm DNA methylation patterns have been reported [8], as well as altered protamine and miRNA expression in the sperm from older men [9]. The clinical significance of this is unclear.

6.3 Effect of Male Age on Conception and Pregnancy Outcomes

Diagnostic semen analysis is itself acknowledged to have limitations in its prediction of male fertility and there are no nomograms to show whether age-related changes in semen quality are likely to be clinically significant. Similarly, with tests of sperm function or measures of sperm genetic integrity, there is little consensus on what these data mean. Recent analysis suggests that a change in semen quality occurs around the age of 40 [4], but it is difficult to be precise and it is more likely that age-related changes to any aspect of semen quality or sperm function are gradual and incremental. For the practising clinician or embryologist it is therefore difficult to conclude whether age-related changes to semen quality, sperm function, or sperm nuclear DNA are truly significant to the probability of natural conception or the success of assisted reproduction. However, given the deterioration in semen quality and increase in sperm DNA damage associated with advancing male age, logic would suggest that male fecundity is likely to reduce as a man gets older. In reality, the effect of male age on fertility is controversial, not least because there is a paucity of studies that have examined this in a robust way.

Perhaps the first one to do so used the Avon Longitudinal Study of Parents and Children (ALSPAC). ALSPAC is a world-leading birth cohort study, charting the health of 14,500 families in the Bristol area (www.bristol.ac.uk/alspac/). A study of 6,524 couples from the cohort examined the effect of male age on time to conception (TTC), which was used as an index of fecundity [10]. The results demonstrated a significant association between advancing male age and length of TTC. A logistic regression model was used to take account of other variables that may have had a significant influence (e.g. female age). After adjustment, paternal age remained highly significantly associated with conception within 6 or 12 months ($p < 0.0001$): the average age of the men who took more than 6 months to impregnate their wives was 31.8 ± 5.75 years compared with 30.8 ± 5.27 years in men who took 6 months or less ($p < 0.0001$). Men who took more than 12 months were also significantly ($p < 0.0001$) older (32.6 ± 5.91 years) than men who took 12 months or less to conceive (30.9 ± 5.32 years). In summary, older men took longer to conceive naturally. An alternative concept is that it is a couple's cumulative age, rather than just paternal age, that defines fertility potential. A retrospective study of 6,188 European women [11] identified a paternal age of 40 years or more to be a risk factor for infertility (TTC >12 months), but only where female age was 35 years or more (odds ratio [OR] 2.99 95% CI: 1.82, 4.91). Similarly, a study of 782 healthy couples observed a decrease in the daily probability of conception where the couple was composed of a woman 35–39 years old and a man in his late thirties or older [12].

As men age, testicular function and metabolism deteriorates [13]. The testis undergoes age-related structural and cellular changes, including loss of volume, narrowing of seminiferous tubules, and a decrease in number of germ cells, Leydig cells, and Sertoli cells. Serum testosterone levels also decrease with age, with resultant effect on the hypothalamic-pituitary-gonadal (HPG) axis. Therefore, whilst age-related changes to semen quality, sperm function, or the quality of sperm DNA may explain decline in male fertility (see above), another plausible explanation is that older men may simply be less interested in sex or suffer increased levels of erectile dysfunction (ED). Both of these will clearly affect TTC and pregnancy rates. For example, in the Massachusetts Male Aging Study (MMAS), sexual function and coital frequency were assessed in 1,290 men. The probability of having severe ED increased three fold and the probability of moderate ED increased two fold between the ages 40 and 70. The annual incidence of ED increased with each decade of age and was 12.4 cases per 1,000 man-years (95% CI: 9.0, 16.9), 29.8 (95% CI: 24.0, 37.0), and 46.4 (95% CI: 36.9, 58.4) for men 40 to 49, 50 to 59, and 60 to 69 years old, respectively [14]. In the same cohort, followed for an average of 9 years, coital frequency was assessed in 1,085 men. After adjusting for baseline sexual function, men engaged in sexual activity on average 6.5 times per month prior to age 40. This frequency decreased by 1 to 2 times per month after age 50 and by another once or twice per month after age 60 [15].

In addition to delay in conception, male age also appears to have an impact on adverse pregnancy outcomes, including pregnancy loss [16]. For example, a prospective study of 5,121 natural conceptions found an adjusted hazard ratio of 1.27 (95% CI: 1.00, 1.6) for first trimester miscarriage for partners of men 35 years and older, compared to those whose partners were younger than 35 years [17]. An analysis of all live and stillbirths in Denmark (1994–2010) identified paternal age as a risk for late pregnancy loss (22+ gestational weeks). Over 75,000 births were fathered by men of more than 40 years old in this large dataset. After meticulous adjustment for maternal age, increasing paternal age was found to significantly increase risk of stillbirth. Compared with offspring of fathers aged 32 years, the risk was 1.23 in offspring of fathers aged 40 years and 1.36 in offspring of fathers aged 50 years [18].

6.4 Effect of Male Age on Outcomes of Assisted Reproduction

One of the first studies to robustly investigate the relationship between male age and outcomes of assisted reproduction examined data from the French National IVF Registry, submitted by 59 IVF centres [19]. By examining the IVF outcomes of 1,938 men on the register whose partners were totally sterile with bilateral tubal occlusion or absence of both tubes, they concluded that the risk of failure to conceive following IVF clearly increased with both maternal and paternal age. However, critically, after taking into account the possibility that the paternal age effect may differ according to maternal age (i.e. generally couples tend to partner with someone of a similar age), they were able to show that once men were older than 40 years of age, the risk of failing to conceive doubled if the female partner was 35 to 37 years old (OR 2.0 [95% CI: 1.1, 3.6]) and increased over five fold if she was above 41 years old (OR 5.74 [95% CI: 2.16. 15.23]). This suggested that there was a male age effect independent of other variables, which influenced the outcome of assisted reproduction. A retrospective study of 17,000 stimulated intrauterine insemination cycles also demonstrated a highly significant effect of paternal age. Following correction for maternal age, a significant reduction in pregnancy rate was seen in couples with older men (12.3% per cycle where paternal age <30 years, 9.3% per cycle where paternal age >45 years; $p<0.001$). Partners of men older than 45 years also had significantly higher miscarriage rates; 32.4% compared with 13.7% in couples with men younger than 30 years ($p < 0.001$) [20].

Further studies using egg donation cycles to control for the influence of maternal age have also examined the association between male age and the outcome of assisted reproduction, but with mixed conclusions. For example, a study of 1,023 men found that there was a significant increase in pregnancy loss and a decrease in live birth rate and blastocyst formation rate in men above the age of 50, but, interestingly, there was no significant difference in implantation rate, pregnancy rate, or measures of early embryo development [21]. This is in contrast to another study that found no effect of male age on the outcome of 1,083 donor oocyte cycles [22]. It is difficult to see how two studies of similar size and design reached such different conclusions and this perhaps reflects why there remains a lack of clarity in this area. Interestingly, neither of these studies discriminated between cycles where fertilisation was achieved through traditional IVF versus intra-cytoplasmic sperm injection (ICSI) and it is possible that the outcome of these treatments may be different. However, a narrative review examining 10 studies involving over 7,000 IVF and ICSI cycles concluded that there was "insufficient evidence to demonstrate an unfavourable effect of paternal age on assisted reproduction technology (ART) outcomes" [23]. Nonetheless, they also noted that most studies were retrospective and there was significant heterogeneity in design, for example, entry criteria and outcome reporting. Certainly paternal age may not be relevant when ICSI and good-quality oocytes are used. A retrospective study of 4,887 donor oocyte cycles showed no effect of male age on biochemical, clinical, ongoing pregnancy rates as well as take-home baby rates, where egg donors were less than 35 years old [24].

The reality is that there remains a lack of well-designed, prospective studies examining the impact of paternal age on ART outcomes, and the literature continues to be contradictory on this point. In recent years, there has been a shift in focus towards understanding the influence of male age on sperm DNA quality and whether this in itself is a critical factor for reproductive outcome, more specifically miscarriage and early pregnancy loss. It is widely acknowledged that there is a general trend for sperm DNA to show more signs of damage as men get older (see above) and meta-analysis shows that there is a relationship between higher damage and early pregnancy loss, at least by some measures of sperm DNA quality [25]. However, there remains a notable lack of consensus and considerable confusion about the best methods to test for sperm DNA damage, as well as how to interpret results [7], so it is perhaps not surprising that there is no clear answer here also (see Chapter 4). However, it has been proposed that the quality of sperm DNA (however it is measured and assessed) may have an important role in determining the health and prospects of any children born and this will be reviewed in Section 6.5.

6.5 Effect of Male Age on Child Health

Continuous division of the male germ cell line results in an increase in frequency of mutations in spermatozoa across the male life course. For example, a longitudinal study of 78 Icelandic parent-offspring trios demonstrated doubling of paternal mutations every 16.5 years, an average of 2 per year [26]. Although rare, paternal age effect (PAE) disorders are autosomal dominant, and caused by mutations in five genes (*FGFR2, FGFR3, HRAS, PTPN11, RET*). PAE disorders are characterised by congenital skeletal deformities and retarded growth, cardiac disorders, skin hyperpigmentation, and cancer susceptibility, and include Apert, Crouzon, Pfeiffer, and Muenke syndromes, achondroplasia, Costello and Noonan syndromes, as well as multiple endocrine neoplasia (MEN) type 2A and type 2B [27].

Age-related genetic and epigenetic changes in spermatozoa are also postulated to cause a variety of other diseases in the resulting offspring. Although "congenital abnormality" is a poorly defined concept, encompassing very heterogeneous conditions both genetically determined and of developmental origin, the association with advanced paternal age (APA) is supported (on the whole) by large data sets. For example, a retrospective cohort study of 5,213,248 subjects (USA birth registrations 1999–2000) assessed the association between paternal age and birth defects [28]. A total of 77,514 birth defects were recorded in this study cohort (1.5%) and multiple logistic regressions were used to estimate the independent effect of paternal age on all birth defects, as well as 21 specific defect groups. In summary, APA was associated with increased risk of heart defects, tracheo-oesophageal fistula, oesophageal atresia, and musculoskeletal abnormalities, as well as Down syndrome and other chromosomal abnormalities. However, the overall risk of birth defect for older fathers was small.

A further study examining the associations between paternal age and birth defects examined data from the National Birth Defects Prevention Study (NBDPS), a large multicenter case-control study (over 15,000 cases) designed to investigate genetic and environmental risk factors for major birth defects in the USA [29]. Paternal age was found to be a significant contributory risk factor for certain birth defects, whereas others were corrected for by maternal age. Elevated odds ratios for each year's increase in paternal age were found for cleft palate (OR 1.02 95% CI: 1.00, 1.04), diaphragmatic hernia (OR 1.04 95% CI: 1.02, 1.06), right ventricular outflow tract obstruction (OR 1.03 95% CI: 1.01, 1.04), and pulmonary valve stenosis (OR 1.02 95% CI: 1.01, 1.04). It is worth noting that whilst the incremental increase in risk per year does not appear large, the difference in odds faced by men several years apart in age is potentially substantial. For example, a 40-year-old father would have twice the odds of having a child with diaphragmatic hernia compared with a child whose father was 20 years old. Moreover, the risk doubles again by age 60. A Danish prospective cohort study of 1,575,521 live-born children born between 1978 and 2004 assessed the relationship between APA and the risk of childhood death in children [18]. Compared to children born to fathers aged 30–34 years, a statistically significant excess risk of death was found for children born to fathers aged 40–44 years and 45+ years old. Increase in paternal age significantly increased the hazard risk of death for children under 5 years old (HR 1.24 [95% CI: 1.0, 1.53] for fathers aged 40–44 years; HR 1.65 [95% CI: 1.24, 2.18] for fathers 45+ years old). This was primarily attributed to fatal congenital anomalies, malignancies, and external causes.

Many studies show a clear epidemiological association between increased paternal age and schizophrenia, autism, and dyslexia. However, although the association is now well established, the underlying mechanisms remain equivocal and are likely due to both: (i) inherited genetic factors in couples where an older male becomes a father; or (ii) *de novo* genetic changes in paternal gametes that arise as a consequence of ageing [30]. This is not specific to assisted reproduction. A population-based study of all individuals (2,615,081) born in Sweden between 1973 and 2001 showed that children whose fathers were over 45 years old had a 3.45 times increased risk of autism, 13.1 times increased risk of attention-deficit /hyperactivity disorder, twice the increased risk of psychosis, 24.7 times increased risk of bipolar disorder, 2.7 times increased likelihood of suicide attempts, and 2.4 times increased risk of substance use problems, compared with offspring born to fathers 20–24 years old [31].

Finally, APA has also been shown to be associated with negative effects on both maternal health as well as those of the offspring. A recent large population-based cohort study of 40,529,905 live births between 2007 and 2016 in the US showed that higher paternal age was associated with an increased risk of premature birth, low birth weight, and low Apgar score [32]. For example, infants born to fathers aged 45 years or older had 14% higher odds of premature birth (OR 1.14, 95% CI: 1.13, 1.15) and 18% higher odds of seizures (OR 1.18, 95% CI: 0.97, 1.44) compared with infants of fathers aged 25 to 34 years. Gestational diabetes was 34% higher (OR 1.34, 95% CI: 1.29, 1.38) in mothers with the oldest partners. To estimate the contribution of APA, the data was recalculated for a scenario in which all fathers were younger than 45 years. In this model, 13.2% of premature births and 18.2% of gestational diabetes were estimated to be specifically attributable to APA.

6.6 Discussion/Conclusions

This chapter has reviewed four aspects of how APA may affect male fertility and the health of any children born. In summary, there seems to be convincing evidence from several studies that there are measurable changes in semen quality, sperm function, and sperm DNA damage as men age and this may underpin, to some extent, the observed male-age-related decline in natural fertility. However, there seems to be less evidence that APA impacts greatly on the outcome of assisted conception, although the studies on which this conclusion is based are not strong. Perhaps the area where there is much more compelling evidence is the relationship between APA and the health of children born to older fathers. APA can contribute to birth defects associated with single gene mutations and chromosomal abnormalities, but is also associated with psychiatric morbidity and may increase the incidence of certain childhood cancers. As such, it is important to consider what these observations mean for clinical practice and how doctors and other healthcare professionals might use this information in their day-to-day work.

First, it is perhaps important to note that there is no universally agreed definition of APA. For example, studies that observe changes of semen quality, or those that show a decrease in natural fertility as men age, tend to suggest that noticeable changes occur around the age of 40. Other studies that investigate health of offspring only determine significant risks at the age of 50 or even 60 years old. Furthermore, many published reviews and commentaries define APA anywhere between 35 and 50 years old, or categorise paternal age into ranges of 5–10 years [33]. In comparison to our understanding of how maternal age impacts on a woman's fertility and the health of her children beyond the age of 35, there is clearly less consensus concerning paternal age. Thus, in the absence of a clear definition, it is difficult for doctors and healthcare professionals to engage patients in a meaningful discussion of reproductive risks associated with male age. Couples should be counselled that age-related changes, and the risks of disorders in offspring, increase continuously over time.

Second, it is noteworthy that there are currently no screening or diagnostic tests that specifically identify the risks of poor reproductive outcome or risk to child health over and above a broad assessment of male age itself. Moreover, given the lack of consensus on what age constitutes APA (see above), it is easy to see why there is an absence of clinical guidelines that propose the use of male age as a cut-off for access to assisted reproduction treatment such as IVF. For example, in the UK, the National Institute for Health and Care Excellence (NICE) 2013 guidelines proposes that women under the age of 40 years be offered three full cycles of IVF and those aged between 40 and 42 be offered a single cycle [34]. However, no mention at all is made regarding the age of the male partner, not even to suggest that doctors highlight that male age may influence the outcome. Male age is only considered for recruitment of sperm donors. The most recent guidelines from the Association of Biomedical Andrologists, the Association of Clinical Embryologists, the British Andrology Society, British Fertility Society, and Royal College of Obstetricians and Gynaecologists [35] recommend that ideally sperm donors should be under the age of 40. This was largely proposed out of concern for the health of any children born, although this has recently been questioned [36].

Finally, there have been several calls over the years to offer various medical solutions to guard against the risks of APA, for the greater good of society. For example, it has been suggested that there should be appropriate health education to promote earlier fatherhood, incentives for young sperm donors, and state-supported universal sperm banking [37]. For the latter, it was argued, that "sperm could be taken (on a voluntary basis) from all young men, with artificial insemination becoming the norm for procreation." However, the paper ignored the fact that for many, given the variable quality of frozen-thawed sperm, intra-uterine insemination (IUI) would not be successful, and this therefore would inevitably lead to an increase in the use of IVF (and/or ICSI) with the associated risks of doing so being incumbent on the female partner.

In conclusion, there is now compelling evidence that APA can directly affect male fertility and the health of children born. However, much more research is required to establish how this information might be used by doctors and other healthcare professionals working in assisted conception.

References

1. Office for National Statistics (2017) *Births by Parents' Characteristics in England and Wales: 2016*. London: Office for National Statistics. www.ons.gov.uk/peoplepopulatio nandcommunity/birthsdeathsandmarria ges/livebirths/bulletins/birthsbyparentschar acteristicsinenglandandwales/2016

2. Khandwala, Y. S., Zhang, C. A., Lud, Y. and Eisenberg, M. L. (2017) The age of fathers in the USA is rising: an analysis of 168,867,480 births from 1872 to 2015. *Hum Reprod* **32**:2110–2116.

3. Johnson, S. L., Dunleavy, J., Gemmell, N. J. and Nakagawa, S. (2015) Consistent age-dependent declines in human semen quality: a systematic review and meta-analysis. *Ageing Res Rev* **19**:22–33.

4. Verón, G. L., Tissera, A. D., Bello, R., Beltramone, F., Estofan, G., Molina, R. I., et al. (2018) Impact of age, clinical conditions, and lifestyle on routine semen parameters and sperm kinematics. *Fertil Steril* **110**:68–75.

5. Almeida, S., Rato, L., Sousa, M., Alves, M. G. and Oliveira, P. F. (2017) Fertility and sperm quality in the aging male. *Curr Pharm Des* **23**:4429–4437.

6. Samavat, J., Natali, I., Degl'Innocenti, S., Filimberti, E., Cantini, G., Di Franco, A., et al. (2014) Acrosome reaction is impaired in spermatozoa of obese men: a preliminary study. *Fertil Steril* **102**:1274–1281.

7. Pacey, A. (2018) Is sperm DNA fragmentation a useful test that identifies a treatable cause of male infertility? *Best Pract Res Clin Obstet Gynaecol* **53**:11–19.

8. Jenkins, T. G., Aston, K. I., Pflueger, C., Cairns, B. R. and Carrell, D. T. (2014) Age-associated sperm DNA methylation alterations: possible implications in offspring disease susceptibility. *PLoS Genet* **10**(7):e1004458.

9. Paoli, D., Pecora, G., Pallotti, F., Faja, F., Pelloni, M., Lenzi, A., et al. (2019) Cytological and molecular aspects of the ageing sperm. *Hum Reprod* **34**:218–227.

10. Ford, W. C., North, K., Taylor, H., Farrow, A., Hull, M. G. and Golding, J. (2000) Increasing paternal age is associated with delayed conception in a large population of fertile couples: evidence for declining fecundity in older men. The ALSPAC Study Team (Avon Longitudinal Study of Pregnancy and Childhood). *Hum Reprod* **15**:1703–1708.

11. de La Rochebrochard, E. and Thonneau, P. (2003) Paternal age >or=40 years: an important risk factor for infertility. *Am J Obstet Gynecol* **189**:901–905.

12. Dunson, D. B., Colombo, B. and Baird, D. D. (2002) Changes with age in the level and duration of fertility in the menstrual cycle. *Hum Reprod* **17**:1399–1403.

13. Gunes, S., Hekim, G. N., Arslan, M. A. and Asci, R. (2016) Effects of aging on the male reproductive system. *J Assist Reprod Genet* **33**:441–454.

14. Johannes, C. B., Araujo, A. B., Feldman, H. A., Derby, C. A., Kleinman, K. P. and McKinlay, J. B. (2000) Incidence of erectile dysfunction in men 40 to 69 years old: longitudinal results from the Massachusetts Male Aging Study. *J Urol* **163**:460–463.

15. Araujo, A. B., Mohr, B. A. and McKinlay, J. B. (2004) Changes in sexual function in middle-aged and older men: longitudinal data from the Massachusetts Male Aging Study. *J Am Geriatr Soc* **52**:1502–1509.

16. Sartorius, G. A. and Nieschlag, E. (2010) Paternal age and reproduction. *Hum Reprod Update* **16**:65–79.

17. Slama, R., Bouyer, J., Windham, G., Fenster, L., Werwatz, A. and Swan, S. H. (2005) Influence of paternal age on the risk of spontaneous abortion. *Am J Epidemiol* **161**:816–823.

18. Urhoj, S. K., Jespersen, L. N., Nissen, M., Mortensen, L. H. and Nybo Andersen, A. M. (2014) Advanced paternal age and mortality of offspring under 5 years of age: a register-based cohort study. *Hum Reprod* **29**:343–350.

19. de La Rochebrochard, E., de Mouzon, J., Thépot, F. and Thonneau, P. (2006) French National IVF Registry (FIVNAT) association. Fathers over 40 and increased failure to conceive: the lessons of *in vitro* fertilisation in France. *Fertil Steril* **85**:1420–1424.

20. Belloc, S., Cohen-Bacrie, P., Benkhalifa, M., Cohen-Bacrie, M., De Mouzon, J., Hazout A., et al. (2008) Effect of maternal and paternal age on pregnancy and miscarriage rates after intrauterine insemination. *Reprod Biomed Online* **17**:392–397.

21. Frattarelli, J. L., Miller, K. A., Miller, B. T., Elkind-Hirsch, K. and Scott, R. T. Jr. (2008) Male age negatively impacts embryo development and reproductive outcome in donor oocyte assisted reproduction technology cycles. *Fertil Steril* **90**:97–103.

22. Whitcomb, B. W., Turzanski-Fortner, R., Richter, K. S., Kipersztok, S., Stillman, R. J., et al. (2011) Contribution of male age to outcomes in assisted reproductive technologies. *Fertil Steril* **95**:147–151.

23. Dain, L., Auslander, R. and Dirnfeld, M. (2011) The effect of paternal age on assisted reproduction outcome. *Fertil Steril* **95**:1–8.

24. Beguería, R., García, D., Obradors, A., Poisot, F., Vassena, R. and Vernaeve, V. (2014) Paternal age and assisted reproductive outcomes in ICSI donor oocytes: is there an effect of older fathers? *Hum Reprod* **10**:2114–2122.

25. Robinson, L., Gallos, I. D., Conner, S. J., Rajkhowa, M., Miller, D., Lewis, S., et al. (2012) The effect of sperm DNA fragmentation on miscarriage rates: a systematic review and meta-analysis. *Hum Reprod* **27**:2908–2917.

26. Kong, A., Frigge, M. L., Masson, G., Besenbacher, S., Sulem, P., Magusson, G., et al. (2012) Rate of *de novo* mutations and the importance of father's age to decrease risk. *Nature* **488**:471–475.

27. Goriely, A. and Wilkie, A. O. (2012) Paternal age effect mutations and selfish spermatogonial selection: causes and consequences for human disease. *Am J Hum Genet* **90**:175–200.

28. Yang, Q., Wen, S. W., Leader, A., Chen, X. K., Lipson, J. and Walker, M. (2007) Paternal age and birth defects: how strong is the association. *Hum Reprod* **22**:696–701.

29. Green, R. F., Devine, O., Crider, K. S., Olney, R. S., Archer, N., Olshan, A. F., et al. (2010) National Birth defects Prevention Study. Association of paternal age and risk for major congenital and anomalies from the National Birth Defects Prevention Study, 1997 to 2004. *Ann Epidemiol* **20**:241–249.

30. Janecka, M., Mill, J., Basson, M. A., Goriely, A., Spiers, H., Reichenberg, A., et al. (2017) Advanced paternal age effects in neurodevelopmental disorders – review of potential underlying mechanisms. *Transl Psychiatry* **31**(7):e1019.

31. D'onofrio, B. M., Rickert, M. E., Frans, E., Kuja-Halkola, R., Almqvist, C., Sjolander, A., et al. (2014) Paternal age at childbearing and offspring psychiatric and academic morbidity. *JAMA Psych* **71**:432–438.

32. Khandwala, Y. S., Baker, V. L., Shaw, G. M., Stevenson, D. K., Lu, Y. and Eisenberg, M. L. (2018) Association of paternal age with perinatal outcomes between 2007 and 2016 in the United States: population based cohort study. *BMJ* **363**:k4372.

33. Wu, C., Lipshultz, L. I. and Kovac, J. R. (2016) The role of advanced paternal age in modern reproductive medicine. *Asian J Androl* **18**:425.

34. National Institute for Health and Clinical Excellence (2013) *Fertility: Assessment and Treatment for People with Fertility Problems.* www.nice.org.uk/guidance/cg156/evidence/full-guideline-pdf-188539453

35. Association of Biomedical Andrologists; Association of Clinical Embryologists; British Andrology Society; British Fertility Society; Royal College of Obstetricians and Gynaecologists (2008) UK guidelines for the medical and laboratory screening of sperm, egg and embryo donors *Hum Fertil* **11**:201–210.

36. Ghuman, N. K., Mair, E., Pearce, K. and Choudhary, M. (2016) Does age of the sperm donor influence live birth outcome in assisted reproduction? *Hum Reprod* **31**:582–590.

37. Smith, K. R. (2015) Paternal age bioethics. *J Med Ethics* **41**:775–779.

The Assessment and Role of Anti-sperm Antibodies

Gary N. Clarke

7.1 Introduction

The primary aim of this chapter is to provide practical, evidence-based information pertinent to the specific detection of anti-sperm antibodies (ASA) in males and females and the assessment of ASA results and their place in fertility evaluation and management. A secondary but equally important aim is to review selected literature which is relevant to understanding why some individuals develop sperm immunity. Third, to focus briefly on whether new research and novel techniques for detecting ASAs might help to refine our understanding of their role in infertility.

7.2 Historical Synopsis

7.2.1 Early Evidence for Immuno-Infertility

Nearly a century ago "clinical trials" involving immunization of women with their partner's semen with the aim of inducing immuno-contraception were conducted [1]. Baskin [2] reported on a study of 20 fertile women immunized 3 times intramuscularly at weekly intervals, with their partner's whole ejaculate. All but one of the women showed sperm immobilizing activity in their serum by one week after the last injection which persisted for up to one year. Only one woman became pregnant after 12 months when the sperm immobilizing activity was no longer detectable in her serum. These trials demonstrated that women could be immunized to develop sperm immobilizing activity, and that this was associated with reduced fecundity.

Obviously, this "trial" would not get past an institutional ethics committee nowadays; however, it was notable from an historical perspective in that it stimulated significant interest in the idea that immunological responses to sperm could be involved in the development of otherwise unexplained infertility, and in the concept of an anti-sperm contraceptive vaccine. The work of Rumke in the 1970s was particularly important in establishing the veracity of immuno-infertility [3]. His work provided a rigorous demonstration of the relationship between delay to conception and the strength or titre of the ASAs in the patient's serum.

7.2.2 Evolution of Sperm Antibody Detection Methodology

Historically, the study of human immuno-infertility was stimulated by reports of the sperm-agglutinating properties of serum from patients presenting with infertility [4–6]. It subsequently became apparent that many of the early studies had significantly overestimated the incidence of sperm antibodies in the infertile population because of their failure to distinguish specific (i.e. antibody-dependent) from non-specific agglutination. Consequently, sperm agglutination assays are no longer acceptable for detection of sperm immunity in the clinical setting.

An important step occurred in 1968, when Isojima and colleagues published a defined protocol for an immunologically specific test for sperm immobilizing antibodies in serum [7]. The sperm immobilization test (SIT) requires the dual presence of sperm-bound antibodies of immunoglobulin class G (IgG) and/or immunoglobulin class M (IgM) and active components of the classical complement cascade. If sufficient antibody and complement components are present then the majority of spermatozoa will be immobilized during a 1 hour incubation at 37°C. The availability of the SIT provided further impetus to the study of immuno-infertility from a research perspective and also significantly improved diagnostic capability in this area. However, a more detailed understanding of the effector mechanisms leading to immuno-infertility necessitated the refinement of specific procedures for detecting and localizing antibodies bound to a patient's spermatozoa. In this regard the development of the mixed anti-globulin reaction (MAR) by Kremer's group provided a relatively simple means of detecting membrane-bound antibodies of IgG class on the surface of motile spermatozoa in semen and was used by this group to make important contributions relating to the role of sperm antibodies in infertility [8]. However, it could not detect antibodies of IgA and IgM classes with equal facility. Thus, there remained a need for a similar type of assay which could be set up in many laboratories for research and routine screening of the patient's semen for sperm-bound antibodies of any of the major immunoglobulin classes.

7.2.3 Development, Validation and Application of the Immunobead Test (IBT)

As described above, sperm immunity was traditionally assessed by observing the sperm agglutinating or immobilizing properties of the patient's serum. However, with the growth of immunological knowledge in the 1970s, it became apparent that circulating antibodies were not necessarily indicative of local antibodies in either titre or immunoglobulin class. Work on the direct IBT was initiated in this laboratory in 1979 and was first presented at the Annual Scientific meeting of the Australian Society for Immunology in 1981 and first published in 1982 [9]. The indirect version of the IBT has since proven to be an excellent test for sperm antibody screening of serum and reproductive tract secretions. A slightly different version of the IBT was developed independently by Bronson's laboratory in New York [10]. The IBT was widely used for both routine diagnostic work and as a research tool. The research group led by Gilbert Haas published evidence that the IBT was more sensitive than radioimmunoassay for sperm antibody detection [11]. Having developed a sensitive and immunologically specific procedure, the next step was to apply it assiduously with the aim of achieving greater understanding of the mechanism by which an immunological reaction to spermatozoa, either in men (autoimmunity) or women (isoimmunity), might cause sub-fertility or infertility. Early studies with the IBT in my laboratory in Melbourne indicated that sperm autoimmunity occurred in approximately 8.5% of the male partners in couples presenting for infertility investigations [12]. The sperm antibodies were predominantly of IgG or IgA classes. IgM class antibodies were rarely detected in semen. In a proportion of men, one immunoglobulin class was obviously dominant, whilst in approximately 50% of men, both classes were equally represented. Approximately 4% of men presenting with infertility had more than 80% of their motile spermatozoa coated with antibodies of IgG and IgA classes. The aim of subsequent work from this laboratory on sperm autoimmunity was to determine whether antibodies of both classes were involved in the detrimental effects on fertility, or whether perhaps IgA, which is present mainly in the form of secretory IgA, might be the main effector molecule.

7.3 Mechanisms by Which Sperm Antibodies Affect Fertility

7.3.1 The Effect of Sperm Antibodies on Sperm Migration through Cervical Mucus

Initial research in this area commenced with a comparison of IBT results with the outcome of the semen-cervical mucus interaction tests [13]. These studies indicated that there was a strong association between the presence of IgA class antibodies and a strong shaking reaction in the semen-cervical mucus contact test (SCMCT), lending support to the hypothesis advanced by Kremer and Jager [14] that IgA class antibodies formed a bridge between spermatozoa and the cervical mucus micellular structure. These bridges tethered the sperm to the mucus framework, preventing normal penetration of the sperm through the mucus. By implication, the operation of this mechanism *in vivo* would ultimately prevent sperm transport to the normal site of fertilization in the ampulla of the fallopian tube.

In females, the uterine cervix is known to be a highly competent mucosal immune site [15], which contains many IgA-positive plasma cells located in the sub-epithelial layers of the endocervix. Most of the IgA in cervical mucus is secretory IgA consisting of two IgA monomers linked by J-chain and secretory piece. The secretory IgA antibodies directed against potential pathogens and occasionally sperm can immobilize the invaders by cross-linking them to the cervical mucus strands, effectively blocking their progress to the upper reaches of the reproductive tract [14]. There are obviously protective mechanisms which normally preclude such immunological reactions to sperm in the majority of women. However, in a small percentage of couples these protective mechanisms are somehow circumvented or disrupted, resulting in local and often circulating ASA production and reduced chances of natural conception. In women with otherwise unexplained infertility, sperm antibody activity has been detected in cervical mucus in more than 10% of cases [16].

Thus, the overall conclusion of these investigations was that IgA was the most important effector molecule leading to inhibition of the normal process of sperm migration through mid-cycle cervical mucus. Although high-titre sperm antibodies will totally block sperm migration through cervical mucus, many patients have intermediate antibody levels which only partially inhibit mucus penetration. Hence, it was vital to determine whether ASAs might affect other aspects of sperm function.

7.3.2 Effects of Sperm Antibodies on *In Vitro* Fertilization (IVF)

Retrospective analysis of IVF results by Clarke and colleagues [17] provided some of the first evidence that ASAs from female serum could inhibit the fertilization of viable human oocytes by human spermatozoa. They observed a fertilization rate of only 15% for patients who had significant titres of IgG and IgA class ASA in their serum, which at that time was used as a supplement in the IVF culture medium, versus 69% for those patients where replacement serum was used during the fertilization culture. Their later results confirmed that very high titre ASA of IgG immunoglobulin class in female serum could effectively inhibit fertilization of fresh human oocytes [18]. Subsequent reports from other laboratories have also indicated that high level ASA can inhibit human fertilization [19–21]. Consequently, it is now generally accepted, at least with strong sperm immunity, that ASA can block sperm functions such as cervical mucus penetration and fertilization and thereby impair fertility.

7.3.3 Post-Fertilization Effects of ASA on Fertility

Definitive studies in various animal models have shown an association between ASA and pre- or post-implantation embryonic degeneration [22]. Why should ASA react with embryos? First, the sperm membrane is integrated as a mosaic into the zygote membrane during the process of fertilization, so that sperm antigens are incorporated, although at relatively low densities, into the developing embryo [23]. Second, embryonic gene expression commencing from the four to eight cell stage results in the synthesis of various developmental antigens which can cross-react with sperm antigens [24]. Consequently, during embryo development and perhaps particularly around the time of blastocyst hatching, there is a chance for the ASA to bind to cross-reacting embryonic antigens and potentially cause embryo degeneration or possibly prevent implantation.

There is also some evidence for post-fertilization effects associated with ASA in humans. Concerning negative effects, Warren Jones reported in 1981 that around 50% of pregnancies conceived in women with ASA subsequently ended in first trimester spontaneous miscarriages [25]. Similar observations have been reported by other groups [16,26]. In the latter study, it was found that 7/16 (44%) of women who miscarried were positive for ASA in their serum, compared with only 2/17 (12%) of women who had successful ongoing pregnancies. Examination of the immunoglobulin classes of the antibodies revealed that IgA was significantly ($p<0.01$) more common in those women who miscarried. The IgA class antibodies in serum may be a marker for local secretory IgA in the female reproductive tract. However, despite the strong evidence in rabbits [27], it is still not known whether IgA class ASA in humans are embryotoxic. In another clinical study [28], it was found that of 173 women referred for a history of three or more consecutive spontaneous miscarriages, there was a significantly higher incidence of sperm immobilizing antibodies when compared with the infertile group. Interestingly, they also observed a higher incidence of ASA in the group of women shown to have an immunological basis for their recurrent miscarriages (e.g. couples sharing at least three HLA determinants, or couples with the female showing a relatively low response to her partner's lymphocytes in mixed lymphocyte culture). Other groups have reported a significant association between ASA and some autoantibodies such as anti-phospholipids, which may be involved in deleterious effects on the foetus. In contrast to the studies cited above, which have reported an association between ASA and recurrent miscarriage, others have not seen a statistically significant association [29]. Further investigations in this area would be useful, particularly focusing on the possible involvement of sub-surface sperm antigens which react with IgA class ASA. It is important to note that sperm antibodies specific for sub-surface antigens are unlikely to be detected by assays such as the IBT or the MAR which are designed to measure reactivity with membrane antigens on motile sperm. It could be very informative to conduct a clinical investigation of IVF patients with repeated implantation failure or early spontaneous miscarriages, using a new generation of highly specific ELISA and immunofluorescence assays in conjunction with the MAR (unfortunately immunobeads are no longer available so the original IBT has become obsolete).

7.4   Possible Causes of Immuno-Infertility

What information is currently available regarding the development of, or predisposing factors for, sperm immunity? In men, sperm auto-immunity often develops after vasectomy or genital trauma or due to cross-reactions with infectious organisms. Observations of potential relevance to understanding the underlying causes of ASA in women include evidence that they are more likely to have detectable sperm antibodies if their male partner also has ASA in his semen [30]. Another important observation was that in about one-third of cases women apparently react only to their partner's sperm antigens, rather than to sperm-specific antigens [31]. This observation requires further investigation because if confirmed, it would indicate that many female patients with immunity to their partner's sperm may be going undiagnosed. Several hypotheses have been proposed in order to explain the origins of sperm immunity and the observed association between male and female sperm immunity in a proportion of couples [32].

7.5   Current Laboratory Procedures for Detection of Sperm Antibodies

There are a few methods which are more suitable for use in the routine diagnostic laboratory, including the MAR, the immunosphere binding assay (IBA) and the SIT. Although there are many ELISA kits available on the market, some of which could prove useful for research applications, I am not convinced that this procedure is suitable for routine screening of patient sera during infertility investigations. I believe that it is indicative that no laboratories report ELISA results for sperm antibody detection in the Australian External Quality Assurance Scheme for Reproductive Medicine (EQASRM). This scheme sends four sample distributions per year and laboratories enrolled for the sperm antibody module receive four serum samples in each distribution. It is vital that any laboratory performing diagnostic sperm antibody tests is enrolled in an appropriate EQA scheme.

For the commercial sperm antibody detection kits it is important to follow the manufacturer's instructions provided with each kit and that any variations are detailed in the laboratory quality system. For "in-house" procedures such as the SIT it is necessary to document any variations from published protocols, to perform internal controls and if possible to participate in an appropriate EQA scheme. The following sections provide extra information relating to particular tests.

7.5.1   Mixed Anti-Globulin Reaction (MAR)

The MAR detects antibodies bound to the surface of motile sperm (Figure 7.1) and can be used in the direct form for detection of antibodies attached to the surface of sperm in the ejaculate, or in an indirect form designed to detect circulating antibodies present in blood serum from the male or female partner. As shown in Figure 7.1, the antibodies are detected by cross-linking of latex beads coated with human immunoglobulin (IgG) to antibodies bound to the surface of motile sperm (an analogous reaction can be used for IgA class sperm

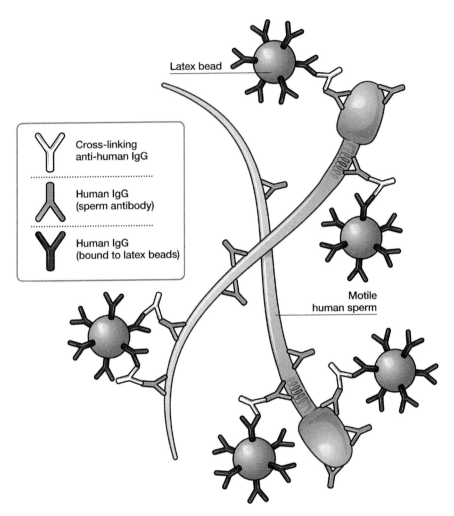

Latex bead

Cross-linking
anti-human IgG

Human IgG
(sperm antibody)

Human IgG
(bound to latex beads)

Motile
human sperm

Figure 7.1 Interactions occurring during a positive MAR for the detection of sperm antibodies of IgG immunoglobulin class on the surface of motile human spermatozoa.

antibodies). The cross-linking is caused by an anti-human immunoglobulin antiserum (anti-globulin). As with any immunological test, it is vital to know that the detection system is effective in detecting sperm antibodies in a known positive sample, and that any nonspecific binding of the latex beads to sperm is minimal as indicated by testing a known negative sample. The positive and negative controls should be performed at regular intervals during the life of each MAR kit (e.g. weekly or fortnightly). An important internal control is to note and record the presence of significant bead-bead clumping during every test. The bead clumping is caused by the added anti-globulin binding specifically to the human immunoglobulin attached to the latex beads and is the same mechanism which causes mixed agglutination between beads and motile sperm coated with sperm antibodies. The vast majority of beads should be in clumps with or without sperm – weak bead clumping indicates that something is not right and should be investigated. If the same thing happens with a repeat test, then perform positive and negative sample controls – if the positive control is weak or negative, this suggests that the kit may have deteriorated during storage (e.g. it may have frozen due to defective refrigeration or become contaminated). If indicated, it may be necessary to open a new kit, test it against the known controls and repeat the patient's test. Some laboratories (e.g. reference or research laboratories) may wish to undertake more rigorous kit evaluation by performing crossed-inhibition tests on new kits. For example, an MAR-IgG kit should show positive controls inhibited by pure human IgG but not by pure IgA or IgM. My laboratory recently performed a crossed-inhibition test using a serum which gave 100% of motile sperm coated with IgA class antibodies on the sperm head. Addition of pure IgA completely inhibited the binding, whereas pure IgG gave no inhibition. This demonstrated the specificity of the kit for detection of antibodies of IgA immunoglobulin class.

Sera which are strongly positive at the initial screening dilution of 1/16 can subsequently be tested at higher dilutions such as 1/256 or 1/4096 in order to obtain a semi-quantitative idea of the strength of the autoantibody (in the male) or isoantibody (in the female). This extra information could be very useful for clinicians in deciding on an assisted reproductive treatment (ART) approach for a patient.

One concern about the MAR kits arises because of the sodium azide used as a preservative in both the latex bead and anti-globulin preparations. The azide is toxic to sperm with variable effect on different samples, with some samples losing nearly all motility when examined after the recommended 3-minute incubation. For this reason I would suggest making an initial examination within 1 minute and if motility has dropped, to commence counting immediately. It would also be helpful if the manufacturers of the kits could investigate alternative and potentially less toxic preservatives such as sodium benzoate, benzyl alcohol or gentamycin sulphate. An interim measure such as reducing the sodium azide concentration to 0.05% could provide significant improvement in this regard.

7.5.2 Immunosphere Binding Assay (IBA)

The IBA is analogous to the original IBT, wherein small latex beads or spheres coated with anti-human immunoglobulin antibodies are washed to remove preservative, then mixed with an equal sized drop of washed human sperm (Figure 7.2). After a short incubation, the percentage of motile sperm with attached immunospheres is determined microscopically. Figure 7.2 depicts the IBA for sperm antibodies of IgA immunoglobulin class; however, analogous interactions can be used for detection of antibodies of either IgG or IgM immunoglobulin classes. The IBA is more time-consuming than the MAR but potentially more sensitive due to the washing steps removing any free immunoglobulin present in the seminal plasma or serum dilution used for screening. This is because in patients who have higher levels of free immunoglobulin in their semen, partial inhibition of the MAR may result.

7.5.3 Sperm Immobilization Test (SIT)

The SIT is an immunologically specific procedure for detection of sperm antibodies because a positive immobilization result requires the simultaneous presence of sperm-bound complement-fixing antibodies (usually IgG or IgM) and complement components in order to breach the cell membrane and cause the sperm to become non-viable

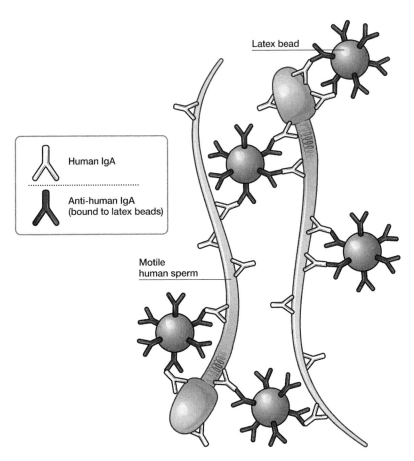

Latex bead

Human IgA

Anti-human IgA
(bound to latex beads)

Motile
human sperm

Figure 7.2 Interactions occurring during a positive IBA for the detection of sperm antibodies of IgA immunoglobulin class bound to the surface of motile human spermatozoa.

and hence nonmotile. We have previously reported excellent agreement between positivity in the SIT and the IBT [33]. The SIT has the advantage of being able to be performed cheaply because it does not require purchase of expensive kits. The SIT could therefore be the assay of choice for laboratories with restricted budgets. The simplest version of the SIT requires only patient and control sera and a normal donor semen sample. The sera must be fresh or frozen soon after collection in order to preserve sufficient complement for the test (it is also possible to add exogenous complement obtained commercially). After thawing the sera, inactivate one aliquot of each serum at 56°C for 30 minutes, then add freshly prepared swim-up sperm, incubate the mixtures at 37°C for 60 minutes and read the motility in each. The ratio of motility in the inactivated aliquot to that in the non-inactivated aliquot is the sperm immobilization index (SI). An SI of 2.0 or more is considered a positive result requiring further testing. In my experience an SI of more than 10 is very significant. In some cases there will be no motility in the non-inactivated aliquot versus more than 90% motility in the complement inactivated aliquot. Sera with a high SI can be retested at higher dilutions to determine the titre of the immobilizing antibody.

7.6 Important Caveats/Suggestions Regarding Testing Procedures

7.6.1 Scoring

Although it is not mentioned in either the SpermMAR or MARScreen instructions, when reading and scoring reactions it is important *not* to count sperm tail-tip binding *and* to score motile sperm as positive only if they have at least two beads bound to their surface, as per the latest edition of the WHO manual [34].

7.6.2 Positive Controls

Seminal plasma can be used as a very appropriate positive control for the direct MAR or IBA. Seminal plasma from men with positive direct MAR or IBA but with low sperm concentration is more likely to contain higher sperm antibody levels because less will have been absorbed onto sperm. The seminal plasma can be aliquoted in 50 µl volumes, thawed on the day of testing, then add an aliquot (5–10 µl) of ASA negative semen containing approximately 2 million motile sperm. Incubate the mixture for 60 minutes at 37°C then test by direct MAR or IBA.

7.6.3 Economical Testing

Expensive kit components can be used for more tests by scaling down. For example, the SpermMAR instructions recommend using 1 µl of each reagent and spreading the mixture under a 24 × 40 mm coverslip. It is possible to scale the volumes down by using a 22 × 22 mm coverslip and thereby get approximately twice as many tests from the same kit.

7.6.4 Mixing of Components

The SpermMAR instructions recommend mixing components with the edge of the coverslip; however, it can be difficult to mix thoroughly with this method. More complete mixing can be obtained by aspirating the mixture in and out of the pipette tip used to dispense the reagent (i.e. as the beads are added to the semen aliquot, then as the antiglobulin reagent is added to the semen-bead mixture). A final gentle mix with the edge of the coverslip can be performed immediately prior to applying the coverslip.

7.6.5 Sperm Washing Medium

The SpermMAR instructions for the indirect test are in my opinion unnecessarily prescriptive regarding the sperm washing medium. They specify to use Earle's balanced salt solution (EBBS, e.g. Sigma-Aldrich E2888) when there is no technical reason to use this particular medium. Any medium which supports human sperm motility and does not contain human immunoglobulins or human serum albumin (as a precaution in case of contamination by immunoglobulins) should be suitable. The instructions for the MARScreen kit take a relatively non-prescriptive approach in just noting that "Sperm washing medium containing 1–5% bovine serum albumin" is required. I believe that this approach could be used for the SpermMAR kit to give laboratories more flexibility.

7.6.6 Alternative Testing Applications

Although not mentioned in the instructions for the SpermMAR or MARScreen kits, both can potentially be used for indirect MAR testing of other reproductive tract fluids such as seminal plasma, cervical mucus and follicular fluid. For example, seminal plasma can be tested by adding an aliquot ($\sim$10 µl) of MAR negative semen containing about 2 million motile sperm to 90 µl of seminal plasma, incubating for 60 minutes at 37°C and then testing by the direct MAR procedure. It is always preferable to obtain a direct MAR result on a patient's semen, but this alternative could be useful when it is not possible to get a reliable direct MAR reading due to poor semen quality.

7.6.7 Protein G Test (PGT)

For some research and trouble-shooting applications, my laboratory has found that Protein G Dynabeads can be used to detect IgG class antibodies on motile sperm. We have developed the following very simple, but effective protocol:

1. Take an aliquot of semen containing approximately 2 million motile sperm (usually between 50 and 300 µl) and add around 3 ml of sperm washing medium (e.g. Tyrode solution containing 0.3% BSA).
2. Centrifuge the mixture at 600 Gmax for 5 minutes at room temperature, aspirate the supernatant and resuspend the sperm pellet in about 50 µl of medium.
3. To perform the test, add 5 µl of Protein G Dynabeads to 5 µl of the washed sperm, mix thoroughly, coverslip (22 × 22 mm) and examine under phase-contrast optics (magnification 200–400×) after 1–2 minutes.
4. Score the results as for the MAR or IBA, keeping in mind the advice given in 1, above.

We have found that the PGT gives positive reactions with known positive samples and that a strong positive reaction was inhibited by pure IgG but not by pure IgA.

Some laboratories may wish to perform a full validation of the PGT against the MAR or IBA and consider using it for routine screening of patients.

7.7 Relevance of Sperm Antibody Results to Patient Management

If the male partner has a high percentage (>75%) of his sperm coated with IgG and/or IgA class antibodies by MAR or IBA, whilst his female partner is negative for sperm antibodies, then the clinician could potentially consider intrauterine insemination of washed sperm to overcome the cervical barrier created when antibody coated sperm encounter cervical mucus. If this approach fails after a few cycles, then consider treatment by ICSI. An identical approach could be considered if the male has a positive SIT in his serum, associated with significant sperm agglutination and/or low sperm motility in his semen, whilst his female partner is negative for SIT in her serum. An exception to the approach outlined above could be considered if the male has 100% of his sperm coated with IgG and or IgA class antibodies or he has a high level of immobilizing antibodies (e.g. SI $\geq$ 10.0) in his serum associated with significant sperm agglutination or low sperm motility in his semen. In the latter situation and depending on the age of the female partner, careful consideration could be given to proceeding straight to ICSI.

7.8   Conclusion

Unfortunately there has been relatively little research interest in sperm immunity in recent years. More refined understanding of the reactivity of the male and female immune system to semen antigenicity may help to explain the etiology of immuno-infertility, but could also have significant implications for the development of immuno-contraceptive vaccines and for the wider understanding of normal pregnancy and its associated pathologies.

References

1. Katsh, S. (1959) Immunology, fertility, and infertility: a historical survey. *Am J Obstet Gynecol* **77(5)**:946–956.

2. Baskin, M. J. (1932) Temporary sterilization by the injection of human spermatozoa. *Am J Obstet Gynecol* **24**:892–897.

3. Rumke, P., Van Amstel, N., Messer, E. N. and Bezemer, P. D. (1974) Prognosis of fertility of men with sperm agglutinins in the serum. *Fertil Steril* **25**:393–398.

4. Rumke, P. (1954) The presence of sperm antibodies in the serum of two patients with oligospermia. *Vox Sang* **4**:135–140.

5. Wilson, L. (1954) Sperm agglutinins in human semen and blood. *Proc Soc Exp Biol Med* **85**:652–655.

6. Franklin, R. R. and Dukes, C. D. (1964) Further studies on sperm-agglutinating antibody and unexplained infertility. *JAMA* **190**:682–683.

7. Isojima, S., Li, T. S. and Ashitaka, Y. (1968) Immunologic analysis of sperm-immobilizing factor found in sera of women with unexplained sterility. *Am J Obstet Gynecol* **101**:677–683.

8. Jager, S., Kremer, J. and van Slochteren-Draaisma, T. (1978) A simple method of screening for antisperm antibodies in the human male. Detection of spermatozoal surface IgG with the direct mixed antiglobulin reaction carried out on untreated fresh human semen. *Int J Fertil* **23**:12–21.

9. Clarke, G. N., Stojanoff, A. and Cauchi, M. N. (1982) Immunoglobulin class of sperm-bound antibodies in semen. In Bratanov, K. (ed.), *Proc Int Symp Immunology of Reproduction*. Bulgaria: Bulgarian Academy of Sciences Press. 482–485.

10. Bronson, R. A., Cooper, G. W. and Rosenfeld, D. L. (1982) Correlation between regional specificity of antisperm antibodies to the spermatozoan surface and complement-mediated sperm immobilization. *Am J Reprod Immunol Microbiol* **2**:222–224.

11. Haas, G. G., D'Cruz, O. J. and De Bault, L. E. (1991) Comparison of the indirect immunobead, radiolabeled, and immunofluorescence assays for immunoglobulin G serum antibodies to sperm. *Fertil Steril* **55**:377–388.

12. Clarke, G. N., Elliott, P. J. and Smaila, C. (1985) Detection of sperm antibodies in semen using the immunobead test: a survey of 813 consecutive patients. *Am J Reprod Immunol Microbiol* **7**:118–123.

13. Clarke, G. N., Stojanoff, A., Cauchi, M. N., McBain, J. C., Speirs, A. L. and Johnston, W. I. (1984) Detection of antispermatozoal antibodies of IgA class in cervical mucus. *Am J Reprod Immunol* **5**:61–65.

14. Kremer, J. and Jager, S. (1992) The significance of antisperm antibodies for sperm-cervical mucus interaction. *Hum Reprod* **7(6)**:781–784.

15. Anderson, D. J. (1996) The importance of mucosal immunology to problems in human reproduction. *J Reprod Immunol* **31**(1–2):3–19.

16. Menge, A. C., Medley, N. E., Mangione, C. M. and Dietrich, J. W. (1982) The incidence and influence of antisperm antibodies in infertile human couples on sperm-cervical mucus interactions and subsequent fertility. *Fertil Steril* **38**:439–446.

17. Clarke, G. N., Lopata, A. and Johnston, W. I. (1986) Effect of sperm antibodies in females on human *in vitro* fertilization. *Fertil Steril* **46**(3):435–441.

18. Clarke, G. N., Hyne, R. V., du Plessis, Y. and Johnston, W. I. (1988) Sperm antibodies and human *in vitro* fertilization. *Fertil Steril* **49**:1018–1025.

19. Yeh, W. R., Acosta, A. A., Seltman, H. J. and Doncel, G. (1995) Impact of immunoglobulin isotype and sperm surface location of antisperm antibodies on fertilization *in vitro* in the human. *Fertil Steril* **63**:1287–1292.

20. Ford, W. C., Williams, K. M., McLaughlin, E. A., Harrison, S., Ray, B. and Hull, M. G. (1996) The indirect immunobead test for seminal antisperm antibodies and fertilization rates at *in-vitro* fertilization. *Hum Reprod* **11**:1418–1422.

21. de Almeida, M., Gazagne, I., Jeulin, C., Herry, M., Belaisch-Allart, J., Frydman, R., et al. (1989) *In-vitro* processing of sperm with autoantibodies and *in-vitro* fertilization results. *Hum Reprod* **4**:49–53.

23. O'Rand, M. G., Irons, G. P. and Porter, J. P. (1984) Monoclonal antibodies to rabbit sperm autoantigens. I: Inhibition of *in vitro* fertilization and localization on the egg. *Biol Reprod* **30**(3):721–729.

24. Menge, A. C. and Naz, R. K. (1988) Immunologic reactions involving sperm cells and preimplantation embryos. *Am J Reprod Immunol Microbiol* **18**(1):17–20.

25. Jones, W. R. (1981) Immunology of infertility. *Clin Obstet Gynaecol* **8**(3):611–639.

26. Witkin, S. S. and David, S. S. (1988) Effect of sperm antibodies on pregnancy outcome in a subfertile population. *Am J Obstet Gynecol* **158**(1):59–62.

27. Menge, A. C. (1970) Immune reactions and infertility. *J Reprod Fertil Suppl* **10**:171–186.

28. Haas, G. G. Jr, Kubota, K., Quebbeman, J. F., Jijon, A., Menge, A. C. and Beer, A. E. (1986) Circulating antisperm antibodies in recurrently aborting women. *Fertil Steril* **45**:209–215.

29. Clarke, G. N. and Baker, H. W. (1993) Lack of association between sperm antibodies and recurrent spontaneous abortion. *Fertil Steril* **59**(2):463–464.

30. Witkin, S. S. and Chaudhry, A. (1989) Relationship between circulating antisperm antibodies in women and autoantibodies on the ejaculated sperm of their partners. *Am J Obstet Gynecol* **161**(4):900–903.

31. Witkin, S. S., Vogel-Roccuzzo, R., David, S. S., Berkeley, A., Goldstein, M. and Graf, M. (1988) Heterogeneity of antigenic determinants on human spermatozoa: relevance to antisperm antibody testing in infertile couples. *Am J Obstet Gynecol* **159**:1228–1231.

32. Clarke, G. N. (2009) Etiology of sperm immunity in women. *Fertil Steril* **91**:639–643.

33. Clarke, G. N., Lopata, A., McBain, J. C., Baker, H. W. and Johnston, W. I. (1985) Effect of sperm antibodies in males on human *in vitro* fertilization (IVF). *Am J Reprod Immunol Microbiol* **8**:62–66.

34. Coper, T. G. (ed.) (2010) *WHO Laboratory Manual for the Examination and Processing of Human Semen*, 5th edition. Geneva: World Health Organization.

FSH Treatment in Male Infertility

Csilla Krausz, Viktória Rosta, and Alberto Ferlin

8.1 Introduction

The regulation of the endocrine and reproductive function of the testis is under the concerted action of gonadotropin-releasing hormone (GnRH) and gonadotropins, such as luteinizing hormone (LH) and follicle-stimulating hormone (FSH). GnRH neurons originate from the olfactory placode from where they migrate through the nasal septum, the cribriform plate to the forebrain, reaching their terminal position in the arcuate nucleus of the hypothalamus. The pulsatile GnRH production starts around the 16th week during foetal development. It is followed by a "mini-puberty" in the first postnatal year, which means the transient activation of the hypothalamic-pituitary-gonadal (H-P-G) axis, leading to a temporary increase of serum testosterone level in the new born baby. After childhood, the reactivation of pulsatile GnRH secretion is the main initiator and regulator of puberty leading to the stimulation of gonadotropin synthesis in the pituitary gland. Both FSH and LH are needed for a quantitatively and qualitatively normal spermatogenesis. FSH directly acts through Sertoli cells to promote germ cell proliferation (mainly spermatogonial mitosis), while LH stimulates testosterone (T) synthesis in Leydig cells, which has a crucial role not only in sperm production but also in the development of secondary sexual characteristics.

The treatment of hypogonadotropic hypogonadism (HH) recapitulates the physiological regulation of the H-P-G axis and is based on the administration of FSH in combination with hCG (long-acting LH analogue). Two types of hCG preparations are available for treatment, urinary-hCG, derived from urine of pregnant women, or recombinant-hCG, derived from genetically manipulated hamster ovary cells by recombinant DNA technology. Similarly, FSH preparations are either extracted and purified from the urine of postmenopausal women, known as hMG (human menopausal gonadotropin, with mainly FSH and some LH activity) and highly purified FSH (hpFSH) with no residual LH activity, or obtained from recombinant *in vitro* technology (rhFSH) [1,2]. All these preparations are equally effective in inducing and maintaining spermatogenesis in patients with HH.

In addition to HH, a relatively new target for FSH monotherapy is idiopathic male subfertility. While the frequency of HH is about 5% in male factor infertility, the proportion of idiopathic cases reaches 40–50%. Given its high clinical impact, there is a growing interest in defining the efficacy of FSH therapy in idiopathic infertile men [3]. In this chapter, we give a clinically oriented description of the use of FSH in the two above-mentioned pathological conditions: HH and idiopathic spermatogenic impairment.

8.2 FSH Treatment in Hypogonadotropic Hypogonadism

Hypogonadotropic hypogonadism (HH) is defined as the consequence of acquired or congenital diseases that affect the hypothalamus and/or pituitary gland, resulting in impaired secretion or defect in the action of the gonadotropin releasing hormone (GnRH) leading to low levels of gonadotropins and testosterone.

8.2.1 Aetiopathogenesis

HH can be acquired (AHH) due to a number of different pathological conditions or congenital (CHH) due to genetic factors (Figure 8.1).

Acquired HH can be of organic or functional origin. Concerning the first group, these are destructive, infiltrative or infectious hypothalamus or pituitary lesions, micro- or macroadenomas of the pituitary gland, empty sella syndrome, encephalic trauma, and pituitary/brain radiation. Functional causes of AHH are related to exhausting exercise, or drug intake (e.g. anabolic steroids, glucocorticoids, antipsychotic agents – which interfere with the dopaminergic system – opioids, androgens) [4]. Nutritional disorders might have a negative effect on hypothalamic GnRH secretion with the consequent HH. A frequent cause of AHH is hyperprolactinemia due to the intake of antipsychotic drugs or hypothyroidism.

Congenital hypogonadotropic hypogonadism (CHH) is a rare and phenotypically heterogeneous condition with an incidence of 1:8,000 in male individuals.

The pathophysiology of CHH may derive from: (i) abnormal differentiation, development or migration of GnRH neurons during foetal development; or (ii) signalling abnormalities that involve neuroendocrine factors necessary for GnRH secretion or responsiveness to the stimulatory effects of GnRH on gonadotrope pituitary cells [5]. From a clinical point of view, CHH can be divided into: (i) Kallmann syndrome (KS), which is associated with

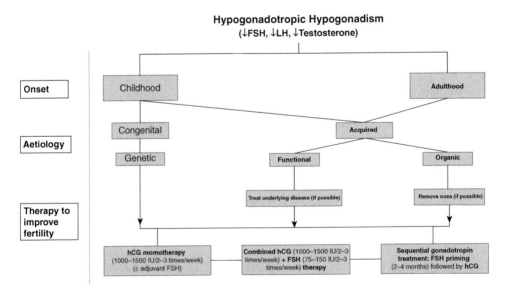

Figure 8.1 Hypogonadotropic Hypogonadism FSH treatment.

decreased sense of smell (anosmia or hyposmia) and other non-olfactory and non-reproductive anomalies/malformations; and (ii) normosmic (nCHH). Phenotypical manifestations common to the two forms are absent or delayed puberty, sparse secondary sexual characteristics, such as absent body hair, high-pitched voice, reduced muscle mass, micropenis, very low testicular volume (<5 ml), and history of cryptorchidism. The clinical appearance depends on the onset of the disease, that is, patients with an infancy onset often have all the above-mentioned severe manifestations, whereas patients with later onset of the disease may have only reduced spermatogenesis and mild hypoandrogenism [6].

CHH is a multifactorial, polygenic disease involving over 35 genes [5,7]. The discovery of novel genes is currently ongoing, thanks to the diffusion of Next Generation Sequencing (NGS) platforms; however, in about 50% of cases the aetiology still remains unknown. A peculiarity of this genetic disease is that CHH does not always follow the classical Mendelian (autosomal dominant, autosomal recessive or X-linked) inheritance pattern. In about 15–20% of cases, a digenic or oligogenic way of transmission has been described, referring to an even more complex mode of transmission. In these cases, the combined effect of heterozygous mutations in more than one gene is responsible for the phenotype. Interestingly enough, different clinical manifestations can be caused by mutations in the same gene (e.g. FGFR1 and PROKR2), indicating that from a genetic point of view a clear-cut distinction between KS and nCHH cannot be always made [6].

8.2.2 Therapy in HH

Discovering the aetiology behind HH is relevant since treatment options may change substantially. For instance, the therapy of AHH is often based on the removal of the noxa and the treatment of the underlying disease such as surgical removal of an adenoma or medical therapy (i.e. substitutive therapy with levotiroxin in hypothyroidism or dopamine agonist in cases of hyperprolactinemia).

In all CHH patients and in those AHH patients in whom the HPG axis cannot be restored, spermatogenesis can be induced by hormone therapy (either long-term pulsatile GnRH administration or subcutaneous gonadotropin injections). With both available therapeutical options, a positive response can be obtained in the majority of affected individuals. However, because of the limitations of GnRH pumps, gonadotropins are much more commonly used in general patient care. The onset and the severity of the neuroendocrine defect is a relatively good predictor for responsiveness. Negative prognostic factors are typical features of childhood onset CHH, such as very low testis volume (TV ≤4 ml), low serum levels of inhibin B, uni- or bilateral cryptorchidism, or micropenis [4]. According to two large studies, predictors for favourable response are larger baseline testicular volume, BMI of less than 30, advanced sexual maturity, the absence of adverse fertility factors and the absence of multiple pituitary hormone deficiency [8,9].

Treatment strategies include exogenous gonadotropins: (i) hCG monotherapy (± adjuvant FSH); (ii) combined hCG + FSH therapy; and (iii) sequential gonadotropin treatment with FSH priming followed by hCG:

1. *hCG monotherapy*: (1,000–1,500 IU/2–3 times/week) is usually advised for individuals with mild HH, thus TV >4 ml and/or no history of cryptorchidism. If the patient remains azoospermic, even after 3–6 months of treatment, FSH supplementation is needed [4,5].

2. *Combined gonadotropin therapy*: with hCG (1,000–1,500 IU/2–3 times/week) and FSH (75–150 IU/2–3 times/week) is the "gold-standard" for patients with pre-pubertal TV (≤4 ml) [4,5].

3. *FSH priming followed by hCG*: appears to be a promising regimen to improve sperm parameters in men with a severe form of CHH. A 2–4 months FSH-priming stimulates Sertoli and spermatogonial cell proliferation with consequent increase of TV and hCG can be added when TV reaches around 8 ml [4,5].

The first signs of an efficient therapy can be observed after 3–6 months, but fertility-induction may take up to 24 months to reach the maximal effect. Especially, CHH patients with cryptorchidism or those with a TV of less than 4 ml require extended courses of treatment, around 18–24 months [10,11]. Similarly, HH men who have been pre-treated with testosterone have a slower achievement of spermatogenesis and of conception in respect to testosterone "naïve" patients [12].

The majority of HH patients will achieve spermatogenesis under gonadotropin treatment and may generate their own biological child. Although sperm count is usually in the range of oligozoospermia, qualitative sperm parameters are normal, allowing a relatively high chance to achieve natural pregnancy. On the other hand, if the sperm parameters are poor, Assisted Reproductive Technology (ART) treatments, such as *in vitro* fertilization (IVF) and intracytoplasmic sperm injection (ICSI), can be performed. In cases of azoospermia, testicular sperm extraction (TESE or micro-TESE) may be offered to the patients with subsequent ICSI.

CHH cases imply the need for genetic testing and genetic counselling in order to inform the couple about the risks of transmission of mutation(s) and about the health consequences on the offspring. However, due to the complexity of the genetic architecture of this disease the prediction of the offspring's phenotype remains difficult. In the case where the mutation is identified, and it follows the Mendelian inheritance mode, preimplantation genetic testing should be advised for the couple. If this is not feasible, during counselling they should be informed about the importance of the screening for "minipuberty" in their offspring. The lack of "minipuberty" will allow an early diagnosis and consequently a timely intervention for pubertal induction in adolescence with consequent improvement of sexual and reproductive function in adulthood.

8.3 FSH Treatment in Idiopathic Male Infertility

8.3.1 Introduction

Idiopathic infertility represents the most commonly observed form of infertility in clinical practice, but unfortunately, rational treatments are lacking. Idiopathic male infertility commonly is represented by oligo-astheno-teratozoospermia (OAT) and the goal of treatment should therefore be the restoration of a quantitative and qualitative normal spermatogenesis. Although ICSI is often regarded as a treatment for infertile men with severe OAT, treatments able to restore the natural fertility would be the primary choice. As FSH acts mainly on the first step of spermatogenesis and represents a successful, rational treatment in HH, it is frequently also offered to men with male normogonadotropic infertility based on the hypothesis that spermatogenesis could be stimulated by increasing gonadotropin levels.

Nevertheless, too often male infertility is not adequately assessed and diagnosed, and there is a general conviction among non-experts that this condition could not be treatable and it is preferable to routinely apply ART. On the other hand, novel strategies for treating male infertility are needed, so that therapies could be converted from empiric into rational therapy. The currently most promising approach to treat male infertility is to stimulate spermatogenesis by FSH treatment. However, it is also clear from many studies published so far that FSH treatment is not indicated for all infertile men, and also in selected patients the effects are not easily predictable. One of the most challenging aspects in this field is, therefore, the identification of the "perfect" patient, that is the patient with the highest probability to respond to treatment. A personalized treatment regimen, which takes into account clinical and genetic factors controlling spermatogenesis, might resemble the most promising approach to this aim [13].

Numerous studies have been published in the last decades, from observational studies, to more recent randomized, multicentre, controlled studies and pharmacogenetic studies [13]. As outlined below, studies differ in patient selection criteria, duration and dosage of therapy, primary and secondary outcome, and have been conducted either with purified FSH (pFSH), highly purified FSH (hpFSH), or recombinant FSH (rhFSH). Therefore, comparison between published data is not immediate, although recent meta-analyses have been performed and guidelines from scientific societies have been produced [3,14].

8.3.2 General Effect of FSH Treatment

In general, the effectiveness of FSH therapy in male-factor infertility has been reported by some authors in terms of significant improvements in sperm quantity/quality and/or pregnancy rates (reviewed in [3,13–16], whereas other authors reported no effect. A meta-analysis by the Cochrane Collaboration [17], only including randomized controlled trials (RCTs), showed that infertile men who received FSH had a significant increase in spontaneous pregnancy rate per couple with respect to patients receiving placebo or no treatment. In another meta-analysis [16], including all available controlled clinical trials, FSH was shown to significantly increase sperm concentration and quality, and spontaneous and ART-related pregnancy rate. A more recent review and meta-analysis [15] on the benefits of medical therapy in couples with idiopathic male subfertility concludes that FSH is among the few empirical therapies with a demonstrated role in improving semen parameters.

Guidelines from the European Academy of Andrology for the management of OAT [14] suggest that treatment with FSH can be offered to selected men from infertile couples (normogonadotropic men with idiopathic oligozoospermia or OAT) in an attempt to improve quantitative and qualitative sperm parameters and pregnancy rate, with low evidence. In a position statement for the Italian Society of Andrology and Sexual Medicine, Barbonetti [3] also suggests the use of FSH to increase sperm concentration and motility in infertile normogonadotropic men with idiopathic oligozoospermia or OAT, with moderate evidence grading.

8.3.3 Selection of Candidate Patients and Predictors of Response

In general, the most important aspect to consider in the clinical practice is not proscribing FSH to all infertile men at random without an adequate diagnostic work-up. It is clear from all published studies that FSH is not effective in all infertile men, neither in all OAT patients. To increase the chance of response to treatment, patient selection is essential (Figure 8.2).

First, FSH treatment is not recommended in azoospermic men (apart from HH cases, as described above) and in men with obstructive/sub-obstructive forms of infertility. Although

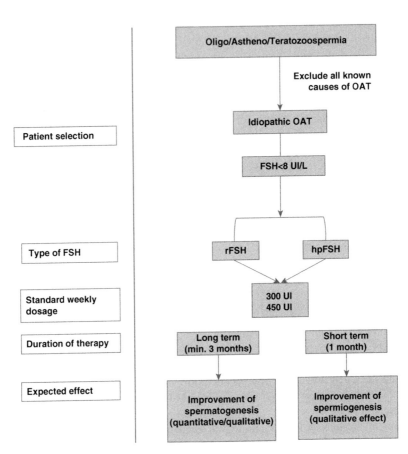

Figure 8.2 Idiopathic infertility FSH treatment.

the rationale not to treat these men is obvious, it implies that diagnostic procedures in infertile men should be applied to clearly distinguish patients with these characteristics from men with secretory (testicular) forms of OAT. Therefore, history, physical examination, reproductive hormone levels, imaging studies, and, when appropriate, genetic studies should be carried out before considering a patient candidate for FSH treatment. One of the most important parameters to identify patients who will certainly not respond to FSH treatment, is the plasma concentration of FSH, taking into consideration that the high levels of this hormone are a strong indicator that primary testicular damage exists, and a further increase of FSH with an exogenous drug is not able to overcome the spermatogenic impairment. Therefore, FSH treatment is suggested only in infertile men with idiopathic oligozoospermia or OAT and normal FSH plasma levels (normogonadotropic) [3,18]. Traditionally, normal FSH levels are considered when up to 8 IU/L.

Obviously, FSH treatment should be considered only when the couple have no female infertility causes. This does not mean that FSH cannot be considered when assisted reproduction techniques are already necessary for the couple, but a comprehensive female evaluation should be performed and the decision on whether to proceed with FSH treatment should be made collegially with the couple, the gynaecologist and andrologist.

Other than sperm count and motility, FSH has been suggested to improve pregnancy (natural and by assisted techniques) by ameliorating sperm chromatin integrity and fertilizing ability [19–22]. Therefore, idiopathic infertile patients exhibiting high values of sperm DNA fragmentation might represent a class of responder men. However, only one RCT had a DNA fragmentation index as the primary endpoint [23], and suggested that the improvement in this parameter is dependent on the p.N680S allele of the FSH receptor (*FSHR*) gene (see Section 8.3.4). While results on sperm DNA fragmentation are therefore encouraging, FSH therapy does not seem to be clearly associated with a reduction of chromosomal aneuploidies [21,24]. Therefore, this parameter, generally assessed by FISH, seems not to be of predictive value.

Other parameters that might be useful in the selection of patients and identification of responders and non-responders might be related to the specific alteration of spermatogenesis underlying oligozoospermia. In fact, low sperm count might be actually due to hypospermatogenesis (reduced number of germ cells) and/or alteration in the maturation process of germ cells (spermatogenic arrest). Two studies, performed by the same research group, demonstrated that the knowledge of the spermatogenic alteration by testicular fine needle aspiration cytology allows predicting the response to FSH therapy in oligozoospermic patients [25,26]. In fact, these studies showed that a pre-treatment testicular cytology characterized by hypospermatogenesis (without associated maturation disturbances) was associated with better response to FSH treatment with respect to hypospermatogenesis associated with partial maturation arrest at the spermatid level. These findings could be interpreted in the light of the demonstration that FSH therapy increased mainly the spermatogonial population [25], therefore being effective in stimulating final sperm production, particularly when the entire process of spermatogenesis is only quantitatively altered.

To overcome the intrinsic difficulties in examining the testicular structure, the same group proposed the analysis of spermatid count in the semen as a marker of maturation disturbance of spermiogenesis [27]. The authors showed that FSH therapy allowed significant improvement in sperm parameters and natural or assisted fertility in patients with lower spermatid count, therefore suggesting the evaluation of this parameter to predict the response to FSH therapy. Validation studies are awaited in order to introduce this parameter into clinical practice.

8.3.4 Dosage, Duration, and Type of FSH

Great discrepancy exists in the literature concerning the dosage and duration of FSH therapy in normogonadotropic infertile men, depending also on the type of FSH prescribed [3]. Considering that the main action of FSH is on the mitotic phases (spermatogonia) of spermatogenesis and that spermatogenesis in humans takes about 72 days, quantitative changes in sperm number in the ejaculate can only be seen after a period of treatment of at least 3 months. Indeed, the majority of studies used a 3-month period of treatment to look at any effect on spermatogenesis induced by FSH. However, the scheme and dosage of treatment vary considerably among the studies, with weekly cumulative doses ranging from "low dose therapy" of no more than 450 IU (e.g. 150 IU three times a week, 75 IU on alternate days, with a range of 150–450 IU/week) to "high dose therapy" of more than 450 IU (e.g. 200 IU on alternate days, 150 IU daily, 300 IU on alternate days, with a range of 600–1,050 IU/week) [3]. No immediate conclusion can be drawn on the efficacy of these different schemes; however, the majority of recent studies agree on 150 IU three times a week.

Duration of FSH therapy also varies in the published studies. Although the great majority evaluated the outcomes (sperm parameter, natural and assisted pregnancy) after a period of 3 months of FSH administration, it is worth noting that studies evaluating the effects on conventional sperm parameters after 4-month-long therapies (both with rhFSH and hpFSH) all reported a significant improvement of the sperm concentration [28–31]. Therefore, from a clinical point of view, these data might suggest prolonging FSH treatment for at least 1 month in those patients not adequately responding after a 3-month period of therapy.

Some studies evaluated qualitative sperm parameters just after 1 month of therapy, based on a putative effect of FSH, also on spermiogenesis and/or the epididymal passage. In particular, one study [22] evaluated the effect of FSH treatment on sperm maturation, expressed in terms of higher sperm hyaluronic acid binding capacity, and found that already after 1 month of FSH this parameter was improved, with a further increase after 3 months of treatment. Therefore, it is hypothesized that FSH could have a double action on both spermatogonia and round spermatids. This double action can be used in different clinical contexts. A long-term (at least 3 months) classic treatment will increase sperm parameters with an ultimate potential benefit on spontaneous pregnancy rate. On the other hand, a 1-month therapy could be indicated prior to ART, with the aim to increase the proportion of functionally mature spermatozoa with consequent higher likelihood of assisted pregnancy.

Meta-analysis did not find significant differences in sperm parameters and pregnancy rates after hpFSH and rhFSH [16]. No study on biosimilar FSH has yet been performed in males.

8.3.5 Prediction of FSH Response by Pharmacogenetics

Polymorphisms in the *FSHR* gene have been demonstrated to influence the expression and/or sensitivity of the receptor for the hormone and polymorphisms in the *FSHB* (coding for the β-subunit of FSH) gene are responsible for the constitutive production of FSH [13]. As a consequence, FSH plasma levels and the reproductive parameters are associated with the individual genotype of these genes both in men and women [13]. The two most common SNPs in the coding region of *FSHR* occur at nucleotides 919 and 2039 in exon 10, in which A/G transitions cause amino acid exchange from threonine (Thr) to alanine (Ala) at codon 307 and from asparagine (Asn) to serine (Ser) at codon 680, respectively [32]. There is a linkage between these polymorphic sites resulting in two major, almost equally common allelic variants in the Caucasian population, Thr307-Asn680 (TN) and Ala307-Ser680 (AS), producing two distinct receptor isoforms [14], leading to three genotypes (TN/TN, TN/AS and AS/AS). In the *FSHB* gene the most common studied SNP is a G/T polymorphism located in the promoter of the gene (−211 bp from the mRNA transcription start site) [32,36]. The combination of G/T SNP can lead therefore to three genotypes: homozygous TT and GG and heterozygous GT.

Based on these findings, four studies have been published so far dealing with the hypothesis that the different genetic polymorphisms in *FSHR* and *FSHB* genes could influence the response to exogenous FSH administration [22,23 33,37]. In particular, two studies [23,33] analysed *FSHR* gene polymorphisms, one the *FSHB* gene [37] and one both genes [22]. Therefore, too few and non-homogeneous data have been published to draw conclusion on the clinical utility of evaluating these polymorphisms in the protocol of FSH treatment, and also because these studies found some discrepancies. In general, however, a pharmacogenetic approach to FSH treatment is very intriguing and promising. Once more data becomes available, the knowledge of the individual genotype could be combined with the other clinical data to obtain a comprehensive view of the predictors to FSH treatment, therefore allowing a better selection and characterization of potential responders and non-responders patients. Furthermore, an FSH treatment scheme (dosage, duration) could be personalized to maximize the response. Patients with the less favourable genotypes could theoretically need higher doses or longer therapy, whereas patients with the most responsive genotypes could benefit also from lower doses and/or standard duration of 3 months.

8.3.6   Conclusions

FSH therapy combined with hCG is a highly successful treatment to induce spermatogenesis in HH. The success rate of FSH treatment in idiopathic male infertility is relatively low in respect to HH. Idiopathic sub/infertility is a heterogeneous etiologic category in which many different, yet unknown genetic/epigenetic, factors are likely to be involved [38]. Since these etiologic factors are not necessarily related to hormonal regulation of spermatogenesis, it is plausible that only a portion of idiopathic OAT men respond to FSH therapy. One of the most challenging aspects of FSH treatment is our ability to predict responsiveness prior to therapy. There is an urgent need for clinical and genetic predictive factors in order to convert FSH treatment in idiopathic infertile men from empiric into rational therapy.

References

1. van Rijkom, J., Leufkens, H., Crommelin, D., Rutten, F. and Broekmans, A. (1999) Assessment of biotechnology drugs: what are the issues? *Health Policy* **47**(3):255–274.

2. Zwart-van Rijkom, J. E., Broekmans, F. J. and Leufkens, H. G. (2002) From HMG through purified urinary FSH preparations to recombinant FSH: a substitution study. *Hum Reprod* **17**(4):857–865.

3. Barbonetti, A., Calogero, A. E., Balercia, G., Garolla, A., Krausz, C., La Vignera, S., et al. (2018) The use of follicle stimulating hormone (FSH) for the treatment of the infertile man: position statement from the Italian Society of Andrology and Sexual Medicine (SIAMS). *J Endocrinol Invest* **41**(9):1107–1122.

4. Swee, D. S. and Quinton, R. (2019) Managing congenital hypogonadotrophic hypogonadism: a contemporary approach directed at optimizing fertility and long-term outcomes in males. *Therap Adv Endo Metab* [Internet], cited 2019 April 11;10.

Available from: www.ncbi.nlm.nih.gov/pmc/articles/PMC6378644/

5. Boehm, U., Bouloux, P-M., Dattani, M. T., de Roux, N., Dodé, C., Dunkel, L., et al. (2015) Expert consensus document: European Consensus Statement on congenital hypogonadotropic hypogonadism: pathogenesis, diagnosis and treatment. *Nat Rev Endocrinol* **11**(9):547–564.

6. Krausz, C. and Riera-Escamilla, A. (2018) Genetics of male infertility. *Nature Rev Urol* **15**(6):369–384.

7. Maione, L, Dwyer, A. A., Francou, B., Guiochon-Mantel, A., Binart, N., Bouligand, J., et al. (2018) Genetics in endocrinology: genetic counseling for congenital hypogonadotropic hypogonadism and Kallmann syndrome: new challenges in the era of oligogenism and next-generation sequencing. *Eur J Endocrinol* **178**(3):R55–R80.

8. Warne, D. W., Decosterd, G., Okada, H., Yano, Y., Koide, N. and Howles, C. M. (2009) A combined analysis of data to

identify predictive factors for spermatogenesis in men with hypogonadotropic hypogonadism treated with recombinant human follicle-stimulating hormone and human chorionic gonadotropin. *Fertil Steril* **92** (2):594–604.

9. Lui, P. Y., Gebski, V. J., Turner, L. et al. (2002) Predicting pregnancy and spermatogenesis by survival analysis during gonadotrophin treatment of gonadotrophin-dificient infertile men. *Hum Reprod* **17**: 625–633.

10. Burris, A. S., Rodbard, H. W., Winters, S. J. and Sherins, R. J. (1988) Gonadotropin therapy in men with isolated hypogonadotropic hypogonadism: the response to human chorionic gonadotropin is predicted by initial testicular size. *J Clin Endocrinol Metab* **66** (6):1144–1151.

11. Büchter, D., Behre, H. M., Kliesch, S. and Nieschlag, E. (1998) Pulsatile GnRH or human chorionic gonadotropin/human menopausal gonadotropin as effective treatment for men with hypogonadotropic hypogonadism: a review of 42 cases. *Eur J Endocrinol* **139**(3):298–303.

12. Liu, P. Y., Baker, H. W. G., Jayadev, V., Zacharin, M., Conway, A. J. and Handelsman, D. J. (2009) Induction of spermatogenesis and fertility during gonadotropin treatment of gonadotropin-deficient infertile men: predictors of fertility outcome. *J Clin Endocrinol Metab* **94**(3):801–808.

13. Schubert, M., Pérez Lanuza, L. and Gromoll, J. (2019) Pharmacogenetics of FSH action in the male. *Front Endocrinol (Lausanne)* **28**(10):47.

14. Colpi, G. M., Francavilla, S., Haidl, G., Link, K., Behre, H. M., et al. (2018) European Academy of Andrology guideline Management of oligo-astheno-teratozoospermia. *Andrology* **6**(4):513–524.

15. Omar, M. I., Pal, R. P., Kelly, B. D., Bruins, H. M., Yuan, Y., Diemer, T., et al. (2019) Benefits of empiric nutritional and medical therapy for semen parameters and pregnancy and live birth rates in couples with idiopathic infertility: a systematic review and meta-analysis. *Eur Urol* **75** (4):615–625.

16. Santi, D., Granata, A. R. and Simoni, M. (2015) FSH treatment of male idiopathic infertility improves pregnancy rate: a meta-analysis. *Endocr Connect* **4**(3): R46–R58.

17. Attia, A. M., Abou-Setta, A. M. and Al-Inany, H. G. (2013) Gonadotrophins for idiopathic male factor subfertility. *Cochrane Database Syst Rev* **23**(8): CD005071.

18. Valenti, D., La Vignera, S., Condorelli, R. A., Rago, R., Barone, N., Vicari, E., et al. (2013) Follicle-stimulating hormone treatment in normogonadotropic infertile men. *Nat Rev Urol* **10**(1):55–62.

19. Colacurci, N., Monti, M. G., Fornaro, F., Izzo, G., Izzo, P., Trotta, C., et al. (2012) Recombinant human FSH reduces sperm DNA fragmentation in men with idiopathic oligoasthenoteratozoospermia. *J Androl* **33**(4):588–593.

20. Ruvolo, G., Roccheri, M. C., Brucculeri, A. M., Longobardi, S., Cittadini, E. and Bosco, L. (2013) Lower sperm DNA fragmentation after r-FSH administration in functional hypogonadotropic hypogonadism. *J Assist Reprod Genet* **30**(4):497–503.

21. Garolla, A., Ghezzi, M., Cosci, I., Sartini, B., Bottacin, A., Engl, B., et al. (2017) FSH treatment in infertile males candidate to assisted reproduction improved sperm DNA fragmentation and pregnancy rate. *Endocrine* **56** (2):416–425.

22. Casamonti, E., Vinci, S., Serra, E., Fino, M. G., Brilli, S., Lotti, F., et al. (2017) Short-term FSH treatment and sperm maturation: a prospective study in idiopathic infertile men. *Andrology* **5** (3):414–422.

23. Simoni, M., Santi, D., Negri, L., Hoffmann, I., Muratori, M., Baldi, E., et al. (2016) Treatment with human, recombinant FSH improves sperm DNA fragmentation in idiopathic infertile men depending on the FSH receptor polymorphism p. N680S:

a pharmacogenetic study. *Hum Reprod* **31** (9):1960–1969.

24. Piomboni, P., Serafini, F., Gambera, L., Musacchio, C., Collodel, G., Morgante, G., et al. (2009) Sperm aneuploidies after human recombinant follicle stimulating hormone therapy in infertile males. *Reprod Biomed Online* **18**(5):622–629.

25. Foresta, C., Bettella, A., Ferlin, A., Garolla, A. and Rossato, M. (1998) Evidence for a stimulatory role of follicle-stimulating hormone on the spermatogonial population in adult males. *Fertil Steril* **69**(4):636–642.

26. Foresta, C., Bettella, A., Merico, M., Garolla, A., Ferlin, A. and Rossato, M. (2002) Use of recombinant human follicle-stimulating hormone in the treatment of male factor infertility. *Fertil Steril* **77**(2):238–244.

27. Garolla, A., Selice, R., Engl, B., Bertoldo, A., Menegazzo, M., Finos, L., et al. (2014) Spermatid count as a predictor of response to FSH therapy. *Reprod Biomed Online* **29** (1):102–112.

28. Ding, Y. M., Zhang, X. J., Li, J. P., Chen, S. S., Zhang, R. T., Tan, W. L., et al. (2015) Treatment of idiopathic oligozoospermia with recombinant human follicle-stimulating hormone: a prospective, randomized, double-blind, placebo-controlled clinical study in Chinese population. *Clin Endocrinol (Oxford, UK)* **83**(6):866–871.

29. Arnaldi, G., Balercia, G., Barbatelli, G. and Mantero, F. (2000) Effects of long-term treatment with human pure follicle-stimulating hormone on semen parameters and sperm-cell ultrastructure in idiopathic oligoteratoasthenozoospermia. *Andrologia* **32**(3):155–161.

30. Paradisi, R., Busacchi, P., Seracchioli, R., Porcu, E. and Venturoli, S. (2006) Effects of high doses of recombinant human follicle-stimulating hormone in the treatment of male factor infertility: results of a pilot study. *Fertil Steril* **86**(3):728–731.

31. Paradisi, R., Natall, F., Fabbri, R., Battaglia, C., Seracchiol, R. and Venturoli, S. (2014) Evidence for a stimulatory role of high doses of recombinant human follicle-stimulating hormone in the treatment of male-factor infertility. *Andrologia* **46**(9):1067–1072.

32. Simoni, M., Gromoll, J. and Nieschlag, E. (1997) The follicle-stimulating hormone receptor: biochemistry, molecular biology, physiology and pathophysiology.*Endocr Rev* **18**(6):739–773.

33. Selice, R., Garolla, A., Pengo, M., Caretta, N., Ferlin, A. and Foresta, C. (2011) The response to FSH treatment in oligozoospermic men depends on FSH receptor gene polymorphisms. *Int J Androl* **34**(4):306–312.

34. Simoni, M., Gromoll, J., Hoppner, W., Kamischke, A., Krafft, T., Stahle, D., et al. (1999) Mutational analysis of the follicle-stimulating hormone (FSH) receptor in normal and infertile men: identification and characterization of two discrete FSH receptor isoforms. *J Clin Endocrinol Metab* **84**(2):751–757.

35. Grigorova, M., Rull, K. and Laan, M. (2007) Haplotype structure of FSHB, the beta-subunit gene for fertility-associated follicle-stimulating hormone: possible influence of balancing selection. *Ann Hum Genet* **71**(Pt 1):18–28.

36. Grigorova, M., Punab, M., Ausmees, K. and Laan, M. (2008) FSHB promoter polymorphism within evolutionary conserved element is associated with serum FSH level in men. *Hum Reprod* **23** (9):2160–2166.

37. Ferlin, A., Vinanzi, C., Selice, R., Garolla, A., Frigo, A. C. and Foresta, C. (2011) Toward a pharmacogenetic approach to male infertility: polymorphism of follicle-stimulating hormone beta-subunit promoter. *Fertil Steril* **96**(6):1344–1349.

38. Krausz, C. (2011) Male infertility: pathogenesis and clinical diagnosis. *Best Pract Res Clin Endocrinol Metab* **25** (2):271–285.

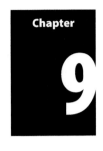

Chapter

9

Antioxidants to Improve Sperm Quality

Elena Martínez-Holguín, Enrique Lledó-García,
Ángel Rebollo-Román, Javier González-García,
José Jara-Rascón, and Carlos Hernández-Fernández

9.1 Introduction

Infertility is defined as a failure of spontaneous conception after one year of regular sexual intercourse in the absence of contraceptive measures [1]. This entity represents a rising medical complaint since one out of eight couples find it difficult to conceive a child for the first time, and up to one in six find it difficult to conceive twice. Currently, 70 million couples of reproductive age suffer from infertility worldwide, accounting for an estimated overall prevalence of 15% [2].

Age remains the leading cause of infertility among women (its incidence abruptly increasing above the age of 35). However, multiple factors including a number of environmental exposures have been identified for the male patient [3]. Reactive oxygen species (ROS) are the result of cellular aerobic metabolism. Physiologic amounts of ROS are required for adequate cell defense against these exposures [4]. However, its excessive accumulation may overcome the natural antioxidant agent concentration levels, thus inducing cellular plasmatic membrane peroxidation, DNA damage, and other oxidative stress deleterious effects [5].

Recently, a number of different studies have linked the excessive accumulation of ROS in seminal liquid to male infertility. Conversely, antioxidant oral supplementation therapy would play a role in counterbalancing the excess of ROS in seminal liquid, thus improving the quality of the sperm of subfertile men [6]. This chapter aims to provide an updated review on this controversial topic.

9.2 Reactive Oxygen Species and Fertility

Aerobic organisms depend on oxygen for vital functions. ROS are the result of this aerobic metabolism [4]. The main source of ROS in the seminal liquid are different oxidative reactions related to the electron transporting chain located at the mitochondrial membrane of the cellular seminal component [7], particularly within the white blood cells [8], producing 1,000-fold more quantity than the remaining cellular populations, but also spermatozoa, and tubular epithelial cells [5].

Physiologic amounts of ROS are required for adequate seminal cellular function. They facilitate spermatozoa chromatin condensation, thus playing an important role in the regulation of germ cell population by inducing apoptosis or enhancing spermatogonia proliferation [9]. In the mature spermatozoon, ROS favor sperm capacitation, acrosome reaction, zona pellucida binding, and sheath stability/mobility; all of them of capital importance for fertility [4,10]. ROS also have an important role as second intracellular messengers for functions other than fertilization [11].

Optimal ROS levels are crucial for cellular defense against a number of different environmental exposures (including pollution, electromagnetic radiation, pesticides, and increased testicular local temperature among others), toxic habits (tobacco and alcohol), lifestyle factors (physical activity and obesity), infections, chronic processes (hypertension and diabetes), and autoimmune diseases [12]. Furthermore, immature spermatozoa and those with altered morphology produce higher amounts of ROS than structurally normal mature spermatozoa, thus decreasing the fertilizing potential of the semen [13]. Hence, different studies have linked ROS seminal levels with male infertility, since abnormally increased ROS concentration values in seminal liquid have been detected in up to 40% of subfertile men [6]. However, although moderately increased ROS concentration values significantly decrease spermatozoa mobility, via adenosine triphosphate (ATP) excessive consumption and phosphorylation reduction of the axonemal proteins encharged for spermatozoa movement, do not seem to alter sperm viability to a greater extent [10].

Varicocele (i.e. varicose dilation of the pampiniform venous plexus of the testes – see Chapter 15) merits special attention. It represents a relatively common anomaly (11.7% of all adult males) and a well-known etiologic factor for infertility in young males, thus being present in 25.4% of men with an abnormal seminal analysis [1]. Although oxidative stress induced by increased local temperature in the testicular environment is still considered the main cause for seminal damage in these men [14], its exact mechanism of action has not been clearly elucidated to date.

9.3 Oxidative Stress and Infertility

Oxidative stress appears as soon as ROS production exceeds the antioxidant agent levels in the sperm, thus inducing cellular plasmatic membrane peroxidation [5]. Spermatozoa plasmatic membranes are rich in polyunsaturated fatty acids with a small proportion of scavenging enzymes [15]. This structural composition provides the cell membrane with flexibility, but makes it vulnerable to ROS-related oxidative damage. Increased ROS levels induce a peroxidation of the lipid chains located at this level, thus producing a loss of integrity that alters the plasmatic membrane permeability, which in turn affects spermatozoa morphology, mobility, and some of its vital functions (i.e. eventually resulting in cell death) [16].

Malondialdehyde (MDA) is the final byproduct of the above-mentioned lipidic peroxidative reactions. Since this metabolite is stable at room temperature, its concentration in semen has been widely used as a diagnostic tool to estimate the degree of oxidative harm to the sperm [17,18]. In this way, MDA seminal concentrations in males suffering from astheno-zoospermia have been shown to be twice as high as those of individuals with normal seminal values. In addition, previous studies have demonstrated that a significant reduction in MDA concentration improves the chance of a successful conception [19].

9.4 The Physiologic Antioxidant System

In aerobic cells, ROS must be adequately counterbalanced by natural plasmatic antioxidant agents to avoid their potential deleterious oxidative effects [5]. The antioxidant physiologic system consists of enzymatic factors (superoxide dismutase, catalase, and glutathione

Table 9.1 Recommended and maximum daily doses of oral supplements of antioxidant [10,61,62]

	Recommended daily dose	Recommended supplementation	Maximum daily dose
Vitamin A	900 mcg	504 mcg	3,000 mcg
Vitamin C	90 mg	200–1,000 mg	2,000 mg
Vitamin E	15 mg	300–600 mg	1,000 mg
Zinc	11 mg	30–40 mg	40 mg
Selenium	55 mcg	100 mcg	400 mcg
L-Carnitine	NR	3,000 mg	3,000 mg
Q10 coenzyme	NR	200–300 mg	12 mg/kg
N-Acetylcysteine	NR	600 mg	NR

NR: Non-referred; mcg: micrograms; mg: milligrams

peroxidase), non-enzymatic factors (coenzyme Q10, L-carnitine, vitamins E and C), micro-nutrients (selenium, zinc, copper), and other factors [19]. The combined interaction between all these elements provides optimal protection against the toxic oxidative effects induced by ROS (Figure 9.1). Likewise, a significant reduction in the antioxidant ability of this system (secondary to the complete absence or even the critical reduction in the seminal concentration of any of the components included) facilitates the accumulation of ROS in the seminal liquid, a fact that explains a detrimental parallel effect on its fertile capacity [19,20]. Conversely, a direct relationship between antioxidant oral therapy and improvement of sperm quality has already been established [2]. The recommended oral supplementation doses for different antioxidant agents are summarized in Table 9.1.

9.4.1 Enzymatic Factors

The most important seminal antioxidant enzymatic system is composed of three enzymes: superoxide dismutase (SOD), catalase (CAT), and glutathione-peroxidase (GPX). Although adequate concentrations of this enzymatic triad are crucial to counterbalance the negative effect of ROS in the seminal liquid, the excessive accumulation of these elements above a critical value may facilitate a paradoxical increase of ROS levels, thus negatively impacting the sperm fertile capacity. For instance, excessive seminal amounts of SOD and CAT may stop acrosome reaction, while excessively high CAT concentration values may prevent local oxidation, thus inhibiting spermatozoa capacitation [21].

9.4.1.1 Superoxide Dismutase

The metallo-enzyme complex SOD consists of three different isoforms that are present in variable concentrations in the cytoplasm and the mitochondrion (SOD-1 and SOD-2) of the cellular compartment, as well as freely dissolved in the seminal liquid (SOD-3). A prostatic origin has been proposed for SOD-1 and SOD-2 [22]. These isoforms are responsible for 75% and 25% of the overall enzymatic activity, respectively. Their intracellular concentrations are modulated according to the presence of different stress conditions (such as

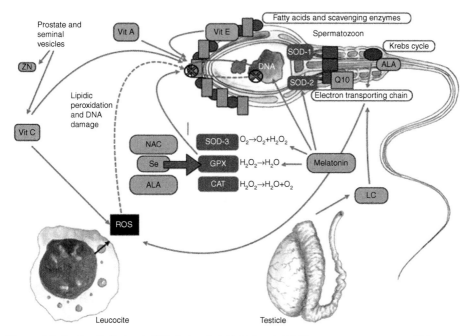

Figure 9.1 Zn: zinc; Vit C: vitamin C, Vit A: vitamin A, Vit E: vitamin E; ROS: reactive oxygen species; SOD: superoxide dismutase; NAC: N-acetyl-cysteine; Se: selenium; ALA: Alpha-lipoic acid; CAT: catalase; Q10: coenzyme Q10; GPX: glutathione peroxidase; LC: L-carnitine.

proinflammatory status), since their main effect is directed to eliminate the free radicals of the superoxide anion. SOD decreases oxidative stress markers, protects spermatozoa from lipidic peroxidation, reduces DNA damage, improves sperm morphology, and plays a role in spermatic mobility [10]. In addition, a number of previous studies have demonstrated a significant reduced activity of SOD complex in the semen of infertile patients when compared to normally fertile individuals [11].

9.4.1.2 Catalase

The antioxidant enzyme, catalase (CAT), although ubiquitous in the organism, is particularly present in the seminal liquid and peroxisomes of the spermatic cells. CAT detoxifies the hydrogen peroxide via splitting this metabolite into innocuous molecular oxygen and water [10]. There is a constant activity of this enzyme in the testicle, so men with asthenoteratozoospermia have lower levels of CAT in the seminal liquid when compared to males with normal sperm. This enzyme level has a positive correlation with spermatic capacitation (via nitrous oxide production), the progressive motility of the sperm, and also to the number of spermatozoa [23].

9.4.1.3 Glutathione Peroxidase

Glutathione peroxidase (GPX) is produced and excreted in the epididymis head [10], and also plays an important role in the defense against oxidative stress by protecting the cell membrane from lipidic peroxidation [24]. This enzyme facilitates a chemical reduction of different organic peroxides (i.e. including hydrogen peroxide), transforming them into inert hydroperoxides (i.e. water). Adequate CAT concentrations in seminal plasma significantly improve different seminal parameters in subfertile patients, including spermatozoa concentration, progressive motility, and normal morphology. Therefore, oral glutathione supplements have been proposed by some authors as a therapy to counteract the deleterious effect of a number of inflammatory andrological conditions [19].

9.4.2 Non-Enzymatic Factors

Non-enzymatic antioxidants can be either a byproduct of endogenous metabolism or directly incorporated from diet, mainly acting as coenzymes for the enzymatic factors previously detailed.

9.4.2.1 Q10-coenzyme

Q10-coenzyme is a vitamin-like liposoluble ubiquinone commonly found in different lipoproteins and the cellular membrane [7]. Most of the Q10-coenzyme in the human body is obtained directly through oral intake from a number of dietary sources including meat, fish, nuts, and vegetable oils [16]. However, a minor proportion of endogenous Q10-coenzyme is synthesized via cholesterol metabolism. Its antioxidant activity relies on adequate seminal concentrations and aims to protect the cell membrane from lipidic peroxidation [16]. As one of the components of the electron transporting chain, it participates in the mitochondrial cell respiration (i.e. dedicated to energy production for tail mobility), thus being found predominantly in the mitochondrial-rich middle zone of the spermatozoon [2,7].

An ordinary Q10-coenzyme oral intake from diet has not been linked to any change in seminal parameters [16]. Nevertheless, numerous studies have analyzed the impact of supplementary oral doses of Q10-coenzyme on different seminal characteristics (Table 9.2). All these clinical trials agree to identify an improvement in overall spermatic concentration and mobility [7,25–27]. However, a recent meta-analysis conducted by Thakur and colleagues [28] found that although spermatic concentration and mobility were significantly improved with 150 mg daily dose of oral Q10-coenzyme supplementation, a parallel increase in pregnancy or live-birth rates was not observed using this strategy.

9.4.2.2 Vitamin C

Ascorbic acid, commonly known as Vitamin C, is a hydrosoluble vitamin showing high antioxidant capacity, with up to 65% of the overall capacity in the semen of fertile men. It is considered the main natural semen antioxidant [29]. It plays a major role in neutralizing hydrogen peroxide, thus preventing DNA oxidative damage and reducing lipidic peroxidation [30]. It also serves other different functions including a role in the synthesis of collagen, proteoglycans, and a number of other components of the intracellular membrane [2]. Vitamin C is mainly excreted in the seminal vesicles, thus being found in high concentrations in the semen (i.e. 10-fold the blood concentration) [19].

Low ascorbic-acid seminal concentrations have been linked to low spermatozoa counts, increased counts of abnormal spermatozoa, and overall reduced mobility. Likewise, a dose-dependent improvement in spermatic mobility following vitamin C oral supplementation

Table 9.2 Summary of the most important literature evidence regarding oral supplementation with antioxidant agents to improve the quality of semen.

Author	Year	Sample	Type of study	Treatment	Time	End-points	Results
Suleiman et al. [17]	1996	110 males with asthenozoospermia	Double-blinded controlled clinical trial	– 300 mg Vit E – Placebo	26 weeks	Spermatic mobility and lipidic peroxidation level	Improvement in mobility in male with asthenozoospermia and reduction of lipidic peroxidation level
Scott et al. [50]	1998	69 males with asthenozoospermia	Randomized double-blinded controlled clinical trial	– 100 mcg Se – 100 mcg Se + 1 mg Vit A +10 mg Vit C + 15 mg Vit C	3 months	Concentration, mobility, morphology and Se in blood	Improvement in mobility
Keskes-Ammar et al. [34]	2003	54 infertile males	Randomized double-blinded controlled clinical trial	– Vit E 400 mg + 225 mcg Se – Vit B	13 weeks	Concentration, mobility, morphology, volume, MDA viability, Vit E and cholesterol in blood	Improvement in mobility
Lenzi et al. [37]	2004	60 males with OAT	Randomized double-blinded controlled clinical trial	–2 g/d LC + 1 g/d LAC	6 months	Concentration, mobility, morphology and volume	Rise in mobile sperm cells and in progressive sperm cell mobility
Cavallini et al. [40]	2004	219 males with oligoastheno-zoospermia + varicocele	Randomized double-blinded controlled clinical trial	– 2 g/d LC + 1 g/d LAC – Placebo	6 months	Concentration, mobility, morphology and testicular volume	Significant rise of spermatic mobility, concentration and morphology. No in varicocele grades IV and V
Greco et al. [30]	2005	64 males with idiopatic infertility and DNA fragmentation.	Double-blinded controlled clinical trial	– 1 g/day Vit E + 1 g/day Vit C – Placebo	2 months	Concentration, mobility, morphology and DNA fragmentation.	DNA damage reduction and improvement in results in patients with previous DNA damage
Balercia et al. [25]	2005	60 males with asthenozoospermia	Double-blinded controlled clinical trial	– 3 g/d LC – 3 g/d LAC – 2 g/d LC + 1 g/d LAC – Placebo	6 months	Concentration, mobility, morphology, volume and total antioxidant capacity	LC and LAC raise progressive sperm cell mobility, and total antioxidant capacity. 9 pregnancy during treatment with LC and 5 after combined treatment

Table 9.2 (cont.)

Author	Year	Sample	Type of study	Treatment	Time	End-points	Results
Ebisch et al. [43]	2005	– 47 fertile males – 40 subfertile males	Double-blinded controlled clinical trial	– 5 mg folic acid + 66 mg Zn – Placebo	26 weeks	Seminal characteristics.	Seminal concentration improvement
Galatioto et al. [36]	2005	42 males with oligospermia	Randomized controlled clinical trial	– 600 mg NAC + Zn + vitamins and minerals – No treatment	3 months	Concentration, mobility, morphology and volume	Rise in perm cell count
Sigman et al. [39]	2006	21 males with asthenozoospermia	Randomized double-blinded controlled clinical trial	– 2 g/d LC + 1 g/d LAC – Placebo	24 weeks	Volume, mobility, concentration, progressive mobility and carnitine levels in semen	No improvement
Tremellen et al. [49]	2007	60 males with morphology, motility or membrane integrity and >25% of sperm cells with DNA fragmentation.	Randomized double-blinded controlled clinical trial	– 6mg/d lycopene + 400 IU Vit E+ 100 mg Vit C +25 mg de Zn+ 26 mcg SE+ 0.5 mg folate, + 1,000 mg garlic – Placebo	3 months	Embryo quality and pregnancy results during IVF-ICSI	Higher success in pregnancy in ICSI vs IVF
Safarinejad et al. [51]	2009	468 males with OAT	Randomized double-blinded controlled clinical trial	– 200 mcg Se – 600 mg NAC – 200 mcg Se + 600 mg NAC – Placebo	30 weeks	Concentration, mobility, morphology, volume, viscosity, liquefaction time and oxidative status.	Improvement in all seminal parameters after Se and NAC administration
Balercia et al. [7]	2009	60 males with asthenozoospermia	Double-blinded controlled clinical trial	– 200 mg Q10 – Placebo	6 months	Concentration, mobility, morphology, volume and total antioxidant capacity	Rise in spermatic mobility in patients that received treatment. 12 spontaneous pregnancies during the study

Author/year	Year	Population	Study type	Intervention	Duration	Outcomes measured	Results
Moslemi et al. [45]	2011	690 males with asthenoteratozoospermia	Non-controlled clinical trial	– 200 mcg Se + 400 IU Vit E	100 days	Seminal characteristics and pregnancy rate	52.6% improvement in sperm cell mobility, morphology or both, and 10.8% of spontaneous pregnancy after oral treatment vs patients with no treatment
Safarinejad et al. [26]	2012	228 males with OAT	Randomized double-blinded controlled clinical trial	– 200 mg Ubiquinone – Placebo	26 weeks	Seminal parameters and total antioxidant capacity	Density, mobility and spermatic morphology improvement vs control group
Hadwan et al. [44]	2012	– 37 infertile males – 37 males with asthenozoospermia	Double-blinded controlled clinical trial	– 220 mg Zn sulphate twice a day	3 months	Quantitative and qualitative semen characteristics	Rise in seminal volume, sperm cell count and spermatic mobility
Abad et al. [58]	2013	20 males with asthenoteratozoospermia	Non-controlled, non-blinded study	– 1500 mg de LC+ 60 mg de VITC+ 20 mg de q10+10 mg de VIT E + 10 mg de ZN,+200 mcg de SE +1 mcg de B12	3 months	DNA fragmentation and seminal characteristics	Reduction of DNA fragmentation. Significant raise in concentration, mobility, vitality and spermatic morphology
Nadjarzadeh et al. [27]	2014	47 males with OAT	Randomized double-blinded controlled clinical trial	– 200 mg q10 – Placebo	3 months	Effects over CAT and SOD	Rise in CAT and SOD level in the seminal liquid with an important positive relation between Q10, CAT, SOD and the normal sperm cell morphology
Haghighian et al. [54]	2015	44 males with asthenozoospermia	Randomized triple-blinded controlled clinical trial	– 600 mg/day ALA – Placebo	12 weeks	Seminal characteristics and oxidative stress markers in semen. Total antioxidant capacity	Rise in sperm cell count, concentration and spermatic mobility. Improvement in total antioxidant capacity and MDA levels

OAT: oligoastheno-teratozoospermia; mcg: micrograms; mg: milligrams; IVF: *in vitro* fertilization; ICSI: intracytoplasmic sperm injection; IU: international units; Se: selenium; Zn: zinc; ALA: Alpha-lipoic acid; LC: L-carnitine; LAC: L-acetyl-carnitine; NAC: N-acetyl-cysteine.

has been demonstrated in smoking males [19]. However, ascorbic acid is quickly oxidized into dehydroascorbate when exposed to an oxidizing environment, so it is difficult for it to retain its antioxidant power for long periods of time [29]. Conversely, reduced concentrations of seminal vitamin C are associated with lower counts of morphologically normal spermatozoa, and hence a role of vitamin C depletion as a risk factor for idiopathic infertility has been suggested [31]. On the contrary, excessive seminal concentrations of ascorbic acid may induce a paradoxical pro-oxidant effect by generating potentially toxic radicals in the presence of a number of different metals, thus raising free-ROS levels [29].

9.4.2.3 Vitamin E

Alpha-tocopherol, known as Vitamin E, is a liposoluble antioxidant commonly present in cellular membranes. Its antioxidant activity is mainly aimed at the inhibition of ROS-mediated lipidic peroxidation [2]. However, a role in capturing and neutralizing hydroxyl- and superoxide-free radicals has been established.

Several trials have been conducted aiming to clarify the beneficial effect on oral supplementation with vitamin E on semen quality (Table 9.1). One of these studies demonstrated improved *in vitro* fertilization rates with a 3-month therapy of oral ascorbic acid (200 mg per day) [32]. In addition, certain efficacy in antagonizing the effects of oxidative stress in men suffering from oligoasthenozoospermia was highlighted by some of these studies [19,33,34]. However, its excessive accumulation may result in a harmful paradoxical pro-oxidant effect [29].

9.4.2.4 Vitamin A

Retinol (and its precursor, beta-carotene), known as Vitamin A, is another liposoluble vitamin with a capital immune-regulatory role. It also serves an antioxidant function by defending sperm cells against oxidative stress and lipidic peroxidation [35]. However, its excessive accumulation may lead to liver cirrhosis [9]. Approximately one-third of the overall diet content is absorbed in the bowel (even boosted with fatty-rich oral intake), although it can also be synthesized endogenously from carotenoids. Low concentrations of retinol and alpha-tocopherol in the seminal liquid have been linked to spermatic dysfunction with important clinical implications for fertility [35]. Conversely, in a recent study by Galatioto and colleagues [36], the use of oral therapy with a multivitamin complex containing vitamin A showed a clear improvement in sperm counts.

9.4.2.5 L-Carnitine

L-Carnitine (LC) (3-amynobutiric-acid or L-acetyl-carnitine (LAC)) are actively excreted in the epididymis (where 2,000-fold higher concentrations compared to blood plasma may be reached) and play an important role in cell metabolism acting as long-chain fatty acid transporters to the mitochondrion, thus providing a fundamental part of the metabolic energy required by the spermatozoon for mobility [2,26]. Therefore, oral supplements of these products have been used with variable outcomes for spermatic mobility enhancement in the treatment of different types of oligoasthenozoospermia (Table 9.1) [26,37–39]. In addition, some authors have suggested a possible indirect antioxidant role of LAC, probably by facilitating the avoidance of membrane lipidic peroxidation. However, its exact mechanism of action remains unknown [40].

9.4.3 Micronutrients

9.4.3.1 Zinc

Although this micronutrient represents the second most abundant metal in the organism, the World Health Organization (WHO) estimated that one-third of the world's population suffers from zinc nutritional deficit [41]. The main source of zinc is in the diet, particularly red meats, fish, and milk. Zinc can be found in more than 200 enzymes involved in cell division, and nucleic (i.e. acids and proteins) biosynthesis [19], thus playing a crucial role in embryonic testicular development and spermatic maturation.

Low zinc blood concentrations have been linked to hypogonadism, incomplete sexual development, and reduced sperm fertilizing capacity [2,42]. Therefore, many studies have been conducted to characterize the role of zinc supplementation in the improvement of seminal parameters of subfertile males [43], observing a variable protective effect in spermatozoa against bacteria and chromosomic damage [44] (Table 9.2).

9.4.3.2 Selenium

This metal represents an essential micronutrient factor for normal testicular development, spermatogenesis, and a number of spermatic functions including mobility [45]. Up to 25 seleno-proteins have been described, most of them helping in sperm formation, maintenance of the structural integrity of the spermatozoon, and testosterone biosynthesis [2]. Selenium deficiency may result in seminiferous epithelium atrophy, alterations in spermatogenesis/epididymal spermatozoon maturation, and testicular volume reduction [46]. A role in free-radical (*in vitro*) detoxification (i.e. via GPX activation) has also been identified, thus protecting cells from oxidative stress [47].

Numerous clinical trials have investigated the effect of selenium supplements in monotherapy and in combination with other substances. Exclusive selenium supplementation showed better spermatic concentration, mobility, and morphology [26,48], while in combination only spermatic mobility seems to be improved [34,49,50] (Table 9.2).

9.4.4 Other Factors

9.4.4.1 N-acetyl-cysteine

N-acetyl-cysteine (NAC) is a natural byproduct of L-cysteine metabolism and precursor of gluthatione, presenting antioxidant properties [51]. NAC possesses an important function in the survival of germ cells in seminipherous tubules, enhances spermatic mobility, and prevents oxidative damage in the DNA.

9.4.4.2 Melatonin

Melatonin is derived from tryptophan, and is synthesized and excreted in the pineal gland. However, it is present in the semen and spermatozoa show membrane receptors for it. This hormone regulates circadian rhythms (i.e. such as sleep–wake and reproductive cycles) [5] and acts as a powerful natural antioxidant, a function that is only enabled through enzymatic (i.e. SOD and GPX) activation. As with other human hormones, melatonin is highly lipophilic, a property that permits its migration through the cell membrane to exert its antioxidant protection over different intracellular structures such as the mitochondrion or nuclear DNA [5]. Numerous studies have demonstrated a positive effect of melatonin supplementation in semen quality improvement, especially in cases of spermatic DNA damage [52,53].

9.4.4.3 Alpha-lipoic Acid

By participating as a cofactor in the Krebs cycle, alpha-lipoic acid (ALA) plays an antioxidant key role in the energy mitochondrion metabolism [54], thus preventing neurodegenerative disease and metabolic syndrome. Exogenous ALA supplementation increases the seminal concentration of this cofactor, thus enhancing its antioxidant properties to fight oxidative stress. In cells and tissues, ALA is reduced into dihydrolipoic acid (DHLA), a metabolite with 7 times higher antioxidant capacity. Both acids neutralize ROS (via metal quelation), thus avoiding lipidic peroxidation [54]. ALA also plays a role in the creation of a protective barrier over the spermatozoon cell membrane indirectly maintaining its structural integrity [55]. According to this observation, different studies performed in animals have demonstrated that after ALA supplementation the percentage of progressive spermatic mobility is higher [56]. Recently, a clinical trial comparing men receiving 600 mg of ALA per day for a 12-week period versus placebo, showed an improvement in spermatic quantity and rapid mobility in the supplementation group [54]. However, excessively high blood concentration levels of this acid favor liver steatosis [57].

9.5 Multi-Antioxidant Complex Therapy

In view of the positive results obtained by numerous studies regarding oral supplementation with different antioxidant agents in monotherapy, a number of research groups focused their efforts on the possible synergic combination of different antioxidant agents, and the impact of these combined complexes on seminal quality parameters. Although variable results were obtained after oral supplementation with different complexes, all these studies agree on the positive effect of oral therapy supplements on different spermatic properties [38,49,58,59]. A complete review on the main studies conducted to date is provided in Table 9.2.

In 2014, Showell and colleagues [6] conducted a systematic review concentrating the evidence of current relevant literature concerning the use of antioxidant therapy for sperm quality improvement in subfertile men, in order to assess its safety and efficacy. This review joined the experience from 48 randomized clinical trials comparing the supplementation with one antioxidant agent in monotherapy or a combination of different antioxidant agents versus placebo, another antioxidant agent/combination, or no treatment at all, including a total of 4,179 males suffering from reduced spermatic motility and lower sperm cell concentration.

The primary endpoint considered was the number of newborn babies after treatment. Secondary endpoints included pregnancy rate, documented side effects, spermatic DNA fragmentation, and sperm cell concentration. The authors stated that although the scientific evidence collected was scarce (i.e. low scientific quality), antioxidant therapy might increase the pregnancy and newborn baby rates (6% vs 11–28%), thus suggesting a role in the improvement of sperm quality of subfertile males. They concluded also that better well-designed, randomized, placebo-controlled clinical trials were required to clarify these outcomes.

Finally, regarding antioxidant treatment for couples under different assisted reproduction therapy, an increase in the live birth rate was detected when they were compared to couples receiving placebo [49,35]. Comparable results were reported by Arhin and colleagues [60]; all the studies included in their review agree to demonstrate that micronutrient supplementation impacts positively when *in vitro* fecundation is used.

9.6 Conclusions

ROS are the resulting byproduct of the cellular aerobic metabolism. Although these radicals play an important role in the cellular defense against a number of potential harmful agents including toxic environmental exposures, proinflammatory conditions, chronic diseases, and different infections, their accumulation in the seminal liquid may overcome the delicate counterbalance provided by the detoxifying capacity of the natural antioxidant system, thus resulting in oxidative stress.

Oxidative stress affects negatively male fertility by inducing a severe cellular membrane lipidic peroxidation and DNA structural damage, which in turn may provoke a detrimental effect on mobility, concentration, and morphologically normal sperm cell amounts. Conversely, different single or combined oral antioxidant supplements have been shown to reduce spermatic DNA lesions, thus positively impacting sperm mobility, morphology, and cell concentration.

However, although there has been a steady increase in available literature regarding this topic in the last ten years, the scientific quality of the most important studies conducted to date remains poor, thus placing oral antioxidant supplementation therapeutic role in a place currently subject to debate. High-quality, well-designed, randomized, and controlled trials, including larger patient samples, are still required to confirm supplementation therapy theoretical beneficial effects on subfertile couples, and set the appropriate profile for a potential candidate to this therapy.

References

1. Jungwirth, A., Diemer, T., Kopa, Z., Krausz, C. and Tournaye, H. (2017) *EAU Guidelines on Male Infertility*. www .uroweb.org 20.06.2018.

2. Ahmadi, S., Bashiri, R., Ghadiri-Anari, A., et al. (2016) Antioxidant supplements and semen parameters: an evidence based review. *Int J Reprod BioMed* 14(12):729–736.

3. Nekonka, P. (2017) Role of trace elements for oxidative status and quality of human sperm. *Balkan Med J* 34:343–348.

4. Gosalvez, J., Tvrda, E. and Agarwal, A. (2017) Free radical and superoxide reactivity detection in semen qualit assessment: past, present, and future. *J Assist Reprod Genet* 34:697–707.

5. Bejarano, I., Monllor, F., Marchena, A. M., et al. (2014) Exogenous melatonin supplementation prevents oxidative stress-evoked DNA damage in human spermatozoa. *J Pineal Res* 57:333–339.

6. Showell, M. G., Mackenzie-Proctor, R., Brown, J., Yazdani, A., Stankiewicz, M. T. and Hart, R. J. (2014) Antioxidants for male subfertility. *Cochrane Database Syst Rev* 12: CD007411.

7. Balercia, G., Buldreghini, E., Vignini, A., Tiano, L., Paggi, F., Amoroso, S., et al. (2009) Coenzyme Q10 treatment in infertile men with idiopathic asthenozoospermia: a placebo-controlled, double-blind randomized trial. *Fertil Steril* 91:1785–1792.

8. Plante, M., de Lamirande, E. and Gagnon, C. (1994) Reactive oxygen species released by activated neutrophils, but not by deficient spermatozoa, are sufficient to affect normal sperm motility. *Fertil Steril* 62:387–393.

9. Calogero, A. E., Condorelli, R. A., Russo, G. I. and La Vignera, S. (2017) Conservative nonhormonal options for the treatment of male infertility: antibiotics, anti-inflammatory drugs, and antioxidants. *Biomed Res Int* 4650182.

10. Wagner, H., Cheng, J. W. and Ko, E. Y. (2017) Role of reactive oxygen species in male infertility: an updated review of literature. *Arab J Urol* **16**:35–43.

11. Hosen, M. B., Islam, M. R., et al. (2015) Oxidative stress induced sperm DNA damage, a possible reason for male infertility. *Iranian J of Reprod Med* **13**:525–532.

12. Agarwal, A., Sharma, R. K., Desai, N. R., Prabakaran, S., Tavares, A. and Sabanegh, E. (2009) Role of oxidative stress in pathogenesis of varicocele and infertility. *Urology* **73**:461–469.

13. Aziz, N., Saleh, R. A., Sharma, R. K., et al. (2004) Novel association between sperm reactive oxygen species production, sperm morphological defects, and the sperm deformity index. *Fertil Steril* **81**:349–354.

14. Harshit, G. and Rajeev, K. (2016) An update on the role of medical treatment including antioxidant therapy in varicocele. *Asian J Androl* **18**:222–228.

15. Linhartova, P., Gazo, I., Shaliutina-Kolesova, A., Hulak, M. and Kaspar, V. (2014) Effects of tetrabrombisphenol A on DNA integrity, oxidative stress, and sterlet (*Acipenser ruthenus*) spermatozoa quality variables. *Environ Toxicol* **1**:1–11.

16. Tiseo, B. C., Gaskins, A. J., Hauser, R., et al. (2017) Coenzyme Q10 intake from foods and semen parameters in a subfertile population. *Urology* **102**:100–105.

17. Suleiman, S. A., Ali, M. E., Zaki, Z. M., el-Malik, E. M. and Nasr, M. A. (1996) Lipid peroxidation and human sperm motility: protective role of vitamin E. *J Androl* **17**:530–537.

18. Moretti, E., Collodel, G., Fiaschi, A. I., et al. (2017) Nitric oxide, malondialdheyde and non-enzymatic antioxidants assessed in viable spermatozoa from selected infertile men. *Reprod Biol* **17**:370–375.

19. Walczak-Jedrzejowska, R., Wolski, J. K. and Slowikowska-Hilczer, J. (2013) The role of oxidative stress and antioxidants in male fertility. *Cent European J Urol* **66**:60–67.

20. Pasqualotto, F. F., Sharma, R. K. and Kobayashi, H. (2001) Oxidative stress in normospermic men undergoing infertility evaluation. *J Androl* **22**:316–322.

21. Lamirande, E., Tsai, C., Harakata, A. and Gagnon, C. (1998) Involvement of reactive oxygen species in human sperm arcosome reaction induced by A23187, lysophosphatidylcholine, and biological fluid ultrafiltrates. *J Androl* **19**:585–594.

22. Peeker, R. Abramsson, L. and Marklund, S. L. (1997) Superoxide dismutase isoenzymes in human seminal plasma and spermatozoa. *Mol Hum Reprod* **3**: 1061–1066.

23. Marzec-Wróblewska, U., Kamiński, P., et al. (2018) Human sperm characteristics with regard to cobalt, chromium, and lead in semen and activity of catalase in seminal plasma. *Biol Trace Elem Res* **Jun 29**.

24. Opuwari, C. S. and Henkel, R. R. (2016) An update on oxidative damage to spermatozoa and oocytes. *Biomed Res Int* **2016**:9540142.

25. Balercia, G., Regoli, F., Armeni, T., et al. (2005) Placebo-controlled double-blind randomized trial on the use of L-carnitine, L-acetylcarnitine, or combined L-carnitine and L-acetylcarnitine in men with idiopathic asthenozoospermia. *Fertil Steril* **84**:662–671.

26. Safarinejad, M. R., Safarinejad, S., Shafiei, N. and Safarinejad, S. (2012) Effects of the reduced form of coenzyme Q10 (ubiquinol) on semen parameters in men with idiopathic infertility: a double-blind, placebo controlled, randomized study. *J Urol* **188**:526–531.

27. Nadjarzadeh, A., Shidfar, F., Amirjannati, N., Vafa, M., Motevalian, S., Gohari, M., et al. (2014) Effect of Coenzyme Q10 supplementation on antioxidant enzymes activity and oxidative stress of seminal plasma: a double-blind randomised clinical trial. *Andrologia* **46**:177–183.

28. Thakur, A. S., Littarru, G. P., Funahashi, I., Painkara, U. S., Dange, N. S. and Chauhan, P. (2015) Effect of ubiquinol therapy on sperm parameters and serum

testosterone levels in oligoasthenozoospermic infertile men. *J Clin Diagn Res* **9**:BC01–BC03.

29. Amidi, F., Pazhohan, A., Shabani Nashtaei, M., et al. (2016) The role of antioxidants in sperm freezing: a review. *Cell Tissue Bank* **17**:745–756.

30. Greco, E., Iacobelli, M., Rienzi, L., et al. (2005) Reduction of the incidence of sperm DNA fragmentation by oral antioxidant treatment. *J Androl* **26**:349–356.

31. Colagar, A. H. and Marzony, E. T. (2009) Ascorbic acid in human seminal plasma: determination and its relationship to sperm quality. *J Clin Biochem Nutr* **45**:144–149.

32. Geva, E., Bartoov, B., Zabludovsky, N., et al. (1996) The effect of antioxidant treatment on human spermatozoa and fertilization rate in an *in vitro* fertilization program. *Fertil Steril* **66**:430–434.

33. Kessopoulou, E., Powers, H. J., Sharma, K. K., Pearson, M. J., Russel, J. M., Cooke, I. D., et al. (1995) A double–blind randomized placebo cross–over controlled trial using the an oxidant vitamin E to treat reac ve oxygen species associated male inferlity. *Fertil Steril* **64**:825–831.

34. Keskes–Ammar, L., Feki-Chakroun, N., Rebai, T., et al. (2003) Sperm oxidative stress and the effect of an oral vitamin E and selenium supplement on semen quality in infer le men. *Arch Androl* **49**: 83–94.

35. Al-Azemi, M. K., Omu, A. E. M, Fatinikun, T. M., et al. (2009) Factors contributing to gender differences in serum retinol and alpha-tocopherol in infertile couples. *Reprod Biomed Online* **19**:583–590.

36. Galatioto, G. P., Gravina, G. L., Angelozzi, G., et al. (2008) May antioxidant therapy improve sperm parameters of men with persistent oligospermia after retrograde embolization for varicocele? *World J Urol* **26**:97–102.

37. Lenzi, A., Sgrò, P., Salacone, P., et al. (2004) Placebo controlled double blind randomized trial on the use of L- carnitine and L-acetyl-carnitine combined treatment in asthenozoospermia. *Fertil Steril* **81**:1578–1584.

38. Garolla, A., Maiorino, M., Roverato, A., Roveri, A., Ursini, F. and Foresta, C. (2005) Oral carnitine supplementation increases sperm motility in asthenozoospermic men with normal sperm phospholipid hydroperoxide glutathione peroxidase levels. *Fertil Steril* **83**:355–361.

39. Sigman, M., Glass, S., Campagnone, J. and Pryor, J. L. (2006) Carnitine for the treatment of idiopathic asthenospermia: a randomized, double-blind, placebo-controlled trial. *Fertil Steril* **85**:1409–1414.

40. Cavallini, G., Ferraretti, A. P., Gianaroli, L., et al. (2004) Cinnoxicam and L-carnitine/ acetyl-L-carnitine treatment for idiopathic and varicocele-associated oligoasthenospermia. *J Androl* **25**:761–770.

41. Khan, M. S., Zaman, S., Sajjad, M., Shoaib, M. and Gilani, G. (2011) Assessment of the level of trace element zinc in seminal plasma of males and evaluation of its role in male infertility. *Int J Appl Bas Med Res* **1**:93–96.

42. Wu, J., Wu, S., Xie. Y., et al. (2015) Zinc protects sperm from being damaged by reactive oxygen species in assisted reproduction techniques. *Reprod Biomed Online* **30**:334–339.

43. Ebisch, I., Pierik, F., De Jong, F., Thomas, C. and Steegers-Theunissen, R. (2006) Does folic acid and zinc sulphate intervention affect endocrine parameters and sperm characteristics in men? *Int J Androl* **29**:339–345.

44. Hadwan, M. H., Almashhedy, L. A. and Alsalman, A. R. S. (2012) (Oral zinc supplementation restore high molecular weight seminal zinc binding protein to normal value in Iraqi infertile men. *BMC Urol* **12**:32.

45. Moslemi, M. K. and Tavanbakhsh, S. (2011) Selenium-vitamin E supplementation in infertile men: effects on semen parameters and pregnancy rate. *Int J Gen Med* **4**:99–104.

46. Camejo, M. I., Abdala, L., Vivas-Acevedo, G., et al. (2011) Selenium, copper and zinc

in seminal plasma of men with varicocele, relationship with seminal parameters. *Biol Trace Elem Res* **143**:1247–1254.

47. Zhang, J., Robinson, D. and Salmon, P. (2006) A novel function for selenium in biological system: selenite as a highly effective iron carrier for Chinese hamster ovary cell growth and monoclonal antibody production. *Biotechnol Bioeng* **20** (95):1188–1197.

48. Safarinejad, M. R. and Safarinejad, S. (2009) Efficacy of selenium and/or N-acetyl-cysteine for improving semen parameters in infertile men: a double-blind, placebo controlled, randomized study. *J Urol* **181**:741–751.

49. Tremellen, K., Miari, G., Froiland, D. and Thompson, J. (2007) A randomised control trial examining the effect of an antioxidant (Menevit) on pregnancy outcome during IVF-ICSI treatment. *Aust N Z J Obstet Gynecol* **47**:216–221.

50. Scott, R., MacPherson, A., Yates, R. W., et al. (1998) The effect of oral selenium supplementation on human sperm motility. *Br J Urol* **82**:76–80.

51. Safarinejad, M. R. and Safarinejad, S. (2009) Efficacy of selenium and/or N-acetyl-cysteine for improving semen parameters in infertile men: a double-blind, placebo controlled, randomized study. *J Urol* **181**:741–751.

52. Espino, J., Bejarano, I., Ortiz, A., et al. (2010) Melatonin as a potential tool against oxidative damage and apoptosis in ejaculated human spermatozoa. *Fertil Steril* **94**:1915–1917.

53. Ortiz, A., Espino, J., Bejarano, I., et al. (2011) High endogenous melatonin concentrations enhance sperm quality and short-term *in vitro* exposure to melatonin improves aspects of sperm motility. *J Pineal Res* **50**:132–139.

54. Haghighian, H. K., Haidari, F., Mohammadi-Asl, J. and Dadfar, M. (2015) Randomized, triple-blind, placebo-controlled clinical trial examining the effects of alpha-lipoic acid supplement

on the spermatogram and seminal oxidative stress in infertile men. *Fertil Steril* **104**:318–324.

55. Azza, M. G. (2010) The protective role of alpha lipoic acid against pesticides induced testicular toxicity – histopathological and histochemical studies. *J Aquacult Res Dev* **1**:1–7.

56. Ibrahim, S. F., Osman, K., Das, S., Othman, A. M., Majid, N. A. and Rahman, M. P. (2008) A study of the antioxidant effect of alpha lipoic acids on sperm quality. *Clinics* **63**:545–550.

57. Kuhla, A., Derbenev, M., Shih, H. Y. and Vollmar, B. (2016) Prophylactic and abundant intake of α-lipoic acid causes hepatic steatosis and should be reconsidered in usage as an anti-aging drug. *Biofactors* **42**:179–189.

58. Abad, C., Amengual, M., Gozálvez, J., et al. (2013) Effects of oral antioxidant treatment upon the dynamics of human sperm DNA fragmentation and subpopulations of sperm with highly degraded DNA. *Andrologia* **45**:211–216.

59. Gopinath, P., Kalra, B., Saxena, A., et al. (2013) Fixed dose combination therapy of antioxidants in treatment of idiopathic oligoasthenozoospermia: results of a randomized, double-blind, placebo-controlled clinical trial. *Int J Infertil Fetal Med* **4**:6–13.

60. Arhin, S. K., Zhao, Y., Lu, X., Chetry, M. and Lu, J. (2017) Effect of micronutrient supplementation on IVF outcomes: a systematic review of the literature. *Reprod Biomed Online* **35**:715–722.

61. Buhling, K. J. and Laakmann, E. (2014) The effect of micronutrient supplements on male fertility. *Curr Opin Obstet Gynecol* **26**:199–209.

62. Ross, A. C., Taylor, C. L., Yaktine, A. L. et al. (2011) *Dietary Reference Intakes for Calcium and Vitamin D. Institute of Medicine (US) Committee to Review Dietary Reference Intakes for Vitamin D and Calcium.* Washington, DC: National Academies Press (US).

The History of Utilization of IVF for Male Factor Subfertility

Gabor T. Kovacs

10.1 Introduction

Up to the 1980s the ability to treat couples with male subfertility was limited. Treatable conditions included gonadotrophin therapy for men with hypogonadotrophic hypogonadism (which is estimated to be present in 1 in 200 infertile men), and the treatment of autoimmunity with high dose steroids with its side effects and complications (i.e. avascular necrosis of the head of the femur) [1]. Obstructive azoospermia could sometimes be treated by epididymal or vasal micro-surgery with moderate results for caudal blockages, but poor results were obtained for proximal blockages, and even if spermatozoa appeared in the ejaculate, pregnancies were rare. Disorders of sexual function could sometimes be treated, and toxic causes (maybe 1 in 500 men) removed [2].

However, about 70% of men who had abnormalities of sperm numbers or quality had no diagnosable cause, and were treated in an uncontrolled way, without evidence of efficacy of any of the following methods [3].

Androgens were used either as rebound therapy where spermatogenesis suppression was hoped to be followed by "rebound" improvement, after the hormone is stopped, or as low-dose testosterone administration, aiming to improve epididymal maturation of sperm [4].

Attempts to improve sperm quantity by increasing gonadotropin secretion by administering clomiphene citrate [5] or injections of gonadotropins [6] were given to "stimulate" spermatogenesis. In men where the presence of infection/inflammation was suspected (raised leucocyte count in the semen), antibiotics and anti-inflammatory drugs were administered. Vitamins and antioxidants, herbs, amino acids, and minerals such as zinc and selenium were also administered empirically, based on a theoretical beneficial effect. Cold testicular douches were also used. Many treatments were recommended on the basis of a report of some quantitative improvement of semen factors, but of course this could always be due to spontaneous improvement, or the phenomenon of "regression towards the mean." Pregnancy rates were not used as an endpoint, so no treatment was evidence based. Artificial insemination with partner's sperm and insemination with donor was widely used.

When the possibility of using IVF in the management of male infertility emerged, there was no longer the need to make a specific diagnosis, nor the need to attempt to improve sperm quality, since only small numbers of spermatozoa were required to fertilize oocytes *in vitro*. It was a casual conversation over sandwiches in the Reproduction Medicine Clinic at Prince Henry's Hospital (a multidisciplinary clinic established in 1977 attended by andrologists, gynaecologiosts, a urologist, and a counsellor), when David de Kretser suggested that maybe males with subfertility and decreased numbers of motile normal sperm could achieve fertilization *in vitro*, where they could not achieve this *in vivo* [7]. This led to

Monash IVF establishing a "Male Factor Group," which David chaired. He took a sabbatical for two months, and selected couples who may have benefited from his large infertility practice. Chris Yates (PhD student and embryologist) became the male factor scientist, Jillian McDonald the nurse co-ordinator, and I was the IVF clinician. Prior to this project, one of the prerequisites for IVF treatment (which at that time was mainly confined to the treatment of tubal disease) was to have a normal semen analysis. Alan Trounson had already attempted to apply IVF to unexplained subfertility [8] and *male factor* was yet another possible application for IVF, where men with low sperm counts, poor sperm motility, and those with an increased percentage of abnormally shaped sperm could all attempt to achieve a pregnancy. The technique used for preparing the sperm for IVF in the Melbourne program at the time is summarised by Alex Lopata [9]:

> Husband's semen was diluted in modified Tyrode's solution and centrifuged. The sperm pellet was diluted again and centrifuged to obtain washed sperm pellet that was free of seminal plasma. A final sperm pellet dilution provided about 600,000 motile sperm in one ml of Tyrode's, supplemented with albumin, was used for inseminating the oocyte.

The aim of *male factor* IVF was to separate the most motile sperm for incubation with the oocytes. Initially the "swim-up" technique was used, followed by a centrifugation–migration technique, with the sperm pellet being re-suspended and motile sperm isolated from uppermost portion of suspension. Later, by adding Ficoll (Pharmacia, Sweden), a density gradient interface was achieved, allowing only motile spermatozoa to pass across it. Albumin columns, glass wool columns, and Percoll gradients were all utilized as sperm selection techniques, aiming to obtain the best sample to add to the oocytes [10].

The use of microdrops for insemination was adopted with low volumes of semen of reasonable quality. It provided good results in mild to moderate male factor subfertility [11,12].

The availability of this technical development led Graeme Southwick (plastic and reconstructive surgeon/microsurgeon) and Peter Temple-Smith (research scientist) to surgically obtain such samples from seminiferous tubules using an operating microscope to recover small numbers of spermatozoa from men with obstructive azoospermia, which could then be used for inseminating oocytes *in vitro* obtained from their partners. The first baby born from sperm microsurgically recovered from a man with obstructive azoospermia after previous vasectomy, then utilizing IVF, was "Baby Joseph" [13].

10.2 Micromanipulation of Oocytes and Sperm

Even with the microdrop technique, many spermatozoa (tens of thousands) were still required. In order to allow smaller numbers of sperm to achieve fertilization, micromanipulation procedures were introduced (Figure 10.1). The two initial assisted fertilization procedures attempted were zona drilling and partial zona dissection (PZD). Unfortunately, although occasional fertilization and pregnancies were reported, neither of these methods was very successful [14,15]. Zona drilling involved making a hole in the zona pellucida of an oocyte, which was then incubated in a sperm suspension. Although this worked well in mice, it did not have much success in humans.

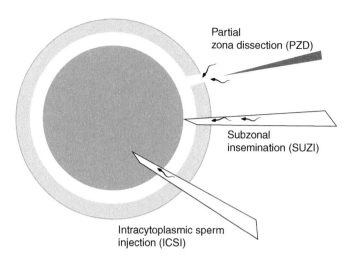

Figure 10.1 Schematic representation of assisted fertilization procedures: PZD, SUZI, and ICSI.

PZD, whereby a mechanical slit was made in the zona pellucida before they were incubated in a sperm suspension, was also attempted. Although fertilization was obtained by this method, monospermic and polyspermic fertilizations were as common as normal fertilization. Although some pregnancies and births occurred, inconsistent results meant that PZD was not widely applied clinically. Around the same time a few case reports were published on the next assisted fertilization procedure: subzonal insemination (SUZI), a micromanipulation technique involving the insertion of a few spermatozoa into the perivitelline space between the zona pellucida and the membrane of the oocyte.

Schematic representation of assisted fertilization procedures: PZD, SUZI, and intracytoplasmic sperm injection (ICSI), is shown in Figure 10.1.

The possibility of using sperm microinjection techniques was suggested as early as 1984 when Alan Trounson wrote, "The possibility of microsurgical fertilization procedures are also being investigated in our laboratory" [16].

The first "Microinjection trial" was commenced at the Infertility Medical Centre (later renamed Monash IVF) in 1987, co-ordinated by Ross Hyne (Figure 10.2).

Trounson and colleagues reported success in mouse oocytes with SUZI [17] and the technique was replicated in humans [18]. Unfortunately, the Minister for Health in Victoria in March 1988 requested that further use of SUZI be suspended (Figure 10.3). With the ban on SUZI in Australia, S. C. Ng who had visited Monash University produced the world's first human birth using SUZI in Singapore in 1988 [19] and several other babies following in Australia and the UK [20–22].

10.3 Two Major Breakthroughs: ICSI and Testicular Sperm Aspiration

ICSI was developed in Brussels at the Centre for Reproductive Medicine of Vrije Universiteit Brussel (VUB), under the supervision of Andre van Steirteghem. He had introduced SUZI into the clinic for patients that had failed several cycles of conventional

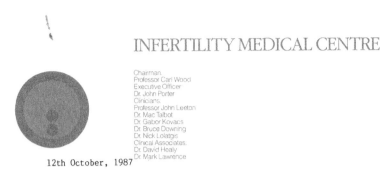

INFERTILITY MEDICAL CENTRE

Chairman.
Professor Carl Wood
Executive Officer
Dr. John Porter
Clinicians.
Professor John Leeton
Dr. Mac Talbot
Dr. Gabor Kovacs
Dr. Bruce Downing
Dr. Nick Lolatgis
Clinical Associates:
Dr. David Healy
Dr. Mark Lawrence

12th October, 1987

Dear IVF/Microinjection Patient,

We plan to commence a research study on whether it is possible to achieve
fertilization by the injection of a single sperm cell into eggs. Any
embryos that are formed will be available for either transfer or freezing.
Patients will be asked if they wish to participate in the study if
they have had poor fertilization results in previous IVF treatment cycles
or if the husband's semen analysis is too poor to be considered for
standard IVF treatment.

The study will involve a new sperm treatment, so if a sufficient number
of motile spermatozoa are available on the day of treatment, patients
will be offered a choice of inseminating either:

1.   One half eggs for IVF. The other half eggs for microinjection.

or

2.   All their eggs for microinjection.

The egg pick-up and IVF will take place at Epworth Hospital, while the
microinjection will take place at the Centre for Early Human Development,
Monash Medical Centre. Husbands will be requested to take the eggs
and spermatozoa for microinjection to the Monash Medical Centre. Embryos
achieved by IVF will be transferred at Epworth Hospital, while embryos
achieved by microinjection will be transferred at Monash Medical
Centre. In case embryos are formed by both treatments, then the couple
would have been asked prior to the egg pick-up which group of embryos
they wish to be put back at transfer and which group they wish to be
frozen.

Arrangements will be made with the husband (and a map provided) for the
transport of the eggs and spermatozoa for microinjection to the Monash
Medical Centre on the day of egg pick-up.

ROSS HYNE
RESEARCH FELLOW   PhD

Figure 10.2 Instructions to patients entering microinjection (SUZI) trial.

IVF. He obtained ethical approval from the VUB Hospital Ethical Committee under the
condition that all pregnancies and children born would be thoroughly followed up, including prenatal diagnosis by either chorionic villous sampling or amniocentesis. Clinical SUZI
was started at VUB in 1990 and a number of pregnancies and births occurred. This was from
sub-zonal insemination of a few spermatozoa, which had been treated prior to enhance the
acrosome reaction [23]. The technical procedure of SUZI is delicate and occasionally one of

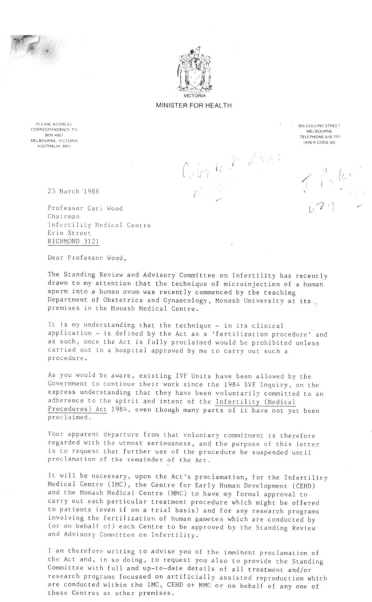

Figure 10.3 Letter from Minister of Health directing the moratorium on microinjection in 1988.

the sperm entered into the cytoplasm of the oocyte. However, in these cases of "failed SUZI," they observed normal fertilization as well as embryo development. He called this procedure ICSI (Figure 10.4). In April 1991, a patient became pregnant after replacing a single ICSI embryo and she delivered on January 14, 1992 [23]. After the initial ICSI observations they continued SUZI and also included ICSI on some oocytes in most cycles. It rapidly became very obvious that the results in terms of fertilization were much more consistent after ICSI

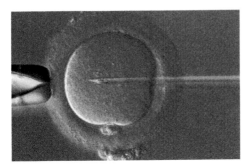

Figure 10.4 One of the first photographs of ICSI; this picture was shown by the late Dame Anne McLaren at meetings (from Prof A. Van Steirteghem, with permission).

than after SUZI, and they obtained ethical approval for ICSI under the same strict protocol, with respect to following up of any pregnancies. After July 1992, the only mechanically-assisted fertilization procedure practiced at VUB was ICSI [24,25]. From late 1992, several ICSI workshops were held at VUB, and they taught many embryologists from around the world, which helped a lot with the dissemination of ICSI worldwide. Andre states that "the VUB's openness to the world in showing ICSI was similar to the approach taken by the Melbourne groups for the introduction of conventional IVF."

A quarter of a century later we recognise that ICSI remains the best treatment for the treatment for severe semen abnormalities, including cryptozoospermia.

ICSI has also been applied to epididymal or testicular spermatozoa in cases of azoospermia, as obtained by testicular needle/open/microsurgical biopsy. Results of ICSI in cases of obstructive azoospermia using epididymal or testicular spermatozoa were similar to the results of ICSI with ejaculated sperm and the results of conventional IVF for female-factor or idiopathic infertility [26–28].

The ICSI technique first came to the general awareness of the Australian scientific community at a Serono Symposium held in Adelaide, in December 1992, when Professor Andre Van Steirteghem presented the Brussels experience and stated that the results were far superior to those achieved with SUZI [29].

The second big breakthrough for the treatment of men with azoospermia was the ability to obtain spermatozoa from the vas deferens or the testes by biopsy, either by a needle biopsy under local anaesthetic, pioneered by Gordon Baker [30], or by open testicular biopsy which has since been further refined by using an operating microscope to identify distended tubules, which were the most likely regions of the tubules from which to harvest small numbers of sperm. This technique was pioneered by Sherman Silber [31] for cases of obstructive azoospermia where there was no vas (congenital bilateral absence of the vasa deferentia); he developed the microepidymal sperm aspiration (MESA) procedure, first with IVF in 1986, and then with ICSI in 1992. They reported that pregnancy and live birth rates were no different from couples with normal sperm counts in the men's ejaculates. They also carried out testicular sperm extraction from men with non-obstructive azooospermia and reported in 1993 that ICSI using testicular non-motile spermatozoa resulted in normal pregnancy and live baby rates; they named the new procedure testicular sperm extraction (TESE) [26]. However, in patients with non-obstructive azoospermia, spermatozoa can only be recovered in half of the men even after testicular biopsy, in spite of using these micro-surgical techniques, and despite often extensive and prolonged searching for spermatozoa.

Sherman still has the original napkin from the surgeon's lounge in Brussels where Paul Devroey wrote this down when they coined the eponym "TESE." This experience also changed the basic science concept of epididymal function. It had been thought that the most motile spermatozoa would be from the most distal region that had traversed through most of the epididymis, but they showed that the opposite was true, and found good motility in the most proximal spermatozoa.

If the biopsy shows germ cell arrest when spermatogenesis ceases at a particular point, for example the primary spermatocyte stage wherein meiosis has not been completed, the chances of finding small areas where sperm are still being produced is very rare.

In the context of IVF, even a very small number of spermatozoa can be successfully used by ICSI and hence sperm samples can be frozen and stored until required for future IVF or ICSI.

Silber and colleagues then used these early pioneering micro-TESE patients to map and sequence the Y chromosome, beginning in 1995, and were the first to discover genes that control spermatogenesis and are deleted in infertile men. This was the now famous DAZ (deleted in azoospermia) gene – an acronym coined by them. They also described the autosomal DAZL gene on chromosome 3, which as it now turns out is the major ancestral universal gene that "licenses" early embryonic stem cells to become germ cells, either spermatozoa or oocytes.

Silber also confirmed the principles of minimal tissue trauma, perfect haemostasis, and pulsatile irrigation with heparinized saline within the scrotum as advocated by the [Fallopian] "tubal microsurgeons" Victor Gomel and Robert Winston.

In summary, IVF with ICSI has become the only effective treatment for many couples with male factor as a component of their subfertility. According to the most recent report on assisted conception in Australia and New Zealand [32], nearly a quarter of all couples treated had either male factor alone (10.7%) or combined female and male factors (12.2%). Consequently, not only is IVF/ICSI an important treatment for male subfertility, but the male factor group are a significant proportion of patients undergoing assisted reproduction.

References

1. Hendry, W. F. (1982) Bilateral aseptic necrosis of femoral heads following intermittent high-dose steroid therapy. *Fertil Steril* **38**:120.

2. Barak, S. and Baker, H. W. G. (2016) *Clinical Management of Male Infertility in Endotext .org*: Male reproduction section.

3. de Kretser, D. (1974) The management of the infertile male. *Clin Obstet Gynaecol* 1:409–427.

4. Lamensdorf, H., Compere, D. and Begley, G. (1975) Testosterone rebound therapy in the treatment of male infertility. *Fertil Steril* 26:469–472.

5. Paulson, D. F., Hammond, C., de Vere, B., White, R. and Wiebe, R. H. (1977) Clomiphene citrate: pharmacologic treatment of hypofertile male. *Urology* 9:419–421.

6. Mroueh, A., Lytton, B. and Kase, N. (1967) Effects of human chorionic gonadotropin and human menopausal gonadotropin (pergonal) in males with oligospermia. *J Clin Endocrinol Metab* **27**:53–60.

7. de Krester, D. (2018) The application of IVF in the management of the infertile male. In Kovacs, G. et al. (eds.) *IVF, The Pioneers' History*. Cambridge UK: Cambridge University Press, 117–179.

8. Trounson, A. O., Leeton, J. F., Wood, C., Webb, J. and Kovacs, G. T. (1980) The investigation of idiopathic infertility by *in vitro* fertilization. *Fertil Steril* **34**:431–438.

9. Lopata, A. and Kovacs, G. (2018) The development of *in-vitro* fertilization in Australia. In Kovacs, G., et al. (eds.) *IVF, the Pioneers' History*. Cambridge UK: Cambridge University Press, 46–65.

10. Yates, C. A., Thomas, C., Kovacs, G. T. and de Kretser, D. M. (1989) Andrology, male factor and IVF. In Wood, C. and Trounson, A. (eds.) *Clinical in Vitro Fertilization*. 2nd edn. Berlin: Springer-Verlag, 95–112.

11. Ombelet, W. (2006) Assisted reproductive technologies. In Schill, W., Comhaire, F. and Hargreave, T. B. (eds.) *Andrology for the Clinician*. Berlin: Springer, 578–584.

12. Svalander, P., Wikland, M., Jakobsson, A. H. and Forsberg, A. S. (1994) Subzonal insemination (SUZI) or *in vitro* fertilization (IVF) in microdroplets for the treatment of male-factor infertility. *J Assist Reprod Genet* **11**:149–155.

13. Temple-Smith, P. D, Southwick, G. J., Yates, C. A., Trounson, A. O. and de Kretser, D. M. (1985) Human pregnancy by *in vitro* fertilization (IVF) using sperm aspirated from the epididymis. *J In Vitro Fert Embryo Transf* 2:119–122.

14. Gordon, J. W., Grunfeld, L., Garrisi, G. J., Talansky, B. E., Richards, C. and Laufer, N. (1988) Fertilization of human oocytes by sperm from infertile males after zona pellucida drilling. *Fertil Steril* 50:68–73.

15. Malter, H. E. and Cohen, J. (1989) Partial zona dissection of the human oocyte: a nontraumatic method using micromanipulation to assist zona pellucida penetration. *Fertil Steril* 51:139–148.

16. Trounson, A. (1984) *In vitro* fertilization and embryo preservation ion. In Trounson, A. and Wood, C. (eds.) *In vitro Fertilization and Embryo*. Edinburgh, UK: Churchill Livingstone, 111–130.

17. Lacham, O., Trounson, A., Holden, C., Mann, J. and Sathananthan, H. (1989) Fertilization and development of mouse eggs injected under the zona pellucida with single spermatozoa treated to induce the acrosome reaction. *Gamete Res* **23**:233–243.

18. Laws-King, A., Trounson, A., Sathananthan, H. and Kola, I. (1987) Fertilization of human oocytes by microinjection of a single spermatozoon under the zona pellucida. *Fertil Steril* 48:637–642.

19. Ng, S. C., Bongso, A., Ratnam, S. S., Sathanansan, H., Chan, C. L. K., Wong, P. O. C., et al. (1988) Pregnancy after transfer of sperm under the zona. *Lancet* 2:790.

20. Lippi, J., Turner, M. and Jansen, R. P. S. (1990) Pregnancies after *in vitro* fertilization by sperm microinjection into the perivitelline space. *46th Annual Meeting of The American Fertility Society, Washington DC. Abstract O-068. Fertil Steril* 54:S29.

21. Lippi, J., Mortimer, D. and Jansen, R. P. S. (1993) Sub-zonal insemination for extreme male factor infertility. *Hum Reprod* 8:908–915.

22. Fishel, S., Antinori, S., Jackson, P., Johnson, J. and Rinaldi, L. (1991) Presentation of six pregnancies established by sub-zonal insemination (SUZI). *Hum Reprod* 6:124–130.

23. Palermo, G., Joris, H., Devroey, P. and Van Steirteghem, A. C. (1992) Pregnancies after intracytoplasmic injection of single spermatozoon into an oocyte. *Lancet* 340:17–18.

24. Van Steirteghem, A. C, Liu, J., Joris, H., Nagy Z., Janssenswillen, C., Tournaye, H., et al. (1993a) Higher success rate by intracytoplasmic sperm injection than by subzonal insemination. Report of a second series of 300 consecutive treatment cycles. *Hum Reprod* 8:1055–1060.

25. Van Steirteghem, A. C., Nagy, Z., Joris, H., Liu, J., Staessen, C., Smitz, J., et al. (1993b) High fertilization and implantation rates after intracytoplasmic sperm injection. *Hum Reprod* 8:1061–1066.

26. Devroey, P., Liu, J., Nagy, Z., Tournaye, H., Silber, S. J. and Van Steirteghem, A. C. (1994) Normal fertilization of human oocytes after testicular sperm extraction and intracytoplasmic sperm injection. *Fertil Steril* **62**:639–641.

27. Silber, S. J., Nagy, Z. P., Liu, J., Godoy, H., Devroey, P. and Van Steirteghem, A. C. (1994) Conventional *in-vitro* fertilization versus intracytoplasmic sperm injection for patients requiring microsurgical sperm aspiration. *Hum Reprod* **9**:1705–1709.

28. Tournaye, H., Devroey, P., Liu, J., Nagy, Z., Lissens, W. and Van Steirteghem, A. (1994) Microsurgical epididymal sperm aspiration and intracytoplasmic sperm injection: a new effective approach to infertility as a result of congenital bilateral absence of the vas deferens. *Fertil Steril* **61**:1045–1051.

29. McLachlan, R. I. (1997) The use of assisted reproductive technology for the treatment of male infertility. In: Kovacs, G. T. (ed.) *The Sub Fertility Handbook: A Clinician's Guide*. Cambridge, UK: Cambridge University Press, 124–138.

30. Mallidis, C. and Baker, H. W. (1994) Fine needle tissue aspiration biopsy of the testis. *Fertil Steril*;**61**:367–375.

31. Silber, S. (2018) History of microsurgery in male (and female) infertility. In Kovacs, G., et al. (eds.) *IVF, the Pioneers' History*. Cambridge, UK: Cambridge University Press, 215–221.

32. Fitzgerald, O., Paul, R. C., Harris, K. and Chambers, G. M. (2018) *Assisted Reproductive Technology in Australia and New Zealand 2016*. Sydney: National Perinatal Epidemiology and Statistics Unit, the University of New South Wales Sydney, p. 7.

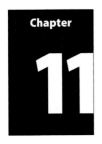

The Case Against Intracytoplasmic Sperm Injection for All

David Mortimer and Sharon T. Mortimer

11.1 Introduction

Unarguably, intracytoplasmic sperm injection (ICSI) is the most significant advance in assisted reproductive technology (ART) for the alleviation of male factor subfertility. However, its use has become increasingly widespread and indiscriminate in ART clinics, extending well beyond the reasons for its necessary application, which are:

- cases of severe male factor subfertility where there is actual evidence for a serious risk of impaired sperm function that would lead to reduced or failed fertilization *in vitro* (also includes autoimmune infertility caused by antibodies directed against the sperm head, and many – although certainly not all – cases of retrograde ejaculation);
- couples in whom conventional *in vitro* fertilization (IVF) has failed due solely to sperm dysfunction, such as failure to acrosome react;
- use of spermatozoa recovered surgically from the male reproductive tract;
- use of spermatozoa that were cryopreserved in finite limited quantities, e.g. prior to chemo- or radiotherapy or prior to vasectomy, or with known poor cryosurvival;
- cases where pre-implantation genetic testing is to be performed for monogenic conditions, and there is a real risk of possible contamination with DNA from spermatozoa still attached to the zona pellucida; and
- with cryopreserved or vitrified oocytes where sperm–oolemma fusion might be compromised.

The proposition for the widespread, even "universal," use of ICSI is based on the commonly held perception among ART clinicians, as well as by numerous embryologists, that ICSI gives a higher fertilization rate than conventional IVF, and that it satisfies their desire to avoid unexpected IVF fertilization failure. In 2000, Fishel and colleagues proposed that ICSI should be used as a first option because it: (i) offered a higher incidence of fertilization; (ii) maximized the number of embryos; and (iii) minimized the risk of complete failure of fertilization for all cases requiring *in vitro* conception [1]. However, they did note that, among other concerns, the then current knowledge of ICSI birth outcomes did not provide the confidence to use it in all cases of IVF for the time being. But a year later, Ola and colleagues concluded that from safety, scientific and economic viewpoints, ICSI should only be used in cases where success of IVF was regarded as unlikely [2].

While wishing to avoid having to explain to a man why his sperm "didn't work" with conventional IVF is perhaps understandable, the indiscriminate, even total, use of ICSI is increasingly being seen as unacceptable, and some jurisdictions have regulated against this approach. For example, an expert Panel Report for the Ontario (Canada) Ministry of Children and Youth Services stated that ICSI should be provided only for individuals where either severe male factor infertility is present, or there is demonstrated fertilization failure in a previous IVF cycle. Clearly, a "poor" semen analysis, even one with several characteristics below the World Health Organization reference values for recently fertile men [3], is not adequate justification for using ICSI.

This chapter investigates the basis for this reasoning, and identifies the risks to which couples are exposed by the unjustified use of ICSI, a debate that has now been raging for two decades [4–7] and is now also extending into considerations of "andrological ignorance," how ICSI has effectively blocked scientific advances in andrology, and how the over-reliance on ICSI has effectively transferred the treatment burden for male factor infertility to the female partner, who is expected to undergo possibly unnecessary controlled ovarian hyperstimulation, oocyte retrieval and embryo transfer procedures [8].

11.2   Does ICSI Have Any Real Benefit in Non-Male Factor Infertility Cases?

11.2.1   Fertilization Rates Are Not Higher Using ICSI

While some studies have reported higher fertilization rates with ICSI than with IVF, a 2003 Cochrane Review concluded that IVF gave better fertilization results than ICSI in couples with male factor subfertility [9]. These authors also noted that pregnancy rates following IVF and ICSI were comparable for couples with non-male subfertility, and also that, if anything, ICSI did not improve on the IVF outcome in these couples.

Analyzing 486 couples without a diagnosis of male factor [10] reported that among the 99 cycles in which ICSI was used (there were no IVF/ICSI "splits") the fertilization rate was lower than among the 598 IVF cycles (61.7% vs 72.9%, $p < 0.001$), and the fertilization failure rate was similar at 4% cf. 3%. Clinical outcomes as measured by positive ß-hCG and live birth rates were not different between the IVF and ICSI treatment cycles (40% cf. 32% and 22% cf. 17%, $p = 0.13$ and 0.24, respectively).

Nyboe Andersen and colleagues [11] and Carrell and colleagues [6] concluded that:

ICSI is invaluable in treating patients with male factor infertility, however, such patients should be evaluated by an andrologist to assure that ICSI is indeed necessary and that broader health concerns are addressed. ICSI may also be indicated in other situations, including the use of cryopreserved oocytes, and in conjunction with PGD, however, the data clearly show no benefit in routine use of ICSI for other patients.

Table 11.1 shows a model analysis of the number of zygotes that would be generated following IVF and ICSI from a "typical" cohort of 13 cumulus–oocyte complexes of which 85% contained MII oocytes by laboratories operating at the "competency" and "benchmark" performance levels, as defined by the Vienna consensus on ART laboratory key performance indicators [12]. In either situation, IVF would generate more zygotes than ICSI (7.8–9.8 vs 6.5–8.4). This represents, on average, between 1.3 and 3.3 fewer zygotes when ICSI is used in a case where IVF would have worked, or a 50% greater outcome for a benchmark IVF lab compared to a competent ICSI lab (9.8 vs 6.5 zygotes). Assuming both labs then had benchmark blastocyst development rates of 60%, the difference would result in two more blastocysts in the IVF lab compared to the ICSI-only lab.

Another situation where ICSI is often perceived to be better practice is in cycles where there are very few oocytes available. This was investigated by Borini and colleagues [13] who

Table 11.1 Model comparing IVF with ICSI in terms of the number of 2PN zygotes generated in a generic typical cycle considering "competency" and "benchmark" laboratory performance levels as per the Vienna Consensus [12].

Parameter	IVF		ICSI	
Number of COCs	13		13	
Number of MII oocytes @ 85%			11.05	
Damaged			Competency (−10%)	Benchmark (−5%)
Inseminated or injected	13		9.95	10.50
Normal fertilization rate	Competency (60%)	Benchmark (75%)	Competency (65%)	Benchmark (80%)
Number of 2PN zygotes	7.80	9.75	6.47	8.40

Note: Normal fertilization rate for IVF is defined as the proportion of 2PN zygotes per cumulus–oocyte complex (COC) inseminated, and for ICSI as the proportion of 2PN zygotes per MII oocyte injected.

found no benefit in using ICSI, and concluded that "Performing ICSI in all cases of IVF is not advantageous, probably only more expensive and time consuming," and commented that "Abandoning IVF appears to be questionable." Considering ICSI for non-male factor infertility in older women, there was still no advantage of ICSI over IVF [14].

11.2.2 What is the Real Risk of Total IVF Fertilization Failure (TIFF)?

Many centres have published a prevalence of TIFF of 5–10%, or even higher, yet others report values of 2% [2]. This discrepancy, and the finding of high rates of TIFF, are the result of two main issues: (i) poor andrological (more correctly, spermatological) evaluation of the male partners; and (ii) poor sperm handling/preparation/capacitation systems that result in impaired sperm function *in vitro*. Centres with these issues create a self-fulfilling prophesy: sperm will show poor function, thereby reducing IVF fertilization rates and causing a high prevalence of TIFF. Although ICSI would eliminate this iatrogenic problem of TIFF due to poor sperm function, what is really needed is just better IVF.

The American Society for Reproductive Medicine (ASRM) has stated that in routine ART for non-male factor infertility the risk of failed fertilization is low, and a similar frequency is found after IVF and ICSI [15]. With optimized IVF lab systems, TIFF rarely exceeds 2–3%, and the Vienna Consensus sets a limit of 5% [12] against a generally established background ICSI fertilization failure rate of 1–2%. Certainly, patients could choose to use ICSI if they found a 1–2% incremental risk of TIFF to be unacceptable, but it would be irresponsible to allow them to believe that the prevalence of TIFF is 10% or higher – although, if it were that high then the lab would not be considered to meet good practice standards [12].

From our own experience [16], after performing a careful assessment of the sperm prior to recommending IVF or ICSI treatment, low fertilization (<25% of eggs inseminated or

Table 11.2 A: Prevalence of low and failed fertilization cases, and B: Stimulation responses in the IVF low and failed fertilization cases. Data from 2006–2014 at Atlantic Assisted Reproductive Therapies, Halifax, NS, Canada [16].

A				B		Fertilization	
Fertilization	IVF	ICSI	P	Stimulation response		0%	1–24%
						(n = 14)	(n = 16)
	n = 830	n = 1129		Normal	5–15 COCs	2	3
Low	16 (1.9%)	34 (3.0%)	0.148	High	>15 COCs	1	8
Failed	14 (1.7%)	27 (2.4%)	0.339	Low	<5 COCs	6	–
					<4 MIIs	7	5

injected) and failed fertilization at IVF can be no greater than levels seen in ICSI cases (1.9% and 1.7% for IVF vs 3.0% and 2.4% for ICSI; Table 11.2-A). More importantly, when analyzing such IVF cases, most abnormal IVF outcomes occurred in cycles with abnormal ovarian stimulation response, either very few mature oocytes or large numbers of oocytes (>15: Table 11.2-B). Key parameters used in the pre-treatment sperm assessment to differentiate these couples into IUI, IVF or ICSI treatment recommendations were: sperm morphology as assessed using the teratozoospermia index (TZI), and not the % normal forms; and the yield from a PureSperm density gradient "trial wash"; and sperm hyperactivation assessed using CASA (Hamilton Thorne IVOS, Beverly, MA, USA) analytical methods which can be found in [17]. Consequently, with adequate sperm pre-assessment, IVF can be recommended with good confidence.

11.2.3 Compromised Embryo Development Following ICSI

An older study reported a significant decrease in blastocyst development in ICSI-derived embryos compared to IVF-derived embryos, including in a limited sibling oocyte study [18], although the blastocyst development rates were low compared to modern-day expectations [12]. This finding complemented an earlier observational study on supernumerary embryo development [19].

In an experimental study on mouse blastocysts generated following IVF, ICSI and ICSI-A (ICSI with artificial oocyte activation using ionophore), Bridges and colleagues [20] found that expression of 197 genes differed between ICSI and IVF, while in blastocysts derived by ICSI-A versus IVF, and ICSI-A versus ICSI, the expression of 132 and 65 genes differed respectively. Classification of the differentially expressed genes into biological pathways revealed consistency to known treatment-induced adverse consequences, including the regulation of metabolic pathways (including cholesterol and lipid metabolism/catabolism), and structural and neural developmental pathways.

11.2.4 Pregnancy and Live Birth Rates are not Higher when Non-Male Factor Cases are Treated using ICSI

A randomized controlled trial showed that ICSI did not offer an advantage over IVF [21]. implantation and clinical pregnancy (fetal heart) rates were higher in the IVF group (30% vs

22%, relative risk 1.35 (95% CI 1.04–1.76) and 33% vs 26%, relative risk 1.17 (95% CI 0.97–1.35), respectively), and mean associated laboratory time was significantly shorter with IVF than with ICSI (22.9 ± 12.1 SD minutes vs 74.0 ± 38.1 minutes; 95% CI for difference 45.6–56.6). These authors concluded that "ICSI offers no advantage over IVF in terms of clinical outcome in cases of non-male factor infertility. Our results support the current practice of reserving ICSI only for severe male-factor problems."

A large registry-based analysis from Australia recently reported that ICSI did not increase the cumulative live birth rate in non-male factor infertility, and that the fertilization rate per oocyte retrieval was lower by ICSI than IVF, 56.2% versus 59.8%, $p < 0.001$ [22] concluding that "These data suggest that ICSI offers no advantage over conventional IVF in terms of live birth rate for couples with non-male factor infertility."

Analysis of data reported to the US National Assisted Reproductive Technology Surveillance System during 1996–2012 revealed that in 317,996 cycles without male factor infertility, ICSI use was associated with lower rates of implantation (23.0% vs 25.2%; adjusted RR 0.93, 95%CI 0.91–0.95) and live birth (36.5% vs 39.2%; adjusted RR 0.95, 95%CI 0.93–0.97) compared to conventional IVF [23]. These authors concluded that "Compared with conventional IVF, ICSI use was not associated with improved post-fertilization reproductive outcomes, irrespective of male factor infertility diagnosis."

Registry data from the USA reveals that in all female age groups younger than 43, cases without diagnosed male factor infertility achieved fewer live births following ICSI compared to IVF [24], confirming the ASRM official statement on ICSI for non-male factor infertility that "Routine use of ICSI for all oocytes does not appear to be justified in cases without male factor infertility or a history of prior fertilization failure" [15].

11.2.5 How Much ICSI is Needed?

From the US National Assisted Reproductive Technology Surveillance System data for 1996–2012, 65.1% of the 1,395,634 fresh IVF cycles used ICSI, although only 35.8% reported male factor infertility [23]. For cycles without male factor infertility, ICSI use increased from 15.4% in 1996 to 66.9% in 2012.

The latest report from the International Committee for Monitoring Assisted Reproductive Technologies (ICMART) [25] reported more than 455,000 ICSI treatment cycles were started in 2010 compared to only 220,000 IVF treatment cycles, with the proportion of ICSI cases ranging from 55% in Asia, through 65% in Europe and 73% in North America, to 86% in Latin America and almost 100% in the Middle East. In Europe, the prevalence of ICSI since 2007 has stabilized to between 65% and 70% [26].

Clearly the application of ICSI has little to do with the prevalence of male factor infertility throughout most of the world. Based on our experience, and that of many centres with which we have been associated over the past 25 years, even though 90% or more of couples might be defined as having a male factor according to current WHO semen analysis reference values, ICSI is typically necessary in no more than about 40% of cases due to a male factor that would be expected to impair sperm fertilizing ability [25,27]. The only exception to this would be for centres that specialize in treating men with spinal cord injuries or have a very specific focus on severe male factor subfertility.

11.2.6 Does using IVF/ICSI "Splits" have any Real Value?

A number of centres employ IVF/ICSI "splits," where the available oocytes are assigned to two groups, one for conventional insemination and the other for ICSI. The rationale is that because these centres' sperm assessments cannot identify those men whose spermatozoa have impaired fertilizing potential, this approach is "easier" than upgrading the diagnostic andrology testing to include sperm functional assessments.

We have even heard some clinicians say that doing "splits" is "easier on the lab," a position that is hard to understand when the practice greatly increases the workload by requiring both IVF and ICSI forms of insemination in each such cycle, with the ICSI component taking far more time than a simple IVF insemination [21].

However, with "splits" it is not uncommon for the "better looking" cumulus-corona-oocyte complexes to be assigned to ICSI, rather than following a proper randomization – creating another self-fulfilling prophesy that (in these cases) ICSI achieves a higher fertilization rate.

11.2.7 Is a "Poor" Semen Analysis Justification for using ICSI?

The limited prognostic value of descriptive semen analysis characteristics has long been known, rendering simple assessments of sperm concentration, motility and even normal sperm morphology (even by properly trained, expert semen analysis technologists) of limited value in defining sperm fertilizing ability. Indeed, the Vienna Consensus recommended that any treatment selection decisions be based only on parameters derived from "trial wash" preparations and not on semen analysis characteristics [12]. Not even sperm morphology was considered sufficiently robust because the current visual evaluation of 200 or 400 spermatozoa used in the vast majority of laboratories to assess "percent normal forms" has such a large uncertainty of measurement that it cannot be considered a reliable predictor for IVF success/failure for individual men.

Moreover, there is no direct equivalence between morphological normality of a spermatozoon and its ability to fertilize an oocyte – or the converse. Many morphologically abnormal spermatozoa fertilize oocytes, and we have routinely employed IVF in men with less than 4% normal forms and achieved normal IVF fertilization rates (albeit so long as the Teratozoospermia Index (TZI) is below the threshold value of 1.80 [17].

11.2.8 Sperm Preparation and Selection Issues

There are well-documented processes of sperm selection *in vivo* during their passage through the female reproductive tract and the oocyte vestments, with the acquisition of fertilizing ability being closely regulated in those spermatozoa that ultimately fertilize oocytes [28–30].

Sperm preparation using a technique that selects properly mature spermatozoa with better functional potential and low levels of DNA damage, and protects them from oxidative damage by reactive oxygen species (ROS) during handling, is essential for both IVF and ICSI. Even though sperm fertilizing ability is unimportant for ICSI, the quality of the male genetic contribution to the embryo is still critical – and perhaps even more so since male factor cases have inherently higher levels of sperm DNA damage.

Sperm selection for ICSI is important to exclude dead spermatozoa that will be undergoing autolysis, and hence at much greater risk of having damaged DNA. Various techniques for selecting "better" spermatozoa have been reported but are not yet in routine clinical use [29,30]. Although there is no specific relationship between sperm phenotype and genotype (beyond diploid spermatozoa having larger heads), men with oligoasthenoteratozoospermia have increased levels of ROS, DNA fragmentation and chromosomal aberrations in their spermatozoa. Because these are the men who will more likely require ICSI to achieve a conception, sperm selection is critical in these cases.

Although sperm-binding to hyaluronic acid has long been proposed as a better means to select spermatozoa for ICSI, a major multi-centre trial in the UK (HABSelect) has now revealed it to be of minimal value [31], so that it now mostly constitutes an unjustifiable "add-on" [32]. While recent developments in electrophoretic sperm separation [33] and sperm migration within microfluidic devices [34] represent possible future enhancements, the best currently available technique for sperm selection for ART procedures in terms of cost and breadth of applicability remains an optimized density gradient separation method [17,35,36].

The use of high optical magnification to select spermatozoa without vacuoles for ICSI (IMSI: intracytoplasmic morphologically selected sperm injection) seems to increase the success rate of ICSI [37], but comes at a high cost, both in terms of the microscopes required and the greatly increased time taken to perform a case (often 1.5–2 hours). Moreover, from the "standard ICSI" fertilization and pregnancy rates reported in these studies, it does seem that IMSI is only of value in extreme cases, which is fortunate as its routine use for all ICSI cases would be enormously expensive in equipment and human resources.

11.3 What Are the Biological Risks Associated with ICSI?

While the increased prevalence of sex chromosome aneuploidy and imprinting disorders in ICSI-derived offspring have been shown to be more related to the higher prevalence of such disorders in couples receiving ICSI treatment, the risk of birth defects associated with ICSI treatment is higher than that following IVF [38]. However, of far greater concern is the accumulating scientific evidence for adverse effects of the ICSI procedure upon the oocyte, the fertilization process, and subsequent embryonic development (reviews: [2,4,5]. In summary:

- During normal fertilization in Eutheria the acrosome is lost prior to sperm–oocyte fusion, and the remaining sperm plasma membrane is incorporated as a patch into the oolemma as part of the fusion process (review: [39]). However, during ICSI, both the intact acrosome and the sperm plasma membrane are inserted directly into the ooplasm. Experiments in mice have shown that the cholesterol content of the plasma membrane of uncapacitated spermatozoa (more specifically, its oxidation by ROS within the ooplasm), and/or the protease(s) contained within the acrosome, can affect sperm chromatin remodelling, leading to DNA damage [40]. Removal of these structures prior to ICSI in this species reduced aberration rates in the resultant embryos to those of IVF-derived embryos.
- Since the sperm plasma membrane is inserted into the ooplasm at ICSI, whatever is bound to its outer surface (including bacteria, viruses and DNA) is also transferred into the ooplasm [41]. Indeed, ICSI-based sperm-mediated gene transfer (SMGT) is a well-established and highly efficient technique for generating transgenic animals [42]. The inadvertent ICSI-mediated transgenesis is a serious risk that must be avoided whenever possible.

- The pattern of sperm-induced Ca^{2+} oscillations during rabbit oocyte activation is different following ICSI compared to normal sperm–oocyte fusion, and this has been associated with impaired blastocyst formation, perhaps due to difficulties in going through cell cycle checkpoints [43]. Studies leading to the first live births following ICSI in the rhesus monkey found abnormal sperm decondensation with the unusual retention of perinuclear structures and the exclusion of the nuclear mitotic apparatus from the decondensing sperm nuclear apex. Male pronuclear remodelling was required before replication of either parental genome, indicating a unique G1-to-S transition checkpoint during zygotic interphase (the first cell cycle). The authors expressed concerns that such irregularities could indicate that ICSI might lead to increased chromosome anomalies as well as DNA damage [44,45]. A study on sibling human oocytes has also shown that the ICSI procedure itself can be detrimental to embryonic development *in vitro* [18].
- Fertilization failure of human oocytes following ICSI is largely due to incomplete oocyte activation, defects in pronuclear apposition, and abnormal sperm head decondensation [43]. Abnormal sperm head decondensation can be due to abnormalities in either the spermatozoon or the oocyte (perhaps as a result of incomplete cytoplasmic maturation, e.g. insufficient glutathione, which is frequently asynchronous with nuclear maturation in oocytes following controlled ovarian hyperstimulation). Sperm-based issues include "super-stabilized" chromatin resulting from zinc deficiency in the seminal plasma, and abnormal chromatin condensation and/or incomplete replacement of histones by protamines during defective spermiogenesis – which is reflected in impaired sperm morphology, a common reason for performing ICSI (review: [39]).
- Finally, in the absence of any serious IVF treatment option, laboratory staff could lose the necessary skills related to the safe handling and processing of spermatozoa. This could then lead to sub-optimal practices and culture conditions, as well as elevated risks of iatrogenic sperm DNA damage and an overall detrimental impact on treatment outcomes, all of which must be avoided when striving for best practice.

11.4 Increased Financial Burden to Patients from ICSI

An economic analysis using UK national data for 1998/1999 revealed that each live birth produced by ICSI cost an extra £2,000 (low cost benefit), and each additional live birth when ICSI was advocated for all cases cost £60,000 (poor cost effectiveness) [2]. Based on UK Government inflation figures, these differential costs equate to £3,366 and £100,992 in 2018 values.

In Canada, where pregnancy rates by IVF and ICSI are equivalent, ICSI typically costs $1,500 extra per treatment cycle, and in 2017 was used in 83.1% of the 15,391 treatment cycles started in women using their own oocytes. With male factor and Preimplantation Genetic Testing cases accounting for just 42.3% of cycles, the extra financial burden of unnecessary ICSI (primarily directly to patients since ART is still mostly in the private sector in Canada) can be estimated at approximately $9.4 M in that year.

Many IVF laboratories' "standard" semen analyses frequently fail to meet the expected minimum standards for accuracy and precision [17]. However, the typical incremental cost in Canada of a comprehensive sperm assessment to include assessments that allow the assignment to conventional IVF with only a 1% or so increased risk of TIFF, compared to the cost of a basic semen analysis, is approximately $200. Compared with the standard ICSI supplement, this would represent an average saving of about $1200 for up to 50% of patient cycles.

11.5 Conclusion: Taking the Best Practice Way Forward

1. ICSI will remain, for the foreseeable future, an essential part of our armamentarium for helping infertile couples with a severe male factor to achieve their goals of a healthy baby.

2. ICSI is not "better" than IVF using any established outcome metric. Indeed, available evidence indicates that ICSI yields fewer embryos per treatment cycle, embryos which may have impaired developmental potential compared to IVF-derived embryos.

3. ICSI costs more than IVF because of the capital cost of ICSI workstations, extra consumables and embryologist time (and IMSI even more so). Most centres identify this cost up-front, but even if a centre charges the same for both treatment modalities, the cost is still higher. If ICSI is not needed, then patients will pay unnecessarily.

4. The argument of universal use of ICSI to avoid low or no fertilization at IVF is a simplistic approach to the issue of managing occult male factor subfertility that cannot be considered best practice. Proper sperm assessments would allow the great majority of patients to undertake IVF with an increased TIFF risk of about 1%; naturally, those who are not prepared to accept this small risk can always choose ICSI, with its associated other risks.

5. The effective transference of the treatment burden for male factor infertility to the female partner via obligate ICSI is increasingly difficult to condone in the modern more gender-aware world.

References

1. Fishel, S., Aslam, I., Lisi, F., Rinaldi, L., Timson, J., Jacobson, M., et al. (2000) Should ICSI be the treatment of choice for all cases of *in-vitro* conception? *Hum Reprod* 15:1278–1283.

2. Ola, B., Afnan, M., Sharif, K., et al. (2001) Should ICSI be the treatment of choice for all cases of *in-vitro* conception? Considerations of fertilization and embryo development, cost-effectiveness and safety. *Hum Reprod* 16:2485–2490.

3. World Health Organization (2010) *WHO Laboratory Manual for the Examination and Processing of Human Semen*. Geneva: World Health Organization.

4. Schatten, G., Hewitson, L., Simerly, C., Sutovsky, P. and Huszar, G. (1998) Cell and molecular biological challenges of ICSI: ART before science? *J Law Med Ethics* 26:29–37.

5. Varghese, A. C., Goldberg, E. and Agarwal, A. (2007) Current and future perspectives on intracytoplasmic sperm injection: a critical commentary. *Reprod Biomed Online*; 15:719–727.

6. Carrell, D. T., Nyboe Andersen, A. and Lamb, D. J. (2015) The need to improve patient care through discriminate use of intracytoplasmic sperm injection (ICSI) and improved understanding of spermatozoa, oocyte and embryo biology. *Andrology* 3:143–146.

7. Evers, J. L. H. (2016) Santa Claus in the fertility clinic. *Hum Reprod* 31:1381–1382.

8. Barratt, C. L. R., De Jonge, C. J. and Sharpe, R. M. (2018) "Man Up": the importance and strategy for placing male reproductive health centre stage in the political and research agenda. *Hum Reprod* 33:541–545.

9. van Rumste, M. M. E, Evers, J. L. H. and Farquhar, C. (2003) Intra-cytoplasmic sperm injection versus conventional techniques for oocyte insemination during *in vitro* fertilisation in couples with non-male subfertility. *Cochrane Database of Systematic Reviews* 2. CD001301

10. Kim, H. H., Bundorf, M. K., Behr, B. and McCallum, S. W. (2007) Use and outcomes of intracytoplasmic sperm injection for non-male factor infertility. *Fertil Steril* **88**:622–628.

11. Nyboe Andersen, A., Carlsen, E. and Loft, A. (2008) Trends in the use of intracytoplasmatic sperm injection marked variability between countries. *Hum Reprod Update* **14**:593–604.

12. ESHRE (2017) Special Interest Group of Embryology and Alpha Scientists in Reproductive Medicine. The Vienna consensus: report of an expert meeting on the development of ART laboratory performance indicators. *Reprod Biomed Online* **35**:494–510.

13. Borini, A., Gambardella, A., Bonu, M, A., et al. (2009) Comparison of IVF and ICSI when only few oocytes are available for insemination. *Reprod Biomed Online* **19**:270–275.

14. Tannus, S., Son, W. Y., Gilman, A., Younes, G., Shavit, T. and Dahan, M. H. (2017) The role of intracytoplasmic sperm injection in non-male factor infertility in advanced maternal age. *Hum Reprod* **32**:119–124.

15. ASRM (2012) The practice committees of the American Society for Reproductive Medicine and Society for Assisted Reproductive Technology. Intracytoplasmic Sperm Injection (ICSI) for non-male factor infertility: a committee opinion. *Fertil Steril* **98**:1395–1399.

16. Mortimer, D., Dufton, M. and MacDonald, J. (2015) *Minimizing Failed and Low IVF Fertilization Rates: Refuting The Concept of "ICSI for All" to Avoid Poor Outcomes*. Halifax, NS: Canadian Fertility and Andrology Society, October 2015. Abstract SC01.

17. Björndahl, L., Mortimer, D., Barratt, C. L. R., Castilla, J. A., Menkveld, R., Kvist, U., et al. (2001) *A Practical Guide to Basic Laboratory Andrology*. Cambridge, UK: Cambridge University Press.

18. Griffiths, T. A., Murdoch, A. P. and Herbert, M. (2000) Embryonic development *in vitro* is compromised by the ICSI procedure. *Hum Reprod* **15**:1592–1596.

19. Shoukir, Y., Chardonnens, D., Campana, A. and Sakka, D. (1998) Blastocyst development from supernumerary embryos after intracytoplasmic sperm injection: a paternal influence? *Hum Reprod* **13**:1632–1637.

20. Bridges, P. J., Jeoung, M., Kim, H., Kim, J. H., Lee, D. R., Ko, C., et al. (2011) Methodology matters: IVF versus ICSI and embryonic gene expression. *Reprod Biomed Online* **23**:234–244.

21. Bhattacharya, S., Hamilton, M. P., Shaaban, M., Khalaf, Y., Seddler, M., Ghobara, T., et al. (2001) Conventional *in-vitro* fertilisation versus intracytoplasmic sperm injection for the treatment of non-male-factor infertility: a randomised controlled trial. *Lancet* **357**:2075–2079.

22. Li, Z., Wang, A. Y., Bowman, M., Hammarberg, K., Farquhar, C., Johnson, L., et al. (2018) ICSI does not increase the cumulative live birth rate in non-male factor infertility. *Hum Reprod* **33**:1322–1330.

23. Boulet, S. L., Mehta, A., Kissin, D. M., Warner, L., Kawwass, J. F. and Jamieson, D. J. (2015) Trends in use of and reproductive outcomes associated with intracytoplasmic sperm injection. *JAMA* **313**:255–263.

24. SART (2016) Society for Assisted Reproductive Technology. SART Clinic Summary Report 2013. www.sartcorsonline.com (membership required for access).

25. Dyer, S., Chambers, G. M., de Mouzon, J., Nygren, K. G., Zegers-Hochschild, F., Mansour, R., et al. (2016) International Committee for Monitoring Assisted Reproductive Technologies world report: Assisted Reproductive Technology 2008, 2009 and 2010. *Hum Reprod* **31**:1588–1609.

26. De Geyter, C., Calhaz-Jorge, C., Kupka, M. S., Wyns, C., Mocanu, E., Motrenko, T., et al. (2018) ART in Europe,

2014: results generated from European registries by ESHRE. *Hum Reprod* **33**:1586–1601.

27. Mortimer, D. (1999) Structured management as a basis for cost-effective infertility care. In Gagnon, C. (ed.) *The Male Gamete: From Basic Science to Clinical Applications*. Vienna, IL, Cache River Press. 363–370.

28. (1995) Sperm transport in the female genital tract. In Grudzinskas. J. G. and Yovich, J. L. (eds.) *Gametes: The Spermatozoon*. Cambridge, Cambridge University Press. 157–174.

29. Franken, D. R. and Bastiaan, H. S. (2009) Can a cumulus cell complex be used to select spermatozoa for assisted reproduction? *Andrologia* **41**:369–376.

30. Sakkas, D., Ramalingam, M., Garrido, N. and Barratt, C. L. (2015) Sperm selection in natural conception: what can we learn from Mother Nature to improve assisted reproduction outcomes? *Hum Reprod Update* **21**:711–726.

31. Miller, D. (2018) *Hyaluronic Acid Binding Sperm Selection for ICSI (HABSelect): Study Outcomes And Conclusions.*, Liverpool, UK: Fertility UK.

32. Harper, J., Jackson, E., Sermon, K., Aitken, R. J., Harbottle, S., Mocanu, E., et al. (2017) Adjuncts in the IVF laboratory: where is the evidence for "add-on" interventions? *Hum Reprod* **32**:485–491.

33. Fleming, S. D., Ilad, R. S., Griffin, A. M., Wu, Y., Ong, K. J., Smith, H. C., et al. (2008) Prospective controlled trial of an electrophoretic method of sperm preparation for assisted reproduction: comparison with density gradient centrifugation. *Hum Reprod* **23**:2646–2651.

34. Quinn, M. M., Jalalian, L., Ribeiro, S., Ona, K., Demirci, U., Cedars, M. I., et al. (2018) Microfluidic sorting selects sperm for clinical use with reduced DNA damage compared to density gradient centrifugation with swim-up in split semen samples. *Hum Reprod* **33**:1388–1393.

35. Mortimer, D. (2000) Sperm preparation methods. *J Androl* **21**:357–366.

36. Mortimer, D. and Mortimer, S. T. (2013) Density gradient separation of sperm for artificial insemination. *Methods Mol Biol* **927**:217–226.

37. Berkovitz, A., Eltes, F., Lederman, H., Peer, S., Ellenbogen, A., Feldberg, B., et al. (2006) How to improve IVF-ICSI outcome by sperm selection. *Reprod Biomed Online* **12**:634–638.

38. Davies, M. J., Moore, V. M., Willson, K. J., Van Essen, P., Priest, K., Scott, H., et al. (2012) Reproductive technologies and the risk of birth defects. *N Engl J Med* **366**:1803–1813.

39. Mortimer, D. (2018) The functional anatomy of the human spermatozoon: relating ultrastructure and function. *Mol Hum Reprod* **24**:567–592.

40. Tateno, H. (2009) Possible causal factors of structural chromosome aberrations in intracytoplasmic sperm injection of the mouse. *Reprod Med Biol* **8**:89–95.

41. Moreira, P. N., Fernández-González, R., Rizos, D., Ramirez, M., Perez-Crespo, M. and Gutiérrez-Adán, A. (2005) Inadvertent transgenesis by conventional ICSI in mice. *Hum Reprod* **20**:3313–3317.

42. Moisyadi, S., Kaminski, J. M. and Yanagimachi, R. (2009) Use of intracytoplasmic sperm injection (ICSI) to generate transgenic animals. *Comp Immunol Microbiol Infect Dis* **32**:47–60.

43. Rawe, V. Y., Olmedo, S. B., Nodar, F. N., et al. (2000) Cytoskeletal organization defects and abortive activation in human oocytes after IVF and ICSI failure. *Mol Hum Reprod* **6**:510–516.

44. Hewitson, L., Dominko, T., Takahashi, D., Martinovich, C., Ramalho-Santos, J., Sutovsky, P., et al. (1999) Unique checkpoints during the first cell cycle of fertilization after intracytoplasmic sperm injection in rhesus monkeys. *Nat Med* **5**:431–433.

45. Hewitson, L., Simerly, C. and Schatten, G. (2000) Cytoskeletal aspects of assisted fertilization. *Semin Reprod Med* **18**:151–159.

Chapter 12

Perinatal Outcomes from IVF and ICSI

Michael Davies

12.1 Introduction

This chapter is a narrative review of the epidemiology of IVF and ICSI as the dominant sub-set of all available assisted reproductive technologies (ART). It is designed to provide the reader with an overview of the principal questions concerning the safety and effectiveness of technologies that have emerged over the last 40 years, from the early years of obscure animal experimentation to become routine medical practice globally for the treatment of infertility. Innovation at the edge of knowledge necessarily involves many steps and occasional leaps based on judgement. The work discussed here focuses on a selected body of literature where the author has confidence in describing the strengths of the research. This is important as much of the relevant literature suffers from serious design imperfections, which in part reflects the limitations of an emerging technology where early available data are partial, fragmented, and related only to short-term and intermediate outcomes. Common weaknesses include small sample size [1,2], pooling of exposure groups [3], or, specifically for case-control studies, retrospective collection of data and questionable appropriateness of controls [1,4,5]. At present, ART is falling short of realising opportunities and obligations to improve the precision and speed of its innovation cycle by not engaging in detailed analyses of clinical data. Nevertheless, with the rapid expansion of ART, we are now in a position to make confident statements on a range of outcomes for both IVF and ICSI, albeit ones that are provisional in the context of future innovation and changing patient characteristics.

12.2 Recent History

The use of assisted reproductive technologies (ART) for the treatment of infertility is increasing dramatically. Globally, more than 7 million babies have been born from assisted conception and this population is now increasing by over 1 million per annum [6]. Australia reflects this international trend; 1 in 25 Australian births are now from ART treatment [7].

In Australia, between 2002 and 2012, the number of ART treatment cycles almost doubled from 35,000 to 65,000 per annum (Figure 12.1). This rapid increase in use of treatments shows limited signs of abating in Australia [7] or internationally [6]. Treatments for infertility range from the simple oral administration of drugs to stimulate ovulation, to more invasive treatments such as IVF and ICSI that involve *in vitro* manipulation of gametes (oocytes and sperm). Data on offspring is only available on births from ART. Since the first IVF birth in 1978, the field of ART has been characterised by continual and rapid innovation, and increasing success in pregnancy and live birth rates (Figure 12.1).

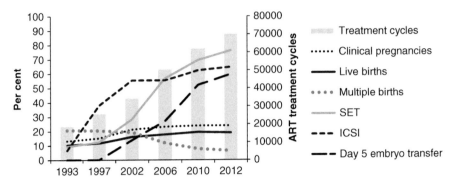

Figure 12.1 Trends in ART treatments and outcomes in Australia and New Zealand, 1993–2012*.
based on annual reports of the Australian and New Zealand Assisted Reproduction Database

However, as ART has expanded, there is also accumulating evidence of adverse health impacts.

Early clinical studies necessarily focused on the short-term outcomes of fertilisation and pregnancy rates. However, we, and others internationally, have demonstrated ART to be associated with increased risks of low birth weight, preterm birth, stillbirth, neonatal death, and major birth defects, and more recently cognitive deficits with the risk of each adverse outcome varying by laboratory and clinical techniques.

Each of these will be discussed in relation to IVF and ICSI based on Australian data, with reference to supporting international work where relevant.

12.3 The South Australian Birth Cohort

We have established a whole population birth cohort, which is a census of all births in South Australia (a State of the Commonwealth of Australia, population 1.6 million) for the period 1986–2002. This includes approximately 327,000 births, including those conceived with ART (~6,500), terminations, and birth defects ascertained to age 5 years (~17,000). These have been linked to all ART treatments, patient diagnoses, and laboratory procedures. This is comprehensive, detailed, representative, and generalisable to other research cites internationally. The cohort is undergoing expansion with plans to eventually become an historical repository covering the entire history of ART technologies and outcomes, including the dramatic expansion of ICSI, the shift to single embryo transfer (SET), routine use of cryopreservation, and changes in embryo culture technology (including extended culture).

12.4 Infertility Patient Records

Details of ART treatment, as defined by the National Health and Medical Research Council (NHMRC) [8], were provided by clinics registered to provide infertility treatment involving embryo manipulation. Greater than 99.99% of ART births were linked to the state birth registry as interstate movements for treatment were rare.

12.5 Perinatal Outcomes

Any ART birth is recorded within the State-wide perinatal collection, which by law requires notification of all live births and stillbirths of at least 20 weeks gestation or 400 g birth weight in South Australia using a standardised notification form (www.health.sa.gov.au/pehs/preg nancyoutcome.htm). Maternal pre-existing medical conditions and conditions in pregnancy are also recorded from the labour ward records onto the notification form. Approximately 20,000 births are recorded annually for South Australia. Notifications of all medical terminations of pregnancy are also required by State law, and those that are induced at 20 weeks gestation or more are included in the perinatal data collection. For completeness, we did not exclude births to women with unknown or out-of-state addresses (0.6% of entire sample, $n = 1,916$).

12.6 Birth Defects

Congenital abnormalities detected at birth or in the neonatal period (within 28 days of birth) are reported by doctors using a standardised Congenital Abnormality Form. The South Australian Birth Defects Register includes information on birth defects (including cerebral palsy) obtained from the perinatal and abortion statistics collections, as well as notifications from multiple sources up to the child's fifth birthday. This is important as only half of major defects are identified at birth (communication, SA Birth Defects Register).

Post-neonatal or "acquired" cerebral palsy cases (i.e. attributed to events occurring after perinatal period) were not included. Birth defects were coded by registry staff independent of birth defect notifications, although blinding of mode of conception by clinical observers issuing notifications was not possible. Prior assessment of the same reporting method in an adjacent jurisdiction revealed no significant reporting bias [9].

Terminations of pregnancy for congenital abnormalities at gestations of less than 20 weeks are reported by law to the Department of Health and included in the State Birth Defects Register. Birth defect diagnoses are validated by cross-referencing of medical reports before being registered, and are coded according to the *British Paediatric Association modification of the International Classification of Diseases, 9th Revision* (ICD-9 BPA), including abnormalities that are structural, biochemical, chromosomal, or other genetic abnormalities. (www .wch.sa.gov.au/services/az/other/phru/birthdefect.html). Minor defects are generally excluded from the register, with the exception of those that require treatment or are disfiguring. Linkage of the ART patient record (used probabilistic matching software) and hand matching (using patient identifiers and birth outcome data) was undertaken. The birth defect data were linked to the perinatal outcomes collection and to the ART pregnancies by a unique accession number for each birth. Hand matching was used to resolve inconsistencies in the patient or birth data between the files, such as family name change for mothers.

Approval for the study was obtained from the ethics committees of the South Australian Department of Health, the University of Adelaide, and the Flinders University of South Australia. As patients were not identified, individual patient consent was not required by the ethics committees.

12.7 Exposures and Outcomes

12.7.1 ART Treatments

We had access to information about all available ART treatments. Each ART conception was classified according to treatment modality: IVF, ICSI, gamete intrafallopian transfer, intrauterine insemination, ovulation induction only, use of donor gametes/embryos, and minimal medical intervention (e.g. women tracking their ovulatory cycles where primary treatment was weight loss); laboratory procedures: culture media type, day of embryo transfer, cryopreservation protocol; and treatment strategy: number of embryos transferred, ovarian stimulation protocol.

12.7.2 Primary Outcomes

- *Adverse perinatal outcomes,* including: stillbirth (fetal death ≥20 completed weeks gestation), birth weight, very low birth weight (<1,500 g), low birth weight (<2,500 g), very preterm birth (<32 completed weeks), preterm birth (<37 completed weeks), post term birth (>41 completed weeks), very small size for gestational age (<3rd percentile), small size for gestational age (<10th percentile), large size for gestational age (>90th percentile), Apgar score (<7 at 5 minutes), and neonatal death.
- *Major birth defect,* which includes a single defect or multiple defects to age 5 years, as defined by the British Paediatric Association modification of the International Classification of Disease (ICD9-BPA), as well as congenital cerebral palsy.
- *Specific classes of birth defects,* including cerebral palsy and the following groups of abnormalities: congenital, cardiovascular, musculoskeletal, urogenital, gastrointestinal, central nervous system, respiratory, chromosomal, metabolic, haematologic, as defined by ICD9-BPA.

12.7.3 Confounders and Covariates

Potential confounding factors include infertility aetiology as documented in ART clinic records, maternal age, parity, foetal sex, year of birth, maternal ethnicity, maternal country of birth, maternal smoking in pregnancy, pre-existing medical conditions, parental occupation (coded to the Australian Standard Classification of Occupations) [10], and postal code indicators of socioeconomic disadvantage from Socio-Economic Indices for Areas [11]. We also have information about pregnancy complications (e.g. gestational diabetes). Whether pregnancy factors are confounders or are on the causal pathway linking ART treatments to adverse outcomes (i.e. mediators) will be considered in the analyses.

12.8 Analysis

The available dataset contained a total of 327,420 births and terminations. After exclusion of births to mothers younger than 20 years (among whom there were only two ART births), there were 308,974 births for analysis. The prevalence of birth defects was compared between the following groups: (i) births as a result of each modality of infertility treatment, including spontaneous pregnancies while a patient was under care; (ii) births as a result of spontaneous pregnancies in women with previous ART birth; (iii) births to women with a history of infertility on their perinatal outcomes record and no history of ART treatment; and (iv) births to women in the general population with no recorded history of infertility or treatment.

Odds ratios (OR) were calculated comparing the prevalence of birth defects between groups using two-tailed *p* values with the aid of SAS statistical software. No adjustment for multiple births was made, except in sensitivity analyses to assess model robustness, as multiple gestation may be considered on the causal pathway between ART exposure and birth defects [9]. Information on the zygosity of twins was not available.

The "crude" estimates include minimal adjustment for the effect of clustering of births within women, using logistic Generalized Estimating Equations. The adjusted analyses included a-priori confounders of maternal age (categorized in 5-year age groups), parity, foetal sex, year of birth, maternal ethnicity, maternal country of birth, and maternal conditions in pregnancy (pre-existing hypertension, pregnancy-induced hypertension, pre-existing diabetes, gestational diabetes, anaemia, urinary tract infection, epilepsy, asthma), maternal smoking in pregnancy, postal code indicators of socioeconomic disadvantage from Socio-economic Indices for Areas [11], and maternal and paternal occupation, coded to the Australian Standard Classification of Occupations [10]. We also pre-specified subgroup analyses for singleton and multiple births, and used pre-specified contrasts to test treatment modality effects (including fresh vs frozen embryo cycles) using the same analytic strategy. There was no adjustment for multiple comparisons.

12.9 Outcomes

There is now a clear body of evidence demonstrating increased risks of poorer perinatal outcomes among ART children [12], with evidence first emerging in 1985 [13]. Historically, the risks have been attributed to an increased prevalence of multiple pregnancies arising in ART, largely due to multiple embryo transfer.

However, relative to natural conceptions, ART singletons have compromised health [12]. Evidence includes our own reports of increased risks of stillbirth (odds ratio [OR] 1.82, 95% CI 1.34–2.48), neonatal death (OR = 2.04 95% CI 1.27–3.26), preterm birth (OR = 1.64, 95% CI 1.46–1.84), low birth weight (OR = 1.98, 95% CI 1.77–2.20), and major birth defects (OR 1.30, 95% CI 1.16–1.45) among singletons conceived with any ART [14,15].

Consistent evidence from individual studies, including registry-based cohort studies [16,17] and meta-analyses has linked assisted conception using *in vitro* fertilisation (IVF) or intra-cytoplasmic sperm injection (ICSI) with an increased risk of birth defects [5, 9,18–21]. The associations between the use of these techniques and birth defects has appeared stronger for singleton than multiple births [4,22].

It is unclear whether the excess of birth defects following IVF and ICSI may be attributable to patient characteristics related to infertility [8], rather than to the treatments, and whether the risk is similar across ART and related therapies [5,23,24].

There is limited understanding of the causes of poor ART outcomes. Parental characteristics related to infertility are likely to contribute to the risk of adverse outcomes including preterm birth and birth defects [12]. Treatment-related factors, particularly mode of fertilisation, have also been proposed [12,25]. Recent meta-analyses confirm that pregnancies resulting from IVF/ICSI have worse perinatal outcomes than natural conceptions [12,26]. However, as both IVF and ICSI comprise a complex set of laboratory and clinical procedures, it is difficult to determine which particular aspects of these treatments are causing poor outcomes. For example, a typical cycle of IVF or ICSI now involves controlled ovulation induction, oocyte retrieval, fertilisation (either IVF or with ICSI), embryo maturation in culture, embryo transfer, and cryopreservation of excess embryos. As a result, there have been calls for research examining the specific factors that are modifiable, rather than implicating IVF or ICSI overall as harmful [27]. The elevated risks associated specifically with one treatment (e.g. ICSI) may also mask reductions in risk over time in other aspects of treatment.

Hence, the current literature is limited by a number of design issues, including the pooling of ART exposure groups, resulting in a lack of specificity in the type, and magnitude of effect, from specific treatment factors.

We have previously demonstrated that the risk of adverse outcomes varies across individual treatment groups. For example, the risk of neonatal death increased further for IVF singletons after fresh embryo transfer (OR = 4.92, 95% CI 2.65–9.11) compared with natural conceptions [7]. Furthermore, singleton ICSI pregnancies were more likely to be complicated by pregnancy-induced hypertension and an increased risk of macrosomia after embryo freezing (OR = 1.54, CI 1.0–2.28), which is consistent with previous studies [28] and may reflect an altered epigenetic signature in the embryo [29]. Risk of major birth defects also varied substantially across treatments, for example the risk was non-significant in IVF singletons but elevated for ICSI (OR = 1.55, 95% CI 1.24–1.94). We showed reduced risks of birth defects after frozen embryo cycles, particularly with ICSI (OR = 1.10, 95% CI 0.65–1.85) [6]. The defects were serious, including cardiac, urogenital, musculoskeletal, and neurological defects.

A limitation of our published work [14,15] is the age of the data, as the most recent births occurred in December 2002. As a result, the findings may not be a reliable guide for contemporary laboratory and clinical practices because the intervening years have seen a number of important changes in culture media, laboratory procedures, clinical practice, and patient infertility diagnosis.

Recent analysis of Nordic birth registry data for the years 1998–2007 [30] identified a steep decline over time in the prevalence of preterm birth among ART singletons (~14–8%), as well as smaller declines in small for gestational age, stillbirth, and infant death (in singletons and twins). The authors suggest that the improvements reflect changes in treatment mix, including greater use of SET, embryo cryopreservation, ICSI, as well as changes in the health profile of couples accessing treatment. However, the Nordic temporal trends were not analysed specifically by these factors, and so the authors could only speculate about their possible impact.

There is also some evidence of improved perinatal outcomes (preterm birth, low birth weight) in more recent ART cohorts examining singleton births from IVF and ICSI [12]. The latest of these cohorts includes ART births until 2006 [31]. Therefore, there is a major gap internationally in knowledge of the safety and effectiveness of ART treatments commonly used in the most recent decade. The extent to which specific changes in ART treatment mix contribute to variation in outcomes in Australia, taking into account patient profile, is unknown. This makes it imperative to create a more contemporary continuously updated dataset, in order to capture the key innovations and changes in practice.

12.10 Recent Innovations

The dramatic rise in the use of ICSI indicates that it is no longer used exclusively for severe semen defects (in ~15% of cases), and now accounts for more than 70% of all treatment cycles globally [32] (Figure 12.1). ICSI improves fertilisation rates, but bypasses a number of biological checkpoints. Recent evidence from Al Kissin's group in Atlanta shows the "take home baby rate" is no better after ICSI, but has worse perinatal outcomes compared to IVF [33]. This confirms that there is a misinformed enthusiasm for ICSI internationally, with recent calls for quantification of the risks of ICSI when used for non-male factor infertility [27].

There are also calls for use of large datasets to examine specific patterns of birth defects associated with ICSI [2] to elucidate underlying mechanisms. Recent studies have indicated a predominance of defects of the cardiovascular, genitourinary, and gastrointestinal systems [2,34], although results have been inconsistent [20]. Existing studies lack statistical power to investigate associations, or to appropriately account for the underlying infertility of couples [26].

Within the last 10 years there has been a significant increase in elective SET, such that now it accounts for the majority (76%) of treatment cycles (Figure 12.1). This practice significantly reduces iatrogenic multiple birth and associated adverse outcomes [30,35,36]. It is important to examine whether the shift to use of SET in Australia has improved perinatal outcomes. First, even though SET is routine in Australia for younger women, multiple embryo transfer still occurs frequently, with twinning still increased fourfold over natural conceptions. In addition, singleton birth after a double embryo transfer (DET) is not benign, as there is evidence that singletons born after SET have higher birth weight than singletons born after DET, and fewer neonatal deaths [30,37].

Consistent with the literature on foetal loss and birth defects [38] we have recently shown that following DET, the presence of a non-progressing foetal co-twin at the 8-week ultrasound (e.g. an empty sac) is associated with a significantly increased risk of major birth defects in the survivor (OR = 2.78), and an overall 18% prevalence of major birth defects [39], which may be due to multiple embryos "cloaking" poor embryos from quality sensing by the endometrium [40]. Therefore, there is a need to further clarify the risks of multiple embryo transfer, particularly when this practice results in a singleton birth, as this is where we observe the defects occurring. We propose that there will be a reduction in the risk of birth defects after elective SET versus DET.

Increasing use of cryopreservation augments SET to reduce multiple pregnancy rates, while also reducing the risk of low birth weight and birth defects, particularly for ICSI [14]. Shifts away from a "slow" freezing method to vitrification whereby the embryo is plunged into liquid nitrogen are occurring, with recent data, particularly from "freeze only" protocols, indicating that children born following the transfer of vitrified embryos may have a higher birth weight when compared with those of fresh or slow frozen embryos [41]. The effect of this technique on perinatal outcomes and birth defects has not been evaluated in detail. The most recent meta-analysis [42] reported that only one study had included congenital abnormalities as an end-point. However, we can now show in our existing dataset (manuscript in preparation) that while cryopreservation is beneficial for defects overall, it does not reduce cardiac defects and may specifically increase the risk of circulatory defects after ICSI (OR = 4.7, CI = 1.89–11.77).

There has been an increased use of extended embryo culture and transfer of blastocysts (i.e. day 5 transfer) to select for longer surviving and potentially euploid embryos [43]. However, this may also alter the pattern of development, where blastocyst transfer is associated with increased monozygotic twinning, which is a risk factor for major adverse outcomes [44,45]. Blastocyst transfer is also associated with an increased risk of birth defects [46,47], which is proposed to occur due to non-physiologic oxygen exposure [48]. Adverse perinatal outcomes were not observed in a recent Australian study [49]; however, birth defects were not examined. Therefore, the impact of day of transfer on perinatal outcomes requires verification, while the risk for birth defects is unclear [12].

Factors in culture media influence fertilisation rates and clinical pregnancy rates, where even small alterations in laboratory parameters result in altered foetal growth *in utero* in animal models [50,51]. Assessment of birth outcomes in humans is scarce and inconsistent. The composition of the culture media for embryo development to the blastocyst stage may alter the birth weight of the babies [52,53], although this finding is not consistent across all studies [54,55]. We have identified that certain brands of culture media were associated with an increased risk of any cardiac defect (OR = 2.56, 1.05–6.23), and of Tetrology of Fallot (OR = 4.16, 1.16–14.9) compared to natural conceptions, controlling for mode of conception and other patient and treatment factors (manuscript in preparation). It is imperative that these and other adverse outcomes are investigated in a contemporary context, as there have been rapid developments in culture media content in the past decade.

12.11 Patient and Treatment Factors

An acknowledged limitation of research on IVF and ICSI outcomes to date has been the difficulty of clearly discerning the independent contribution of patient and treatment factors for adverse outcomes. We are certainly aware that both patient and treatment factors play a critical role in treatment success. However, the obverse is not clear, in part because many of the causes for adverse events in natural conception are unknown, and for events in early pregnancy, unobservable. Second, many of the treatment factors have not been subject to randomisation on a scale that is amenable to the study of infrequent events such as birth defects. It may even be unethical to do so, which means that few studies are appropriately designed for adverse events. Nevertheless, there are precedents for using a multiple alternative number of strategies to identify likely causal relationships, as for instance, there is no RCT of lung cancer and smoking and yet we have a consensus that the relationship is causal. An initial strategy is to use statistical adjustment where, for example, we observed major reductions in the risk of birth defects after adjustment for maternal factors for IVF but not for ICSI [14]. This indicated that maternal factors played a major role for IVF. Further adjustment for infertility aetiology could not eliminate the excess risk of birth defects for ICSI.

A second strategy was to consider fresh versus frozen transfers, where the patient population is largely the same with regard to patient characteristics. Cryopreserved embryos had a lower risk of birth defects, which is indicative of a treatment effect, possibly related to embryo survivorship or the adverse effects of hyperstimulation on the endometrium. However, women with multiple embryos available for freezing may also be healthier, which may result in residual confounding. A third strategy is to use sibling comparisons where the mode of conception varies between siblings. This was used by us to determine that the sibling conceived by ART had an elevated risk of birth defects compared to the naturally conceived sibling [56], which is consistent with a treatment effect. We can also compare patient responses to different treatments where the underlying patient biology is not expected to differ between groups. For instance, we have reported that for IVF, increasing obesity and cigarette smoking are both risk factors for birth defects in natural conceptions and for IVF, but neither are for ICSI [57]. This suggests that ICSI conceptions interact with maternal biology in a distinct but as yet unknown fashion. Comparison with animal data is a further way of identifying potential pathways. Extending the current example, ICSI in particular has been linked to placental inflammation and oxidative stress in a mouse model [58] and altered methylation signatures in the human [59].

12.12 Summary

ART emerged as a "breakthrough" technology that was translated from animal production without the benefit of a pre-existing knowledge base in humans. A series of further changes in techniques have occurred in the absence of high-quality evidence about efficacy and safety, focusing instead on pregnancy and live birth rates [60–62]. This is because of the difficulties in undertaking large, well-controlled studies in this area with adequate sample size, and long-term follow-up, including infrequent but critically important and costly outcomes [27]. As a consequence, there is a lack of reliable contemporary evidence on safety and effectiveness, to inform ART research, policy, and practice internationally.

We propose that there is a hierarchy of risk associated with contemporary treatment strategies, and the challenge is to identify the safest, minimal treatment strategy of known conception benefits before considering riskier and more invasive options. Hence, many adverse events following ART are entirely preventable, as they reflect under-informed patient and clinical choices. For instance, the use of multiple embryo transfer is entirely discretionary, and while Australia has made great progress, multiple births are still elevated several-fold. In many countries, including the USA, about half of ART babies are born from multiple gestations, which we have shown quadruples the risk of congenital cerebral palsy to 9/1,000 births [14]. The additional iatrogenic suffering of the afflicted individual and the immediate family comes at a massive cost. Birth defects are the major cause of infant death and contribute to long-term disability in survivors. Defects occur at up to nearly double the population rate for specific ART treatments, such as fresh-cycle ICSI at 9.9%. This can potentially be halved through use of frozen IVF cycles [14].

More adverse events are linked to modifiable laboratory or clinical practices with established impacts on foetal development (culture media, cryopreservation, drug type and dose) that require detailed feedback on relevant health outcomes during their innovation cycle.

Outcomes such as very preterm birth and very low birth weight are potentially catastrophic and often result in significant family distress. They are also extremely expensive in terms of immediate medical costs as well as long-term care that may be required due to the presence of major disabilities. For instance, estimates of the cost of neonatal intensive care are $2,000–$3,000 per day, with a course of care for a very premature baby at around $300,000 [63]. As the risk of very preterm birth is doubled in ART singletons (occurring in around 2%) [15], this equates to a cost of approximately $600,000 per 100 ART births. Prematurity and poor growth are also early indicators of vulnerability for conditions, including poorer metabolic health and intellectual disability [64].

12.13 The Future

Rapid change in patient and clinical behaviour is feasible. Clinicians and patients have demonstrated a strong willingness to change practice in line with emerging evidence, such as the voluntary adoption of single embryo transfer (SET) in Australia. However, further changes in practice and consumer behaviour are stymied by critical knowledge gaps and confusion over the magnitude and sources of risk [64].

We have a demonstrated capacity to follow individual gametes through fertilisation, embryo and foetal development, birth, and into childhood. We recognise a need to extend population cohorts to examine contemporary treatments, and increase the precision of our observations to inform specific clinical changes. Further developments are feasible to quantify critical perinatal risks across a compendium of all treatment options, past and present, within a single, whole of population cohort. This is potentially feasible using refinements to administrative data repositories, such as the Australian and New Zealand Assisted Reproduction Database (ANZARD) or those held by the Society for Assisted Reproductive Technology (SART, USA) or Human Fertility and Embryo Authority (HFEA, UK). High-quality research data form a valuable independent replication site for critical outcomes and treatment modalities.

References

1. Kurinczuk, J. J., Hansen, M. and Bower, C. (2004) The risk of birth defects in children born after assisted reproductive technologies. *Curr Opin Obstet Gynecol* **16**:201–209.

2. Kurinczuk, J. J. and Bower, C. (1997) Birth defects in infants conceived by intracytoplasmic sperm injection: an alternative interpretation. *BMJ* **315**:1260–1265; discussion 5–6.

3. El-Chaar, D., Yang, Q., Gao, J., et al. (2009) Risk of birth defects increased in pregnancies conceived by assisted human reproduction. *Fertil Steril* **92**:1557–1561.

4. Reefhuis, J., Honein, M. A., Schieve, L. A., Correa, A., Hobbs, C. A. and Rasmussen, S. A. (2009) Assisted reproductive technology and major structural birth defects in the United States. *Hum Reprod* **24**:360–366.

5. Rimm, A. A., Katayama, A. C., Diaz, M. and Katayama, K. P. (2004) A meta-analysis of controlled studies comparing major malformation rates in IVF and ICSI infants with naturally conceived children. *J Assist Reprod Genet* **21**:437–443.

6. Mansour, R., Ishihara, O., Adamson, G. D., et al. (2014) International Committee for Monitoring Assisted Reproductive Technologies world report: Assisted Reproductive Technology 2006. *Hum Reprod* **29**:1536–1551.

7. Macaldowie, A., Wang, Y., Chughtai, A. and Chambers, G. (2014) *Australia's Mothers and Babies 2012*. Sydney, NSW: AIHW National Perinatal Statistics Unit.

8. NHMRC (2007) *Ethical Guidelines on the Use of Assisted Reproductive Technology in Clinical Practice and Research 2004* (revised in 2007). Canberra: NHMRC.

9. Hansen, M., Kurinczuk, J. J., Bower, C. and Webb, S. (2002) The risk of major birth defects after intracytoplasmic sperm injection and *in vitro* fertilization. *Hum Reprod* **346**:725–730.

10. ABS. Australian Standard Classification of Occupations (1990) *ASCO First Edition. Occupation Definitions*. Canberra: ABS.

11. ABS (2006) *Census of Population and Housing. Socio-economic Indices for Areas (SEIFA)*. Canberra: ABS.

12. Pinborg, A., Wennerholm, U. B., Romundstad, L. B., et al. (2013) Why do singletons conceived after assisted reproduction technology have adverse perinatal outcome? Systematic review and meta-analysis. *Hum Reprod Update* **19**:87–104.

13. Lancaster, P. A. (1985) Obstetric outcome. *Clin Obstet Gynaecol* **12**:847–864.

14. Davies, M. J., Moore, V. M., Willson, K. J., et al. (2012) Reproductive technologies and the risk of birth defects. *New Eng J Med* **366**:1803–1813.

15. Marino, J. L., Moore, V. M., Willson, K. J., et al. (2014)Perinatal outcomes by mode of assisted conception and sub-fertility in an Australian data linkage cohort. *PloS one* **9**: e80398.

16. Kallen, B., Finnstrom, O., Nygren, K. G. and Olausson, P. O. (2005) *In vitro* fertilization (IVF) in Sweden: risk for congenital malformations after different IVF methods. *Birth Defects Res A Clin Mol Teratol* **73**:162–169.

17. El-Chaar, D., Yang, Q., Gao, J., et al. (2008) Risk of birth defects increased in pregnancies conceived by assisted human reproduction. *Fertil Steril* **92**(5):1557–1561.

18. Hansen, M., Bower, C., Milne, E., de Klerk, N. and Kurinczuk, J. J. (2005)

Assisted reproductive technologies and the risk of birth defects–a systematic review. *Hum Reprod* **20**:328–338.

19. Schieve, L. A., Rasmussen, S. A. and Reefhuis, J. (2005) Risk of birth defects among children conceived with assisted reproductive technology: providing an epidemiologic context to the data. *Fertil Steril* **84**:1320–1324; discussion 7.

20. Lie, R. T., Lyngstadaas, A., Orstavik, K. H., Bakketeig, L. S., Jacobsen, G. and Tanbo, T. (2005) Birth defects in children conceived by ICSI compared with children conceived by other IVF-methods; a meta-analysis. *Int J Epidem* **34**:696–701.

21. Zhu, J. L., Basso, O., Obel, C., Bille, C. and Olsen, J. (2006) Infertility, infertility treatment, and congenital malformations: Danish national birth cohort. *BMJ*:**333**:679.

22. Lambert, R. D. (2002) Safety issues in assisted reproduction technology: the children of assisted reproduction confront the responsible conduct of assisted reproductive technologies. *Hum Reprod* **17**:3011–3015.

23. Schieve, L. A., Rasmussen, S. A., Buck, G. M., Schendel, D. E., Reynolds, M. A. and Wright, V. C. (2004) Are children born after assisted reproductive technology at increased risk for adverse health outcomes? *Obstet Gynecol* **103**:1154–1163.

24. Lambert, R. D. (2003) Safety issues in assisted reproductive technology: aetiology of health problems in singleton ART babies. *Hum Reprod* **18**:1987–1991.

25. Maheshwari, A., Pandey, S., Shetty, A., Hamilton, M. and Bhattacharya, S. (2012) Obstetric and perinatal outcomes in singleton pregnancies resulting from the transfer of frozen thawed versus fresh embryos generated through *in vitro* fertilization treatment: a systematic review and meta-analysis. *Fertil Steril* **98**:368–77e1–9.

26. Hansen, M. and Bower, C. (2014) The impact of assisted reproductive technologies on intra-uterine growth and birth defects in singletons. *Semin Fetal Neonatal Med* **19**:228–233.

27. Barnhart, K. T. (2013) Assisted reproductive technologies and perinatal morbidity: interrogating the association. *Fertil Steril* **99**:299–302.

28. Pinborg, A., Henningsen, A. A., Loft, A., Malchau, S. S., Forman, J. and Andersen, A. N. (2014) Large baby syndrome in singletons born after frozen embryo transfer (FET): is it due to maternal factors or the cryotechnique? *Hum Reprod* **29**:618–627.

29. Whitelaw, N., Bhattacharya, S., Hoad, G., Horgan, G. W., Hamilton, M. and Haggarty, P. (2014) Epigenetic status in the offspring of spontaneous and assisted conception. *Hum Reprod* **29**(7):1452–1458.

30. Henningsen, A. A., Gissler, M., Skjaerven, R., et al. (2015) Trends in perinatal health after assisted reproduction: a Nordic study from the CoNARTaS group. *Hum Reprod* **30**(3):710–716.

31. Sazonova, A., Källen, K., Thurin-Kjellberg, A., Wennerholm U-B. and Bergh. C. (2012) Obstetric outcome in singletons *after in vitro* fertilization with cryopreserved/thawed embryos. *Hum Reprod* **27**:1343–1350.

32. Macaldowie. A., Wang. Y., Chambers. G. and Sullivan. E. (2012) *Assisted reproductive technology in Australia and New Zealand 2010*. Canberra: AIHW.

33. Boulet. S. L., Mehta. A., Kissin. D. M., Warner. L., Kawwass. J. F. and Jamieson. D. J. (2015) Trends in use of and reproductive outcomes associated with intracytoplasmic sperm injection. *JAMA* **313**:255–263.

34. Tararbit. K., Houyel. L., Bonnet. D., et al. (2011) Risk of congenital heart defects associated with assisted reproductive technologies: a population-based evaluation. *Eur Heart J* **32**:500–508.

35. van Heesch. M. M., Evers. J. L., Dumoulin. J. C., et al. (2014) A comparison of perinatal outcomes in singletons and multiples born after *in vitro* fertilization or intracytoplasmic sperm injection stratified for neonatal risk criteria. *Acta Obstet Gynecol Scand* **93**:277–286.

36. Toshimitsu. M., Nagamatsu. T., Nagasaka. T., et al. (2014) Increased risk of pregnancy-induced hypertension and operative delivery after conception induced by *in vitro* fertilization/intracytoplasmic sperm injection in women aged 40 years and older. *Fertil Steril* **102**(4):1065–1070.

37. Okun, N. and Sierra, S. Genetics Committee: Special Contributors (2014) Pregnancy outcomes after assisted human reproduction. *J Obstet Gynaecol Can* **36**:64–83.

38. Pinborg, A., Lidegaard, O. and Andersen, A. N. (2006) The vanishing twin: a major determinant of infant outcome in IVF singleton births. *Br J Hosp Med (Lond)* **67**:417–420.

39. Davies, M. J., Rumbold, A. R., Whitrow, M. J., et al. (2016) Spontaneous loss of a co-twin and the risk of birth defects after assisted conception. *J Dev Orig Health Dis* **7**:678–684.

40. Teklenburg, G., Salker, M., Molokhia, M., et al. (2010) Natural selection of human embryos: decidualizing endometrial stromal cells serve as sensors of embryo quality upon implantation. *PloS one* **5**: e10258.

41. Liu, S. Y., Teng, B., Fu, J., Li, X., Zheng, Y. and Sun, X. X. (2013) Obstetric and neonatal outcomes after transfer of vitrified early cleavage embryos. *Hum Reprod* **28**:2093–2100.

42. AbdelHafez, F. F., Desai, N., Abou-Setta, A. M., Falcone, T. and Goldfarb, J. (2010) Slow freezing, vitrification and ultra-rapid freezing of human embryos: a systematic review and meta-analysis. *Reprod Biomed online* **20**:209–222.

43. Vega, M., Breborowicz, A., Moshier, E. L., McGovern, P. G. and Keltz, M. D. (2014) Blastulation rates decline in a linear fashion from euploid to aneuploid embryos with single versus multiple chromosomal errors. *Fertil Steril* **102**:394–398.

44. Kanter, J. R., Boulet, S. L., Kawwass, J. F., Jamieson, D. J. and Kissin, D. M. (2015) Trends and correlates of monozygotic twinning after single embryo transfer. *Obstet Gynecol* **125**:111–117.

45. Wright, V., Schieve, L. A., Vahratian, A. and Reynolds, M. A. (2004) Monozygotic twinning associated with day 5 embryo transfer in pregnancies conceived after IVF. *Hum Reprod* **19**:1831–1836.

46. Pinborg, A., Henningsen, A. K., Malchau, S. S. and Loft, A. (2013) Congenital anomalies after assisted reproductive technology. *Fertil Steril* **99**:327–332.

47. Kallen, B., Finnstrom, O., Lindam, A., Nilsson, E., Nygren, K. G. and Olausson, P. O. (2010) Blastocyst versus cleavage stage transfer in *in vitro* fertilization: differences in neonatal outcome? *Fertil Steril* **94**:1680–1683.

48. Gardner, D. K. (2016) The impact of physiological oxygen during culture, and vitrification for cryopreservation, on the outcome of extended culture in human IVF. *Reprod Biomed Online* **32**:137–141.

49. Chambers, G. M., Chughtai, A. A., Farquhar, C. M. and Wang, Y. A. (2015) Risk of preterm birth after blastocyst embryo transfer: a large population study using contemporary registry data from Australia and New Zealand. *Fertil Steril* **104**:997–1003.

50. Zander-Fox, D., Lane, M. and Hamilton, H. (2013) Slow freezing and vitrification of mouse morula and early blastocysts. *J Assist Reprod Genet* **30**:1091–1098.

51. Banwell, K. M., Lane, M., Russell, D. L., Kind, K. L. and Thompson, J. G. (2007) Oxygen concentration during mouse oocyte *in vitro* maturation affects embryo and fetal development. *Hum Reprod* **22**:2768–2775.

52. Kleijkers, S. H., van Montfoort, A. P., Smits, L. J., et al. (2014) IVF culture medium affects post-natal weight in humans during the first 2 years of life. *Hum Reprod* **29**(4):661–669.

53. Eskild, A., Monkerud, L. and Tanbo, T. (2013) Birthweight and placental weight; do changes in culture media used for IVF matter? Comparisons with spontaneous pregnancies in the corresponding time periods. *Hum Reprod* **28**:3207–3214.

54. Vergouw, C. G., Kostelijk, E. H., Doejaaren, E., Hompes, P. G. A., Lambalk, C. B. and Schats, R. (2012) The influence of the type of embryo culture medium on neonatal birthweight after single embryo transfer in IVF. *Hum Reprod (Oxford, UK)* **27**:2619–2626.

55. Carrasco, B., Boada, M., Rodriguez, I., Coroleu, B., Barri, P. N. and Veiga, A. (2013) Does culture medium influence offspring birth weight? *Fert Steril* **100**:1283–1288.

56. Davies, M. J., Moore, V. M. and Haan, E. A. (2012) Reproductive technologies and the risk of birth defects reply. *New Eng J Med* **367**:875–876.

57. Davies, M. J., Rumbold, A. R., Marino, J. L., et al. (2017) Maternal factors and the risk of birth defects after IVF and ICSI: a whole of population cohort study. *BJOG: Int J Obstet Gyn* **124**:1537–1544.

58. Raunig, J. M., Yamauchi, Y., Ward, M. A. and Collier, A. C. (2011) Placental inflammation and oxidative stress in the mouse model of assisted reproduction. *Placenta* **32**:852–858.

59. Nelissen, E. C., Dumoulin, J. C., Daunay, A., Evers, J. L., Tost, J. and van Montfoort, A. P. (2013) Placentas from pregnancies conceived by IVF/ICSI have a reduced DNA methylation level at the H19 and MEST differentially methylated regions. *Hum Reprod* **28**:1117–1126.

60. Allen, V. M., Wilson, R. D. and Cheung, A. (2006) Pregnancy outcomes after assisted reproductive technology. *J Obstet Gynaecol Can* **28**:220–250.

61. Medical Advisory Secretariat (2006) *In vitro* fertilization and multiple pregnancies: an evidence-based analysis. *Ont Health Technol Assess Ser* **6**:1–63.

62. Myers, E. R., McCrory, D. C., Mills, A. A., et al. (2008) *Effectiveness of Assisted Reproductive Technology (ART). Evid Rep Technol Assess (Full Rep)* 1–195.

63. Petrou, S., Eddama, O. and Mangham, L. (2011) A structured review of the recent literature on the economic consequences of preterm birth. *Arch Dis Childhood Fetal Neonatal Edn* **96**:F225–232.

64. Hart, R. and Norman, R. J. (2013) The longer-term health outcomes for children born as a result of IVF treatment. Part I: General health outcomes. *Hum Reprod Update* **19**:232–243.

Chapter 13

Artificial Insemination with Partner's Sperm for Male Subfertility

Willem Ombelet

13.1 Introduction

Infertility is a universal health issue and it has been estimated that 8–12% of couples worldwide are infertile, with 9% currently cited as the probable global average and remarkably similar between more and less developed countries [1].

Assisted reproductive technologies (ART) are considered as an established therapy for the treatment of infertility in a multitude of clinical conditions. They embrace a wide scope of techniques of which intrauterine insemination (IUI), *in vitro* fertilization (IVF), and intra-cytoplasmic sperm injection (ICSI) are the most popular.

IUI is easy to learn, requires less equipment, and is less expensive and less invasive than IVF/ICSI, with a reasonable success rate within three or four cycles. It is associated with reduced psychological burden and the couple compliance is usually good with a low drop-out rate. In addition, the risk of ovarian hyperstimulation syndrome (OHSS) is reduced and the rate of multiple pregnancies is also lower when performed with natural cycles, clomiphene citrate, or low-dose Human Menopausal Gonadotropins (HMG) stimulation protocols. It is a safe and easy treatment with minimal risks and monitoring.

Nevertheless, the use of AIH (artificial insemination with homologous sperm) as a first-line treatment in case of unexplained and mild/moderate male infertility remained controversial until very recently. This was caused by a lack of prospective randomized trials and large prospective cohort studies as a result of the low budget linked to IUI when compared to the budget associated with other methods of assisted reproduction such as IVF and ICSI. Therefore, large multicentre trials organized by the pharmaceutical industry are not available on the IUI scene, for obvious reasons.

To find out which couples can benefit from AIH in case of male infertility we need to investigate the power of different semen parameters in predicting success after AIH. Huge differences in methodology in semen analysis worldwide make it difficult to draw some conclusions, although the World Health Organization tried to standardize the performances of semen analysis and related procedures in order to reduce variation in the results obtained. A literature search on this topic remains frustrating due to the ongoing lack of standardization in interpretation of semen results.

Based on the results of an ESHRE Capri workshop in 2009, IUI was considered to be a poor substitute for IVF and responsible for a significant rate of high-order multiple births. The recommendations were made in the absence of proper trials and live birth data were not available [2]. It was also not mentioned that the high rate of multiple pregnancies was mostly seen outside Europe and due to the use of high doses of gonadotrophins, especially in the USA.

The NICE guidelines [3] recommended that IUI should not be used in cases of unexplained and moderate male subfertility. According to these guidelines "expectant management was recommended as the first line option and IUI has a very limited value in infertility care." It is well known that the NICE guidelines were being constructed by using the data of a few studies with obvious shortcomings and not taking into account the HFEA data showing an UK average pregnancy rate of 13% per cycle for IUI in 2011 and 2012 [4–7]. Ignoring these guidelines, surveys performed in the UK showed that 96% of fertility clinics continued to offer IUI – despite the NICE recommendations [8, 9].

Since then, a number of excellent randomized trials have been published supporting the value of IUI in unexplained and mild/moderate male subfertility cases. In a multicentre randomized noninferiority trial in the Netherlands, the effectiveness of IVF with single embryo transfer or IVF in a modified natural cycle was compared with the effectiveness of IUI-OS (ovarian stimulation) with a healthy live birth as the main outcome parameter [10].

IUI-OS seemed to be noninferior compared to the two alternative strategies of IVF, with a reasonably and comparable low multiple birth rate. By investigating the direct healthcare costs in the same cohort of patients, IUI turned out to be the most cost-effective strategy for heterosexual couples with mild male factor or unexplained infertility with a poor prognosis of becoming pregnant through normal coitus [11].

Farquhar and colleagues [12] published the results of an RCT in which 201 couples with 3–4 years unexplained infertility were randomized to receive three cycles of IUI or expectant management. A live birth rate of 31% with IUI and 9% with expectant management was observed, a threefold difference in outcome.

According to the literature it is obvious that we are over-using IVF to treat unexplained and moderate male infertility. Evidence-based data in 2019 clearly indicate that promoting IVF and ICSI to result in pregnancy "as quick as possible" ignores the advantages of IUI completely in cases of mild or moderate male factor infertility.

13.2 Factors Influencing AIH Outcome in Male Subfertility

Many different factors can influence the success rates in IUI programmes. We give an overview of the most important factors associated with AIH outcome.

13.2.1 Semen Quality

As mentioned before, there is a worldwide lack of standardization in interpretation of semen samples. Despite the use of various external quality control systems and the WHO laboratory manuals to improve the value of semen examinations, the results remain poor. Consequently, the value of semen parameters in predicting ART outcome is difficult to interpret when reviewing the literature.

We performed a structured review to investigate the threshold levels of sperm parameters above which IUI pregnancy outcome is significantly improved or the cut-off values reaching substantial discriminative performance in an IUI programme [13].

In 20 selected articles, the IMC (Inseminating Motile Count or the number of motile sperm inseminated) was cited as an important predictive parameter, in 8 out of 20 studies a cut-off value of 1 million was mentioned, in 4 studies between 1 and 2 million, and in 5 studies the authors calculated a threshold value of 5 million. Sperm morphology using strict criteria was the second-most cited sperm parameter. In 11 out of 15 studies, 4% normal forms were reported as the best cut-off value. When utilizing these cut-off values of sperm

Table 13.1 According to a structured review [13], the success rate of AIH is improved with a morphology score of more than 4% normal forms, an IMC of more than 1 million, a TMSC of more than 5 million, and an initial total motility of more than 30%

Sperm morphology using strict criteria	**>4 %**
Inseminating Motile Count (IMC)	**>1 million**
Total Motile Sperm Counts (TMSC)	**>5 million**
Total Motility in native sample (TM)	**>30 %**

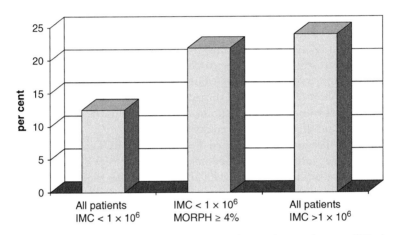

Figure 13.1 Cumulative live birth rate after three inseminations (IUIs) with partner's semen (IMC = Inseminating Motile Count; Morph = sperm morphology using strict criteria) [14].

morphology and IMC, there is poor sensitivity for predicting who will conceive but a high specificity for predicting failure to conceive with IUI. The TMSC (Total Motile Sperm Count before sperm washing) was also reported to be an important predictive parameter in 10 papers, with a cut-off value of 5 million in 5 papers and 10 million in 5 papers [13] (Table 13.I).

Already in 1997 we published the results of a study examining the predictive value of sperm parameters in an AIH programme. We observed that an IMC of 1 million was at a reasonable threshold level above which IUI can be performed with acceptable pregnancy rates. Overall, sperm morphology and IMC were of no prognostic value using ROC curve analysis. Sperm morphology turned out to be a valuable prognostic parameter in predicting IUI success if the IMC was less than 1 million (area under ROC curve: 77.6%). The cumulative live birth rate (CLBR) after three IUI cycles was 13.6% if the IMC was less than 1 million, significantly different from the group with an IMC of less than 1 million (22.4%, $p < 0.05$). Considering only patients with IMC of less than 1 million and sperm morphology more than 4%, the CLBR was 21.9%, comparable with the CLBR of all cycles with a normal semen sample or an IMC of more than 1 million [14] (Figure 13.1). The proposed algorithm for male subfertility we have used in our centre since 1998 is shown in Figure 13.2.

Merviel and colleagues [15] reported the data of a retrospective analysis of 1,038 AIH cycles performed between 2002 and 2005 in a single university medical centre, aiming to

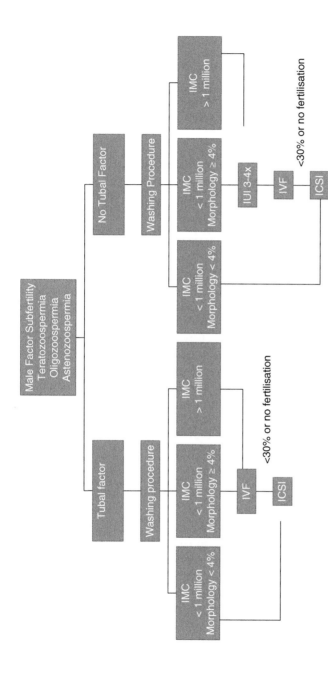

Figure 13.2 Proposed algorithm for male subfertility treatment at the Genk Institute for Fertility Technology since 1998 [14].

determine the predictive factors for pregnancy after AIH. According to their results, a TMSC of 5 million or more could be used as a threshold value above which AIH is more successful.

According to Lemmens and colleagues [16], AIH is especially relevant for couples with moderate male factor infertility. They observed a positive relationship for less than or equal to 4% of morphologically normal spermatozoa (odds ratio [OR] 1.39) and a moderate IMC (5–10 million; OR 1.73). Low IMC values showed a negative relation (≤1 million; OR 0.42). In the multivariable model, however, the predictive power of these sperm parameters was rather low. These data were based on the results of a retrospective, observational study with logistic regression analyses of 4,251 first AIH cycles in 1,166 couples visiting the fertility laboratory for their first AIH episode.

Comparable results were obtained in a prospective cohort study of 1,401 AIH cycles in 556 couples in our AIH programme in Genk [17]. Univariate statistical analysis revealed female and male age, male smoking, female body mass index, ovarian stimulation, and inseminating motile count (IMC) as covariates significantly influencing CPR (clinical pregnancy rate) per cycle. Multivariate GEE analysis (generalized estimating equations) revealed that the only valuable prognostic covariates included female age, male smoking, and infertility status (i.e. primary/secondary infertility). IMC showed a significant curvilinear relationship, with first an increase and then a decrease in pregnancy rate, with the best results for an IMC of between 5 and 10 million [17].

Moolenaar and colleagues [18] made use of a computer-simulated cohort of subfertile women to examine the cost-effectiveness of AIH compared to IVF and ICSI. The base-case calculation was centred on a 30-year-old woman with a regular menstrual cycle, normal fallopian tubes, and a partner with a pre-wash TMSC between 0 and 10 million. A 30-year-old woman was selected because previous studies of pregnancy probabilities according to pre-wash TMSC were based on couples in whom the woman had a mean age near 30 years. Three different treatment options were investigated: AIH with and without controlled ovarian stimulation, IVF, and ICSI. The main outcome was expected live birth; secondary outcomes were cost per couple and the incremental cost-effectiveness ratio. If only cost per live birth is considered for each treatment, above a pre-wash TMSC of 3 million, AIH seemed to be less costly than IVF and below a pre-wash TMSC of 3 million, ICSI is less costly.

13.2.2 Male Age

Increased male age seems to be associated with a decline in semen volume, sperm motility, and sperm morphology but not with sperm concentration. Semen parameters start to decline after 35 years of age. Male fertility was found to decrease substantially in the late 30s and continues to decrease after age 40 [19]. Nevertheless, in contrast to female fertility, male fertility is maintained until very late in life. Age-dependent decrease of fertility in couples is usually attributed to female ageing, which makes studies on a male age effect difficult. In addition to female age, other confounders such as reduced coital frequency and an increasing incidence of erectile dysfunction may play an important role as well. It seems that for natural conception, paternal age has a limited effect whenever the female partner is young. Time to pregnancy is longer with advancing age of men. However, when the female partner too is of age, then a synergistic adverse effect of paternal age is observed.

The more invasive the treatment, the less important the effect of male age; success rates of IVF or ICSI are not affected by male age. On the other hand, the success rate of intra-uterine insemination (IUI) is affected by male age, probably because IUI requires sperm of much higher quality compared to IVF and ICSI [19]. According to the actual literature, paternal age has no impact on IUI success rates as long as the female partner is less than 35 years.

On the other hand, oxidative stress-induced mtDNA damage and nuclear DNA damage in ageing men may put them at a higher risk for transmitting multiple genetic and chromosomal defects. Paternal age above 40 years seems to be a risk factor for spontaneous abortion.

13.2.3 Oxidative Stress

A number of factors are responsible for the low pregnancy rates seen with IUI, including oxidative stress. Oxidative stress occurs when there is excessive generation of reactive oxygen species (ROS) and/or underproduction of protective enzymatic and nonenzymatic antioxidants. ROS, at low levels, are essential for facilitating complex cellular redox inter-actions and modifying biological molecules, for example, DNA, proteins, and lipids in various cellular organelles. Low levels of ROS can also enhance the ability of human spermatozoa to bind with the zonae pellucida, an effect that is hampered by the addition of the antioxidant vitamin E. Low concentrations of hydrogen peroxide (H_2O_2), when incubated with spermatozoa, can stimulate sperm capacitation and induce spermatozoa to undergo the acrosome reaction and fuse with other types of ROS (e.g. nitric oxide and superoxide anion (O_2) can also promote sperm capacitation and the acrosome reaction) [20].

High levels of seminal ROS are present in 40–80% of unselected infertile men. Seminal ROS commonly occurs in men with varicocele, leukocytospermia, and/or idiopathic infertility. The main sources of ROS are immature sperm and seminal leukocytes [20].

Bungum and colleagues [21] examined the relationship between the results of sperm chromatin structure assay (SCSA) and the outcome of IVF, ICSI, and intrauterine insemi-nation. A total of 387 intrauterine insemination (IUI) cycles were included. SCSA results were expressed as DNA fragmentation index (DFI). Clinical pregnancy rate and delivery rate were significantly higher in the group with DFI less than or equal to 30% than in patients with DFI of more than 30%. In the latter group, the results of ICSI were significantly better than those of IVF.

According to a systematic review performed by Cho and Agarwal [22], current evidence supports the association between high SDF (sperm DNA fragmentation) and poor repro-ductive outcomes for natural conception and intrauterine insemination.

13.2.4 Semen Preparation Techniques

Sperm preparation techniques (SPTs) should isolate and select sperm cells with intact functional and genetic properties, including normal morphology, minimal DNA damage, and intact cell membranes with functional binding properties [23]. Sperm processing techniques are used to prepare a concentrated volume of highly motile sperm. The handling of semen samples during these procedures may result in excessive generation of ROS. There are two commonly used techniques: density-gradient centrifugation (DGC) and the swim-up technique. The first technique uses centrifugation to separate fractions of spermatozoa based upon their motility, size, and density. The mature, leukocyte-free spermatozoa are separated from the immature immotile sperm and are then centrifuged. However, the process of centrifugation itself can provoke leukocytes to generate high levels of ROS. Double-density gradient centrifugation is especially associated with high levels of ROS. Reducing the centrifugation time rather than the centrifugation force can minimize the generation of ROS and may assist in retrieval of the highest proportion of mature sperm.

The other technique used to prepare semen for IUI is the swim-up technique, in which highly motile sperm are separated based on their natural ability to migrate against gravity. This technique may be inappropriate for semen samples that contain a high concentration of ROS producer cells such as leukocytes, and immature and damaged spermatozoa [23]. A Cochrane review did not find any significant differences in pregnancy rates between these two techniques in the setting of AIH [24].

On the other hand, Ricci and colleagues [25] showed that the DGC technique resulted in higher recovery rates of total motile, progressive motile, and viable sperm than the swim-up technique. Because the most harmful effects of ROS on sperm are seen in motility and viability, it seems plausible that DGC is associated with the least amount of ROS. Unfortunately, no studies have directly assessed the impact of these techniques on ROS generation and the relationship to IUI outcomes.

To conclude, there is insufficient evidence to recommend any specific SPT at this moment. Novel sperm selection methods based on sperm surface charge or nonapoptotic sperm selection show promising results. Selection based on sperm surface charge did not lead to any improvement in fertilization rates or embryo quality following ICSI. The zeta potential method was reported in one study to increase fertilization, implantation, and pregnancy rates, although not significantly.

Nonapoptotic sperm selection by Magnetic Activated Cell Sorting (MACS) resulted in spermatozoa with higher motility and less apoptosis, higher embryo cleavage, and higher pregnancy rates. Fertilization or implantation rates were not higher. More evidence is needed before using them routinely in AIH programmes [23].

13.2.5 Ovarian Hyperstimulation

The rationale behind IUI is increasing the number of available motile spermatozoa at the site of fertilization. In addition to increase the number of spermatozoa, one can also increase the number of available oocytes by applying ovarian hyperstimulation. With the use of hyperstimulation one might also overcome subtle cycle disturbances, and increase the accuracy of timing of the insemination. On the other hand, applying hyperstimulation increases the probability of achieving multiple pregnancies. Therefore, ovarian hyperstimulation in IUI programmes should be applied when proven effective only [26].

AIH in combination with (mild) ovarian hyperstimulation seems effective in couples with mild male subfertility defined as an average total motile sperm count above 10 million and more than 0.8 million motile sperm after preparation [26].

When ovarian hyperstimulation is applied one should strive after the occurrence of two follicles (using mild stimulation starting with 50–75 IU FSH per day) and gonadotrophins are the drugs of first choice.

13.2.6 Number of IUIs per Cycle

The current available evidence suggests a time frame in which the insemination can be performed from 12 to 36 hours after hCG injection. Most of the national and international guidelines advise a single IUI per cycle. However, double insemination may be the answer when more dominant follicles, which rupture at different time intervals, are available due to ovarian hyperstimulation [27].

Data from the literature show that repeating the insemination procedure after 12 or 24 hours in the same cycle is not effective in couples suffering from unexplained subfertility [28]. For male subfertility, one study reported a positive effect of double insemination. In a prospective randomized study, 1,257 COH-IUI cycles were performed, including 776 cycles with mild or moderate male factor infertility and 494 cycles with idiopathic infertility [29]. According to their results, double IUI increases the pregnancy rate significantly in patients with male factor infertility, and single IUI acts as efficient as double IUI in patients with idiopathic or unexplained infertility.

We believe that more randomized controlled trials are needed to confirm the outcome results of this latter study.

13.3 HPV Infections and IUI Outcome

A meta-analysis of Xiong and colleagues [30] of eight articles, providing data on 1,955 participants, suggest that human papillomavirus (HPV) infection of semen is a risk factor for male fertility abnormality with an OR of 3.02 (95% CI: 2.11–4.32; $I^2 = 6.9\%$). Sensitivity analysis revealed that the results of this study were robust. According to this analysis it is clear that HPV infection of semen represents a risk factor for male fertility abnormality and subsequently can influence AIH outcome results.

In another study it was shown that the presence of the HPV in semen impact seminal parameters and sperm DNA quality in white European men seeking medical help for primary couple's infertility [31]. In this cross-sectional study, complete demographic, clinical, and laboratory data from 729 infertile men were analysed. The overall rate of HPV positivity was 15.5%. Sperm progressive motility was significantly lower ($P = 0.01$) while SDF values were higher ($P = 0.005$) in HPV+ men compared to those with no HPV. HR (high risk) HPV+ men had a significantly lower sperm progressive motility and higher SDF values than those with a negative HPV test.

Another cross-sectional study included a cohort of 430 males. Overall, HPV was detected in 14.9% (64/430) of semen samples. In this study an association between HPV presence in semen and impairment of semen quality could not be found [32].

In a prospective non-interventional multi-centre study of 732 infertile couples undergoing 1,753 AIH cycles with capacitated sperm, it was recently reported that women inseminated with HPV-positive sperm had 4 times less clinical pregnancies compared to women who had HPV-negative partners. HPV prevalence in sperm was 12.5%/cycle. Detection of HPV-virions in sperm was associated with a negative IUI outcome, and according to these results, HPV screening in semen should be part of the routine examination and counselling of infertile couples [33].

13.4 Immunologic Male Infertility

Immunologic male infertility is considered an important issue among fertility specialists. The problem is recognized as difficult to treat, and the results of IUI programmes are stated to be poor.

In developed countries the most important origin of ASAs (antisperm antibodies) is probably vasectomy. More than 80% of vasectomized males develop ASAs during the first year following their operation. In most cases it concerns IgGs which are considered to be less harmful. Nevertheless, even IgAs are frequently found in these males, considering that this type of ASA interferes more powerfully with fertility. Immunological infertility can, however, be found in several other clinical situations such as torsion of the testis, varicocele, testicular trauma, and orchitis [34].

The choice of the most appropriate treatment for the individual couple with immunologic male infertility is often a difficult one, especially in couples after vasectomy reversal. Although it is widely accepted that in severe cases of immunologic male infertility (>80% antibody coated), ICSI has to be recommended, but AIH can play a particular role in the treatment of this situation with reasonable results [35].

There is a need for a good pretreatment tool predicting the success rate of *in utero* insemination in couples with immunologic male infertility. The IMC may have a unique value as a prognostic tool, since it reflects the motile sperm available for insemination. Nevertheless, at this moment no studies are available confirming this theory.

13.5 Conclusive Remarks

- IUI should be used as a first-line treatment in cases of moderate male subfertility, provided more than 1 million motile spermatozoa are available after washing and at least one tube is patent.
- The success rate of AIH is improved with a morphology score of more than 4% normal forms, a TMSC of more than 5 million, and an initial total motility of more than 30%.
- The influence of sperm parameters on AIH outcome is influenced by other parameters such as female age and number of follicles obtained after ovarian stimulation.
- Men with a female partner above 35 years should be informed that increasing paternal age (40 years and above) has a potential negative impact on IUI success rates.
- Concerning sperm preparation, the DGC is shown to be superior to swim-up and wash techniques, with an improvement of morphological normal spermatozoa with grade A motility and normal DNA integrity, reduced concentrations of ROS and leucocytes, etc.
- Concerning clinical outcome (pregnancy rates) after AIH, there is no clear evidence of which Sperm Preparation Test is superior.
- Double IUI results in higher pregnancy rates compared with single IUI in couples with male factor subfertility.
- IUI in combination with (mild) ovarian hyperstimulation seems effective in couples with mild male subfertility defined as an average total motile sperm count above 10 million.
- High sperm DNA damage is associated with low IUI pregnancy rates.
- Screening for antisperm antibodies before the start of IUI could be of use.

References

1. Boivin, J., Bunting, L., Collins, J. A. and Nygren, K. G. (2007) International estimates of infertility prevalence and treatment-seeking: potential need and demand for infertility medical care. *Hum Reprod* 22:1506–1512.

2. ESHRE Capri Workshop Group (2009) Intrauterine insemination. *Hum Reprod Update* 15:265–277.

3. NICE (2013) *Fertility Problems: Assessment and Treatment*. London. Available at: www.nice.org.uk/guidance/cg156?unlid=86583397720167208641.

4. Bhattacharya, S., Harrild, K., Mollison, J., Wordsworth, S., Tay, C., Harrold, A., et al. (2008) Clomifene citrate or unstimulated intrauterine insemination compared with expectant management for unexplained infertility: pragmatic randomised controlled trial. *BMJ* 337:a716.

5. Reindollar, R. H., Regan, M. M., Neumann, P. J., et al. (2010) A randomized clinical trial to evaluate optimal treatment for unexplained infertility: the fast track and standard treatment (FASTT) trial. *Fertil Steril* 94:888–899.

6. HFEA (2015) *Latest UK Fertility Treatment Data and Figures: 2011–2012*. Available at: www.hfea.gov.uk/104.htlm

7. Wordsworth, S., Buchanan, J., Mollison, J., Harrild, K., Robertson, L., Tay, C., et al. (2011) Clomifene citrate and intrauterine insemination as first-line treatments for unexplained infertility: are they cost-effective? *Hum Reprod* 26:369–375.

8. Bahadur, G., Homburg, R., Muneer, A., Racich, P., Alangaden, T., et al. (2016) First line fertility treatment strategies regarding IUI and IVF require clinical evidence. *Hum Reprod* 31:1141–1146.

9. Kim, D., Child, T. and Farquhar, C. (2015) Intrauterine insemination: a UK survey on the adherence to NICE clinical guidelines by fertility clinics. *BMJ Open* 5:e007588.

10. Bensdorp, A. J., Tjon-Kon-Fat, R. I., Bossuyt, P. M. M., Koks, C. A. M., Oosterhuis, G. J. E., et al. (2015) Prevention of multiple pregnancies in couples with unexplained or mild male subfertility: randomised controlled trial of *in vitro* fertilisation with single embryo transfer or *in vitro* fertilisation in modified natural cycle compared with intrauterine insemination. *BMJ* 350:g7771.

11. Tjon-Kon-Fat, R. I., Bensdorp, A. J., Bossuyt, P. M. M., Koks, C., Oosterhuis, G. J. E., Hoek, A., et al. (2015) Is IVF-served two different ways more cost-effective than IUI with controlled ovarian hyperstimulation? *Hum Reprod* 30:2331–2339.

12. Farquhar, C. M., Liu, E., Armstrong, S., Arroll, N., Lensen, S. and Brown, J. (2018) Intrauterine insemination with ovarian stimulation versus expectant management for unexplained infertility (TUI): a pragmatic, open-label, randomised, controlled, two-centre trial. *Lancet* 391 (10119):441–450.

13. Ombelet, W., Dhont, N., Thijssen, A., Bosmans, E. and Kruger, T. (2014) Semen quality and prediction of IUI success in male subfertility: a systematic review. *Reprod Biomed Online* 28:300–309.

14. Ombelet, W., Vandeput, H., Van de Putte, G., Cox, A., Janssen, M., Jacobs, P., et al. (1997) Intrauterine insemination after ovarian stimulation with clomiphene citrate: predictive potential of inseminating motile count and sperm morphology. *Hum Reprod* 12:1458–1463.

15. Merviel, P., Heraud, M. H., Grenier, N., Lourdel, E., Sanguinet, P. and Copin, H. (2010) Predictive factors for pregnancy after intrauterine insemination (IUI): an analysis of 1,038 cycles and a review of the literature. *Fertil Steril* 93:79–88.

16. Lemmens, L., Kos, S., Beijer, C., Brinkman, J. W., van der Horst, F. A., van den Hoven, L., et al. (2016) Semen Section of the Dutch Foundation for Quality Assessment in Medical Laboratories. Predictive value of sperm morphology and progressively motile sperm count for pregnancy outcomes in intrauterine insemination. *Fertil Steril* 105:1462–1468.

17. Thijssen, A., Creemers, A., Van Der Elst, W., Creemers, E., Vandormael, E., Dhont, N. and Ombelet, W. (2017) Predictive value of different covariates

influencing pregnancy rate following intrauterine insemination with homologous semen: a prospective cohort study. *Reprod Biomed Online* 34:643–472.

18. Moolenaar, L. M., Cissen, M., de Bruin, J. P., Hompes, P. G. A., Repping, S. and van der Veen,F., et al. (2015) Cost-effectiveness of assisted conception for male subfertility. *Reprod Biomed Online* 30:659–666.

19. De Brucker, M. and Tournaye, H. (2014) Factors influencing IUI outcome: male age. In Cohlen, B. J. and Ombelet, W. (eds.) *Intra-Uterine Insemination: Evidence-Based Guidelines for Daily Practice.* Boca Raton, FL: CRC Press, Taylor & Francis Group, 35–38.

20. Hamada, A., Agarwal, A. and Oehninger, S. (2014) Oxidative stress IUI outcomes. In Cohlen, B. J. and Ombelet, W. (eds.) *Intra-Uterine Insemination: Evidence-Based Guidelines for Daily Practice.* Boca Raton, FL: CRC Press, Taylor & Francis Group, 97–104.

21. Bungum, M., Humaidan, P., Axmon, A., Spano, M., Bungum, L., Erenpreiss, J., et al. (2007) Sperm DNA integrity assessment in prediction of assisted reproduction technology outcome. *Hum Reprod* 22:174–179.

22. Cho, C. L. and Agarwal, A. (2017) Role of sperm DNA fragmentation in male factor infertility: A systematic review. *Arab J Urol* 16:21–34.

23. Nijs, M. and Boomsma, C. M. (2014) Factors influencing IUI outcome: semen preparation techniques. In Cohlen, B. J. and Ombelet, W. (eds.) *Intra-Uterine Insemination: Evidence-Based Guidelines for Daily Practice.* Boca Raton, FL: CRC Press, Taylor & Francis Group, 49–54.

24. Boomsma, C. M., Heineman, M. J., Cohlen, B. J. and Farquhar, C. (2004) Semen preparation techniques for intrauterine insemination. *Cochrane Database Syst Rev* 3:CD004507.

25. Ricci, G., Perticarari, S., Boscolo, R., Montico, M., Guaschino, S. and Presani, G. (2009) Semen preparation methods and sperm apoptosis: swim-up versus gradient-density centrifugation technique. *Fertil Steril* 91:632–638.

26. Cohlen, B., Tur, R. and Buxaderas, R. (2014) Factors influencing IUI outcome: ovarian hyperstimulation. In Cohlen, B. J. and Ombelet, W. (eds.) *Intra-Uterine Insemination: Evidence-Based Guidelines for Daily Practice.* Boca Raton, FL: CRC Press, Taylor & Francis Group, 77–81.

27. Cantineau, A. and Cohlen, B. (2014) Factors influencing IUI outcome: Timing and number of inseminations per cycle. In Cohlen, B. J. and Ombelet, W. (eds.) *Intra-Uterine Insemination: Evidence-Based Guidelines for Daily Practice.* Boca Raton, FL: CRC Press, Taylor & Francis Group, 67–73.

28. Liu, W., Gong, F., Luo, K. and Lu, G. (2006) Comparing the pregnancy rates of one versus two intrauterine inseminations (IUIs) in male factor and idiopathic infertility. *J Assist Reprod Genet* 23:75–79.

29. Bagis, T., Haydardedeoglu, B., Kilicdag, E. B., Cok, T., Simsek, E. and Parlakgumus, A. H. (2010) Single versus double intrauterine insemination in multi-follicular ovarian hyperstimulation cycles: a randomized trial. *Hum Reprod* 25:1684–1690.

30. Xiong, Y. Q., Chen, Y. X., Cheng, M. J., He, W. Q. and Chen, Q. (2018) The risk of human papillomavirus infection for male fertility abnormality: a meta-analysis. *Asian J Androl* 20:493–497.

31. Boeri, L., Capogrosso, P., Ventimiglia, E., Pederzoli, F., Cazzaniga, W., Chierigo, F., et al. (2019) High-risk human papillomavirus in semen is associated with poor sperm progressive motility and a high sperm DNA fragmentation index in infertile men. *Hum Reprod* 34:209–217.

32. Luttmer, R., Dijkstra, M. G., Snijders, P. J., Hompes, P. G., Pronk, D. T., Hubeek, I., et al. (2016) Presence of human papillomavirus in semen in relation to semen quality. *Hum Reprod* 31:280–286.

33. Depuydt, C., Donders, G., Verstraete, L., Vanden Broeck, D., Beert, J., Salembier, G., et al. (2019) Infectious human Papillomavirus virions in semen reduce

clinical pregnancy rates in women undergoing intra-uterine insemination. *Fertil Steril* **111**:1135–1144.

34. Verheyden, B. (2014) Immunologic male infertility. In Cohlen, B. J. and Ombelet, W. (eds.) *Intra-Uterine Insemination: Evidence-Based Guidelines for Daily Practice*. Boca Raton, FL: CRC Press, Taylor & Francis Group, 21–25.

35. Ombelet, W., Vandeput, H., Janssen, M., Cox, A., Vossen, C., Pollet, H., et al. (1997) Treatment of male infertility due to sperm surface antibodies: IUI or IVF? *Hum Reprod* **12**:1165–1170.

Obstructive Azoospermia: Is There a Place for Microsurgical Testicular Sperm Extraction?

Ahmad Aboukhshaba, Russell P. Hayden, and Peter N. Schlegel

14.1 Introduction

Obstructive pathology is a common cause of male factor infertility, affecting up to 40% of men presenting with azoospermia [1]. A wide variety of etiologies can result in obstructive azoospermia (OA), ranging from iatrogenic to infectious to congenital causes. Today's reproductive urologist has a multiple of treatment options to offer patients faced with a diagnosis of OA. We believe that reconstruction remains the gold standard for the appropriately selected couple, whereas a staged operative plan is required should sperm retrieval prove necessary. Just as important as facility resources and provider experience, a treatment plan must also consider the risks, benefits, and success rates of any planned intervention. Careful counseling and objective consideration of existing data will guide the urologist to a tailored treatment plan. In the review below, we will present the advantages and disadvantages for the various therapeutic options that can be employed for OA. Special attention will be paid to microdissection testicular sperm extraction (microTESE), as it serves as an important rescue procedure in difficult cases and is overall underutilized for the OA population.

14.2 Reconstruction Versus Sperm Retrieval

OA can now be successfully treated with a number of treatment options, ranging from definitive reconstruction to the myriad of sperm retrieval techniques (Table 14.1). Prior to the widespread use of intracytoplasmic sperm injection (ICSI), the only options for men with OA were vasovasostomy (VV) and/or vasoepididymostomy (VE). Before the ICSI era during the 1980s and 1990s, significant effort was spent optimizing both of these techniques. In experienced hands, it can now be expected that post-operative patency rates will approach at least 85% for a primary VV [2]. Outcomes following reconstruction have typically been reported as clinical pregnancy within a short term of follow-up, ranging up to 53% at 2 years post-procedure [3]. Success rates diminish if the patient requires a bilateral VE. It is difficult to predict which individuals may require bilateral VE, and just as important, how proximally along the epididymis a surgeon must anastomose the vas deferens. Though published outcomes still favor reconstruction in these scenarios, it is necessary to realize that fertility potential is a function of anastomosis location, with clinical pregnancy rates dropping precipitously for a VE near the efferent ducts.

Table 14.1 Advantages and disadvantages of various treatment options for obstructive azoospermia

Treatment	Advantages	Disadvantages
Reconstruction: Vasovasostomy (VV) and Vasoepididymostomy (VE)	• Allows for natural conception • Reestablishes a reliable sperm source for couples desiring multiple future children • Cost-effective • May obviate the need for fertility procedures in the female partner	• Reconstruction may not be technically feasible based on intra-op findings • Late failure may occur • It may take several months for sperm to return to the ejaculate
Percutaneous epididymal sperm aspiration (PESA)	• Office-based procedure, requiring only local anesthesia • Operating microscope and microsurgical skills are not required	• Inability to visualize and control bleeding • Usually cannot cryopreserve • Unable to visualize and select for tubules with high-quality sperm • Relatively high rate of failure
Testicular sperm aspiration (TESA) and Percutaneous testis biopsy (percBx)	• Office-based procedure, requiring only local anesthesia • Operating microscope and microsurgical skills are not required	• Inability to visualize and control bleeding • Usually cannot cryopreserve • Relatively high rate of failure
Microsurgical epididymal sperm aspiration (MESA)	• Allows for control of bleeding • Visualization of tubules allows for sampling of high-quality sperm • Typically yields enough sample for cryopreservation	• Usually requires general anesthesia • An operating microscope and microsurgical training are required • Moderate rate of failure • Incurs the cost of an operating room

Table 14.1 (cont.)

Treatment	Advantages	Disadvantages
Conventional testicular sperm extraction (TESE)	• Possible to conduct in the office under local anesthesia • Operating microscope and microsurgical skills are not required • High rate of success • Usually allows for cryopreservation	• May be difficult to recognize and control bleeding from intratubular vessels • Relatively high rate of intratesticular hematoma
Microdissection testicular sperm extraction (micro-TESE)	• High rate of success • Usually allows for cryopreservation • Minimal intratesticular dissection will be required for OA • Least risk for intratesticular hematoma • Particularly suited if the patient has concomitant defects of spermatogenesis	• General anesthesia is required • An operating microscope and microsurgical training are required • Incurs the cost of an operating room • Difficult to coordinate with female procedures for "fresh" ART cycles

Reconstruction has been shown to be cost-effective compared to upfront sperm retrieval for the purposes of ICSI [4,5]. Undertaking VV or VE may obviate the need for future procedures in the female partner, and as a result, prevent complications that are associated with assisted reproductive technology (ART) and the accompanying risk of negative perinatal outcomes. For couples that desire multiple children, reconstruction is particularly beneficial as it offers an established and reliable source of future sperm. Although data is limited regarding the long-term safety of ICSI, natural conception following VV or VE maintains the putative adaptations of natural fertilization of the oocyte, selecting against sperm that are suboptimal. To date, preliminary data suggests that ICSI is reasonably safe, at least in regard to the risks of congenital malformation and early childhood development [6]. Time will tell if the initial ICSI generation maintains comparable health outcomes to their naturally conceived peers.

For couples that face a significant female factor, reconstruction may not be the best initial option. One recent study established the kinetics of male reproductive potential following VV and VE [7]. It can take more than 6 months following reconstruction for sperm to return to the ejaculate in sufficient numbers, a duration that may be unacceptable for situations involving advanced maternal age. Additionally, certain clinical characteristics of the male partner will serve as contraindications to reconstruction, as is the case for congenital bilateral absence of the vas deferens. Nevertheless, a discussion of the risks and benefits of VV/VE is necessary in most couples presenting with OA, which is reflected in the most recent committee opinion by the American Society of Reproductive Medicine [8]. As always, treatment decisions must be adjusted to the individual needs and wishes of the couple.

14.3 Sperm Retrieval: Staged Intervention

The reproductive urologist can utilize a multitude of techniques and anatomical sources for sperm should the treatment plan progress to sperm retrieval. Appropriate pre-operative counseling of the male partner will include a description of these various techniques, success rates, risks, and benefits. Since no single surgical approach is ideal for all patients with OA, options for management including a staged approach should be outlined at the time of informed consent. Generally speaking, it is our opinion that microTESE should be used primarily as a back-up procedure in the event initial retrieval attempts fail.

We believe that the operative plan should ideally begin with an attempted retrieval from the epididymis. Early data for OA, in which use of epididymal sperm for assisted reproduction was compared against testicular sperm, suggested some limited benefit of epididymal sperm for ICSI outcomes, although cases were not directly matched [1]. However, in one of the largest OA cohorts where sperm source was evaluated, van Wely and colleagues demonstrated a statistically significant difference in live birth rates favoring an epididymal source [9]. In their retrospective analysis, 280 men who underwent microsurgical epididymal sperm aspiration (MESA) obtained a live birth rate of 39% compared to 24% in men who required testicular sperm extraction (TESE). After adjusting for maternal age and ovarian reserve, their data demonstrated an odds ratio of 1.82 (CI 1.05–3.67) supporting the use of MESA-derived sperm. It is possible that the MESA approach, where the epididymis is searched microscopically and the most promising regions of the epididymis are aspirated, provides for optimal sperm quality.

Although van Wely and colleagues obtained good results using MESA, percutaneous approaches remain a viable option for the initial technique in a staged operative plan. Percutaneous epididymal sperm aspiration (PESA) allows for office-based retrievals under local anesthetic, eliminating the costs and logistics of the operating room and anesthesia. A percutaneous approach is useful if a fresh sample is required for ART, or in the unexpected situation of a male partner unable to produce a semen sample. PESA does not require microsurgical equipment or microsurgical training. In a large series of 146 men, Esteves and colleagues were able to retrieve motile sperm with PESA alone in 78% of cases [10]. As a rescue, they preferred testicular sperm aspiration (TESA), which was successful in all but four patients. However, percutaneously retrieved sperm does not allow selection of the best region of epididymal sperm. Authors have suggested that percutaneously retrieved epididymal sperm may have increased sperm DNA fragmentation, thereby risking worse reproductive outcomes [11].

PESA is an initial option in sperm retrieval, if one accepts the limitation of sperm quality discussed above. If resources and timing permits, however, we recommend MESA for obtaining epididymal sperm. In terms of complications, open techniques tend to be safer than percutaneous approaches since bleeding can be recognized and controlled, thereby minimizing the risk of post-operative hematoma [8]. Another advantage of MESA is the direct visualization of the epididymis. It is common to observe under magnification macrophage-laden tubules that should be avoided, as sperm from these locations will often carry significant DNA fragmentation and will usually lack motility. It is also apparent that in obstructed systems, the macrophage concentration increases as one progresses distally along the epididymis. With PESA the surgeon is blinded to optimal tubule selection, whereas during MESA the yellowish tubules associated with poor sperm quality can easily be avoided [9]. An additional consideration is the ability to cryopreserve sperm following MESA. In the PESA series conducted by Esteves and colleagues, only 27% of cases yielded enough specimen to allow for freezing [10]. MESA reliably produces enough sperm to allow for cryopreservation, a notable advantage since most couples will require at least two cycles of IVF for one live birth. Thus, MESA will avoid subsequent sperm retrieval procedures, allows for optimal epididymal tubule identification for high-quality sperm, and offers the ability to escalate the operative intervention should TESE prove necessary. Although PESA can fall back on percutaneous testis sampling, these procedures expose the patient to the same risk of hematoma as PESA, although typically more reliable in terms of successful sperm retrieval in OA [11,12].

The role of microTESE becomes significant for the atypical presentation of nonobstructive azoospermia when the initial workup suggests OA. The seminal study by Schoor and colleagues established that a follicle-stimulating hormone (FSH) of less than 7.6 mIU/mL, in combination with a testicular long-axis dimension of at least 4.6 cm, predicted OA in 96% of cases, and will accurately diagnose nonobstructive azoospermia with a rate of 89% [13]. These preoperative rubrics have effectively eliminated the use of diagnostic testis biopsy in modern practice. However, it is apparent that approximately 1 in 20 men considered to have OA by these criteria will actually harbor a defect in sperm production. The initial presentation may further be clouded by accompanying risk factors for OA. For example, bilateral inguinal hernia repair is a common presenting history, and can be a cause for iatrogenic injury of both vasa. Unfortunately, other findings on physical examination, such as epididymal fullness or induration, are highly subjective, depend heavily on examiner experience, and perform poorly diagnostically for the average practitioner's exam. Both men with nonobstructive azoospermia, and the approximate 15% of cases of OA secondary to obstruction at the rete testis, may have "flat" epididymides when examined by an experienced practitioner [1]. In both of these scenarios an epididymal source will fail, necessitating a testicular procedure.

Most men with impaired sperm production, low FSH, and preserved testicular size will have a form of maturation arrest on histology. Hung and colleagues conducted a retrospective case review of nonobstructive azoospermia evaluated at a single institution [14]. They identified 26 men out of 600 who demonstrated uniform maturation arrest, an FSH below 7.6 mIU/mL, and normal testis volume. The resulting rate of 26/600 (4.3%) was consistent with the earlier work conducted by Schoor and colleagues [13]. In another series by Tsai and colleagues, a normal FSH and testis volume was observed in 38% of cases when focusing only on patients with maturation arrest [15]. Given these data, it is clear that any high-volume reproductive urologist will periodically encounter occult maturation arrest despite a pre-operative diagnosis of OA. It is our opinion that these men benefit most from microTESE as compared to conventional TESE due to the maximal exposure for sampling favorable seminiferous tubules. Although a meta-analysis conducted by Deruyver and colleagues failed to demonstrate a statistical difference in sperm retrieval rates for maturation arrest comparing conventional TESE versus microTESE, it is notable that all included studies documented higher retrieval rates for the microTESE arm [16]. All of the included studies were unfortunately underpowered, with an average cohort of 30 maturation arrest subjects. Appropriately powered studies have yet to be conducted to differentiate the ideal TESE technique for this subpopulation. Just as important as sperm retrieval success, conventional TESE carries an increased complication rate compared to microTESE, a perspective that will be addressed in Section 14.4 of this chapter. For these reasons, we often prefer microTESE as the backup intervention should MESA fail to produce adequate quality or number of sperm.

14.4 Safety of Testis Sampling Techniques

Testicular sperm retrieval rates approach 100% in cases of OA with otherwise intact spermatogenesis [9,17]. When planning a staged intervention, the reproductive urologist must plan accordingly to maximize the success of any testicular backup procedure. As stated previously, percutaneous techniques such as TESA and testis percutaneous biopsy (percBx) carry a small risk of hematoma [8]. Several groups have adopted TESA given the perception of less invasiveness. To obtain adequate numbers of sperm, however, multiple passes of a needle are typically required. In an animal model addressing the safety of TESA, Shufaro and colleagues performed seven punctures of the left testis with a 23-gauge needle under negative pressure [18]. In the contralateral testis, a conventional TESE was performed. Surprisingly, TESA resulted in widespread architectural changes within the testicle, decreased spermatogenesis, and significant volume loss. Conversely, in testicles subjected to TESE, the associated changes observed in the TESA arm were only present in 10% of the remaining testicular parenchyma. Though such drastic changes are not typically seen clinically, diffuse scarring can be encountered during microTESE following a prior TESA attempt, especially when a mapping technique was utilized.

Similar concerning results are also apparent on radiographic studies of post-TESA testicles. In one small prospective series, intratesticular lesions were observed on ultrasound following TESA in 6.6% of cases, all of which resolved after 9 months [12]. Perhaps of more concern, 11% of men in this series experienced signs and symptoms consistent with intratesticular hematoma. Intratesticular hematoma is particularly harmful as it elevates parenchymal pressures given the noncompliant tunica albuginea, essentially causing a potential compartment syndrome [19]. In a contemporary TESA cohort published by Zhu and colleagues, an unacceptable hematoma rate of 5.3% was observed in 76 men who were concomitantly taking a PDE5 inhibitor [20]. Interestingly, the same group documented no hemorrhagic complications in 428 men who were not exposed to a PDE5 inhibitor. The cause of this discrepancy is unclear. Nevertheless, it is apparent that TESA carries a real risk of post-procedure bleeding while simultaneously precluding reliable cryopreservation [21].

The desire to limit invasiveness has also driven many providers to favor conventional TESE over microTESE [22]. Another perceived advantage of conventional TESE is the ability to perform the procedure under local anesthesia, whereas microTESE is less well tolerated by patients in this setting [23]. Practically speaking, it is our opinion that conventional TESE should not be routinely used in this setting because of the small but real intratesticular effects of the procedure.

As stated previously, we prefer microTESE if time and resources permit. Although conventional TESE may seem less invasive, the procedure can suffer from inadequate intratesticular hemostasis. In conventional TESE, a 5 to 10 mm incision is made in the tunica albuginea, through which seminiferous tubules are herniated via gentle pressure. The testicular sample is often sharply excised using fine scissors, and hemostasis is obtained thereafter using bipolar cautery. It is underappreciated that intertubular arteries will retract within the testis after the biopsy. These transected vessels may not be accessible to the superficial cauterization TESE exposure allows. Additionally, these vessels may spasm following the insult, presenting the surgeon with a false sense of adequate hemostasis. The end result is an elevated risk of intratesticular hematoma. In microTESE, intratubular vessels are directly visualized and can be addressed without difficulty. An equatorial incision in the tunica albuginea is created under magnification, providing for a relatively avascular plane. For cases of OA, we have found an incision of 2 to 3 cm is usually adequate to allow for appropriate exposure (as opposed to 3 to 4 cm that is often required for nonobstructive azoospermia). In our opinion, the difference in morbidity between a 5 mm and a 3 cm equatorial incision of the tunica albuginea is minor. However, the morbidity of intratesticular hemorrhage is significant, as it is painful and will negatively impact future testis function [19,21].

Multiple groups have attempted to delineate the risk profile of conventional versus microTESE. In an early series by Schlegel and Su, 64 patients were followed with serial ultrasounds after conventional TESE [24]. At 3 months post-procedure, 82% of men had sonographic signs of resolving hematoma and inflammation. Following a duration of 6 months, the initial findings were replaced by linear fibrosis and calcification. More concerning, two patients had testicular atrophy following multiple biopsies, with one patient suffering complete devascularization. In a subsequent report, one group documented bilateral testis atrophy in a patient due to ischemia following multiple TESE biopsies, obligating the individual to lifelong testosterone replacement [17]. These early experiences, along with disappointing sperm retrieval rates, provided the motivation for the development of microTESE [25].

To directly compare conventional TESE and microTESE, Amer and colleagues conducted both procedures (one technique for each side) in a cohort of 100 men [26]. Again, using serial ultrasounds, an intratesticular hematoma rate of 58% versus 15% was observed at 1 month for conventional and microTESE, respectively. Furthermore, microTESE resulted in significantly less tissue removal (4.6 vs 53 mg). In a similar study, Okada and colleagues documented significant testicular volume loss, defined as more than 2 cc, in 25% of men undergoing multiple TESE biopsies as opposed to 2.5% for microTESE [26]. Through a subsequent meta-analysis comparing the two procedures, microTESE resulted in higher sperm retrieval rates, fewer hematomas, less intratesticular fibrosis, and tended to preserve more testis volume [16]. Anecdotally, Silber and colleagues observed smoother and less symptomatic convalescence following microTESE, likely as a result of less intratesticular pressure secondary to hematoma [19].

In terms of Leydig cell function, multiple groups have documented testosterone kinetics in men with nonobstructive azoospermia following TESE. There have been no large series documenting androgen levels in patients with OA following microTESE or any other sperm retrieval attempt. In a contemporary meta-analysis conducted by Eliveld and colleagues, spanning 15 studies that included various testicular retrieval procedures, testosterone levels did diminish below baseline before full recovery at 18 months [27]. When interpreting these data, it is important to recall that men undergoing microTESE for nonobstructive etiologies tend to have moderately extensive, possibly bilateral tissue dissections to identify rare foci of sperm production. These patients are also prone to hypogonadism, and so will likely present worse androgen levels post-procedure than individuals with a diagnosis of OA. This prediction is supported by the data of Eliveld and colleagues, in which Klinefelter's Syndrome resulted in worse androgen recovery rates when compared to individuals with less severe nonobstructive azoospermia phenotypes [27]. In OA, microTESE will produce sufficient samples with unilateral interventions with relatively minimal tissue dissection. Additionally, these men presumably have normal Leydig cell function, and so are unlikely to have clinically meaningful changes in testosterone levels post-procedure due to increased reserve.

14.5 Conclusions

Due to advances in ART and sperm retrieval techniques, men with OA have an excellent prognosis for achieving paternity. In the correctly selected couple, reconstruction of the male reproductive tract remains the gold standard for natural conception. However, with the growing trend in developed nations to delay family building, reproductive specialists are facing ever-increasing time constraints due to advanced maternal age. The popularity of sperm retrieval for use in ICSI is a direct reflection of these societal changes. In OA, a staged operative plan must be established before any intervention to maximize sperm retrieval success while minimizing damage to the male reproductive system. Many providers now routinely offer percutaneous techniques, as they appear less invasive, have reasonable success rates, and can be performed with limited time and resources. However, we argue that staged open procedures should be pursued when possible. MESA followed by microTESE offers the highest chance of success, while simultaneously allowing for cryopreservation of ample sperm for subsequent cycles. The key to these microscopic techniques is the ability to obtain meticulous hemostasis, which will translate to less ultimate damage to gonadal function. In the above review, a case for the utilization of microTESE in OA is presented. We strongly encourage providers who offer these procedures to critique the primary data for themselves, and in terms of rescue testicular interventions, to reconsider the notion of "less invasive" treatment options for our mutual patient population.

Acknowledgments

Salary support provided by Frederick J. and Theresa Dow Wallace Fund of the New York Community Trust, The Robert S. Dow Foundation, and the Irena and Howard Laks Foundation.

References

1. Miyaoka, R. and Esteves, S. C. (2013) Predictive factors for sperm retrieval and sperm injection outcomes in obstructive azoospermia: do etiology, retrieval techniques and gamete source play a role? *Clinics (Sao Paulo, Brazil)* **68**(Suppl 1):111–119.

2. Baker, K. and Sabanegh, E., Jr. (2013) Obstructive azoospermia: reconstructive techniques and results. *Clinics (Sao Paulo, Brazil)* **68**(Suppl 1):61–73.

3. Bolduc, S., Fischer, M. A., Deceuninck, G. and Thabet, M. (2007) Factors predicting overall success: a review of 747 microsurgical vasovasostomies. *Can Urol Assoc J /Journal de l'Association des urologues du Canada* **1**:388–394.

4. Heidenreich, A., Altmann, P. and Engelmann, U. H. (2000) Microsurgical vasovasostomy versus microsurgical epididymal sperm aspiration/testicular extraction of sperm combined with intracytoplasmic sperm injection. A cost-benefit analysis. *Eur Urol* **37**:609–614.

5. Lee, R., Li, P. S., Goldstein, M., Tanrikut, C., Schattman, G., Schlegel, P. N. (2008) A decision analysis of treatments for obstructive azoospermia. *Hum Reprod (Oxford, UK)* **23**:2043–2049.

6. Rumbold, A. R., Moore, V. M., Whitrow, M. J., Oswald, T. K., Moran, L. J., Fernandez, R. C., et al. (2017) The impact of specific fertility treatments on cognitive development in childhood and adolescence: a systematic review. *Hum Reprod (Oxford, UK)* **32**:1489–1507.

7. Farber, N. J., Flannigan, R., Li, P., Li, P. S. and Goldstein, M. (2018) The kinetics of sperm return and late failure following vasovasostomy or vasoepididymostomy: a systematic review. *J Urol* **201** 241–250.

8. ASRM (2008) Sperm retrieval for obstructive azoospermia. *Fertil Steril* **90**: S213–218.

9. van Wely, M., Barbey, N., Meissner, A., Repping, S. and Silber, S. J. (2015) Live birth rates after MESA or TESE in men with obstructive azoospermia: is there a difference? *Hum Reprod (Oxford, UK)* **30**:761–766.

10. Esteves, S. C., Lee, W., Benjamin, D. J., Seol, B., Verza, S., Jr. and Agarwal, A. (2013) Reproductive potential of men with obstructive azoospermia undergoing percutaneous sperm retrieval and intracytoplasmic sperm injection according to the cause of obstruction. *J Urol* **189**:232–237.

11. Steele, E. K., McClure, N., Maxwell, R. J. and Lewis, S. E. (1999) A comparison of DNA damage in testicular and proximal epididymal spermatozoa in obstructive azoospermia. *Mol Hum Reprod* **5**:831–835.

12. Westlander, G., Ekerhovd, E., Granberg, S., Lycke, N., Nilsson, L., Werner, C., et al. (2001) Serial ultrasonography, hormonal profile and antisperm antibody response after testicular sperm aspiration. *Hum Reprod (Oxford, UK)* **16**:2621–2627.

13. Schoor, R. A., Elhanbly, S., Niederberger, C. S. and Ross, L. S. (2002) The role of testicular biopsy in the modern management of male infertility. *J Urol* **167**:197–200.

14. Hung, A. J., King, P. and Schlegel, P. N. (2007) Uniform testicular maturation arrest: a unique subset of men with nonobstructive azoospermia. *J Urol* **178**:608–612; discussion 612.

15. Tsai, M. C., Cheng, Y. S., Lin, T. Y., Yang, W. H. and Lin, Y. M. (2012) Clinical characteristics and reproductive outcomes in infertile men with testicular early and late maturation arrest. *Urology* 80:826–832.

16. Deruyver, Y., Vanderschueren, D. and Van der Aa, F. (2014) Outcome of microdissection TESE compared with conventional TESE in non-obstructive azoospermia: a systematic review. *Andrology* 2:20–24.

17. Okada, H., Dobashi, M., Yamazaki, T., Hara, I., Fujisawa, M., Arakawa, S., et al. (2002) Conventional versus microdissection testicular sperm extraction for nonobstructive azoospermia. *J Urol* 168:1063–1067.

18. Shufaro, Y., Prus, D., Laufer, N. and Simon, A. (2002) Impact of repeated testicular fine needle aspirations (TEFNA) and testicular sperm extraction (TESE) on the microscopic morphology of the testis: an animal model. *Hum Reprod (Oxford, UK)* 17:1795–1799.

19. Silber, S. J. (2000) Microsurgical TESE and the distribution of spermatogenesis in non-obstructive azoospermia. *Hum Reprod (Oxford, UK)* 15:2278–2284.

20. Zhu, Y. T., Hua, R., Quan, S., Tan, W. L., Chu, Q. J. and Wang, C. Y. (2018) Scrotal hemorrhage after testicular sperm aspiration may be associated with phosphodiesterase-5 inhibitor administration: a retrospective study. *BMC Urology* 18:8.

21. Donoso, P., Tournaye, H. and Devroey, P. (2007) Which is the best sperm retrieval technique for non-obstructive azoospermia? A systematic review. *Hum Reprod Update* 13:539–549.

22. Franco, G., Scarselli, F., Casciani, V., De Nunzio, C., Dente, D., Leonardo, C., et al. (2016) A novel stepwise micro-TESE approach in non obstructive azoospermia. *BMC Urology* 16:20.

23. Alom, M., Ziegelmann, M., Savage, J., Miest, T., Kohler, T. S. and Trost, L. (2017) Office-based andrology and male infertility procedures-a cost-effective alternative. *Trans Androl Urol* 6:761–772.

24. Schlegel, P. N. and Su, L. M. (1997) Physiological consequences of testicular sperm extraction. *Hum Reprod (Oxford, UK)* 12:1688–1692.

25. Schlegel, P. N. (1999) Testicular sperm extraction: microdissection improves sperm yield with minimal tissue excision. *Hum Reprod (Oxford, UK)* 14:131–135.

26. Amer, M., Ateyah, A., Hany, R. and Zohdy, W. (2000) Prospective comparative study between microsurgical and conventional testicular sperm extraction in non-obstructive azoospermia: follow-up by serial ultrasound examinations. *Hum Reprod (Oxford, UK)* 15:653–656.

27. Eliveld, J., van Wely, M., Meissner, A., Repping, S., van der Veen, F. and van Pelt, A. M. M. (2018) The risk of TESE-induced hypogonadism: a systematic review and meta-analysis. *Hum Reprod Update* 24:442–454.

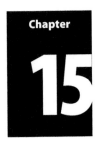

Chapter

15

Should Varicocele Be Operated on Before IVF?

Shannon H. K. Kim and Victoria Nisenblat

15.1 Introduction

The management of varicoceles is one of the most controversial areas in urology and reproductive medicine. Varicoceles are the most common correctable cause of male infertility. Although a large body of evidence supports the adverse effects of varicoceles on fertility, the evidence on improved fertility after repair is not consistent. Assisted reproductive technologies (ART) can often overcome poor sperm quality and quantity. Intracytoplasmic sperm injection (ICSI) requires only a single sperm to be injected into an egg. It is not uncommon to encourage the couples with male factor infertility to proceed with ART without giving an opportunity for evaluation and management of potentially correctable causes. While opinions are divided about the role of varicocele repair in management of male infertility, it is even less clear whether varicocele should be addressed within the framework of ART. In this chapter we explore the question whether repair of varicocele benefits couples undergoing ART. We describe the anatomy of varicocele to provide a background for its etiology and overview the putative mechanisms for varicocele-induced infertility. Next, we discuss the diagnostics of varicocele and methods of repair. We then present an unbiased coverage of the literature on the clinical implications of varicocele repair in the context of fertility. Finally, we address the limitations of the current evidence and reflect on ongoing uncertainties.

15.2 Anatomy and Etiology

A varicocele is defined as a pathologic dilatation of the pampiniform venous plexus of the testis. The pampiniform plexus is a network of small veins that drain the testis and epididymis and ascend within a spermatic cord. The surrounding fasciomuscular layer of the spermatic, cremasteric fasciae and the cremasteric muscle assist in perfusion of the cord. The veins of the pampiniform plexus merge into the spermatic (testicular) veins as they pass the inguinal canal. In the abdomen, the left and right spermatic veins travel retroperitoneally alongside the spermatic artery on each side and vary in their drainage pattern. The left spermatic vein ascends vertically, travels posteriorly to the descending colon and drains into the renal vein at a right angle, which raises the hydrostatic pressure of the left spermatic vein. The renal vein then courses between the aorta and superior mesenteric artery to join the inferior vena cava. The right spermatic vein ascends more horizontally, is 8–10 cm shorter and drains directly into the inferior vena cava at an oblique angle. Infrequently, the right spermatic vein drains into the right renal vein, mimicking the left-side pattern. The valves are absent in up to 40% in the left and in 23% in the right spermatic vein, and this further compromises the upward blood flow. While a single spermatic vein drains each testis in most men, an accessory vein is present in 13% of men on the left and in 2% on the right side [1].

The mechanism of varicocele development involves a complex interplay of venous and intra-abdominal pressure, venous valvular function and gravitational force. The factors that favor high drainage pressure and thus predispose to left-sided varicocele, include the failure of the fasciomuscular venous pump of the spermatic cord, the longer length of the left spermatic vein, its right-angle entry into the left renal vein, the nut-cracker compression of the left renal vein between superior mesenteric artery and aorta and the absences or incompetence of valves in the testicular veins. Varicoceles are more prevalent in taller men due to the increased length of venous drainage, although there are no clearly defined height cut-offs predisposing to development. In addition, spermatic vein duplication and anastomoses between the spermatic vein and systemic circulation also play a role and may be responsible for varicocele recurrence after spermatic vein ligation or embolization. Less commonly, varicoceles result from external compression by renal or retroperitoneal tumors or from vena cava malformations [1].

The higher occurrence of varicoceles among first-degree relatives suggests the possibility of a genetic component. However, this is an under-researched area and the pattern of inheritance or genes implicated in the condition remains unclear [2].

Taken together, it is evident that the anatomy of testicular venous drainage predisposes to the development of left-sided varicoceles. Isolated varicoceles on the right or rapidly progressing new onset varicoceles warrant the exclusion of an abdominal or retroperitoneal mass with appropriate imaging.

15.3 Epidemiology

Varicoceles are a dynamic progressive condition, exhibiting varying prevalence with age. Varicoceles are rarely seen in pre-pubertal boys but become more prominent after 10–14 years of age due to the increased venous drainage of the developing testes. The prevalence of varicoceles increases from 0.8% in 2–6 years old boys to 11% by the age of 11–19 years, ranging between 4 and 35% in adolescents [3]. In the general adult population, the prevalence of varicoceles ranges from 4.4 to 22.6%, averaging around 15% and reaches up to 42% in elderly men. In men presenting for evaluation of infertility, varicoceles are 2–3 times more common, affecting 19–45% of the evaluated men [1]. In men with secondary infertility, the prevalence of varicoceles has been reported to be raised to 70–80%, but this observation has not been consistently confirmed across the studies. Subclinical varicoceles have been found in 55–70% of infertile men, although these estimates have been reported only by small-sized heterogeneous studies [4].

Whilst varicoceles are considered predominantly a left-sided condition, bilateral clinically apparent varicoceles are reported in 1–30% of the affected men and in up to 59% of adolescents. One study reported that the rate of bilateral subclinical varicoceles in infertile adults may be as high as 80%. Isolated right-sided varicoceles are rare, affecting fewer than 5% of men diagnosed. As stated above, this flags the possibility of sinister pathology causing a mass effect compressing the venous tract [1,4].

15.4 Pathophysiology

Varicoceles impair testicular function by affecting both Sertoli and Leydig cells. This results in negative effect on semen parameters, ultrastructural features of sperm, testicular steroidogenesis and testicular growth. The pathophysiology of varicoceles remains a question and there is no single theory to explain its effect. It is also unclear why fertility is affected in some men but not others, implying the multifactorial nature of the condition. The proposed pathologic mechanisms are largely derived from animal studies and include oxidative stress, heat stress, testicular hypoperfusion, increased apoptosis and impaired steroidogenesis [1,5].

15.4.1 Oxidative Stress

Reactive oxygen species (ROS) are the end products of oxygen metabolism that are deactivated and eliminated by a series of antioxidant defense mechanisms. Disruption to the oxidant-antioxidant balance leads to mitochondrial dysfunction and an accumulation of ROS with subsequent oxidative DNA damage and multiple cellular aberrations. An excess of ROS has been associated with reduced sperm motility, abnormal sperm morphology and compromised sperm DNA integrity, all of which may lead to morphological or functional sperm abnormalities and subsequently to impaired fertilization. The raised levels of ROS in the seminal fluid of men with varicocele have been demonstrated to decline after varicocele repair. Some men with a varicocele presenting with infertility have been shown to have abnormal semen parameters and increased sperm DNA damage. These factors may lead to decreased pregnancy rates both in spontaneous conception and following ART treatments. Varicocelectomy, on the other hand, has been shown to improve sperm parameters and decrease the DNA fragmentation index. It has been proposed that assessment of ROS and DNA fragmentation can be used as a prognostic marker in subfertile men with a varicocele. Clinical utility of these tests is still limited by a lack of standardized laboratory methods and an undetermined decision threshold for most assays [1].

15.4.2 Heat Stress

Spermatogenesis is a temperature-sensitive process, requiring a scrotal temperature of 35–36°C. Varicoceles result in a rise of the scrotal temperature by 2.6°C due to regurgitation of warm blood from the abdomen and dilatation of the engorged scrotal veins. Exposure to scrotal heat may induce testicular heat stress. There is a well-described association between heat and dysfunction within the temperature-sensitive Leydig, Sertoli and germ cells. At a molecular level, heat stress is known to increase oxidative stress markers, accelerate apoptosis and impair function of key enzymes involved in DNA replication, namely topoisomerase I and DNA polymerase [1,5]. The effect of heat stress on testicular function is well recognized in men with cryptorchidism. Febrile illness has also been shown to transiently affect sperm concentration and progressive motility commencing within a few weeks of a febrile episode for a period of several months. Scrotal cooling, on the other hand, has been shown to improve semen parameters in small uncontrolled studies [6].

15.4.3 Toxin Accumulation and Testicular Hypoperfusion

Impaired venous drainage in men with a varicocele results in the stasis of blood, which may initiate activation of trapped white cells and increase the release of ROS. Blood stasis may also lead to low tissue perfusion with subsequent hypoxia, ischemia and impaired function. Stagnation of blood within the testicular microcirculation and ischemic changes within the testes have been confirmed on testicular biopsies in men with a varicocele. High levels of hypoxia-inducible factor 1 (HIF1), known to regulate tissue response to hypoxia, have been observed in the testicular vein in varicoceles. Improvement in testicular blood flow has been demonstrated after varicocelectomy. In animal models with an induced varicocele, administration of vascular endothelial growth factor (VEGF), known to counteract hypoxic changes of tissue hypoperfusion, led to markedly decreased rates of apoptosis and improved testicular function similarly to that observed after varicocelectomy. Likewise, supplementation with Polydeoxyribonucleotide (PDRN), an anti-inflammatory and angiogenic agent, improved spermatogenesis in experimental varicoceles in rats. Little is known about the effect of these agents on testicular function in men, hence their role in treatment is not established [1,5].

15.4.4 Apoptosis

Apoptosis, or programmed cell death, is well described in association with varicoceles and plays an important role in varicocele-induced infertility. Reduced expression of the anti-apoptotic proteins Neuronal Apoptosis Inhibitory Protein (NAIP) and Survivin, as well as decreased spermatogenesis have been observed in animal models of varicocele. Elevated levels of apoptotic markers have been observed in seminal fluid and in testicular tissues of men with varicoceles. Moreover, the expression of molecular mediators of apoptosis is increased in patients with varicoceles with compromised spermatogenesis. Apoptosis can be triggered by a variety of injurious stimuli including but not limited to heat stress, oxidative stress and testis hypoperfusion. Conversely, varicocele repair results in up-regulation of genes encoding anti-apoptotic proteins [5].

15.4.5 Impaired Steroidogenesis

Varicoceles have been linked with testicular fibrosis, featured by collagen deposition in the tubular basement membrane, blood vessels and interstitial tissue. Improvement of testicular histology has been shown after varicocelectomy. *In vitro* studies clearly demonstrate direct consequences of varicoceles on the viability and function of Leydig cells, which are responsible for testosterone production and maintaining normal intra-testicular testosterone concentrations required for spermatogenesis. There is well-documented association between varicoceles and low testosterone levels. Numerous animal studies show that varicoceles are associated with low intra-testicular testosterone and enzymatic dysfunction at several stages of steroidogenesis. Improvement in testicular histological changes and significant increases in testosterone levels have been observed after varicocele repair. This implies that the hypogonadism in men with varicoceles may be reversible. These observations have been supported in human studies that demonstrate improvement in serum testosterone levels after varicocelectomy [1,5].

15.4.6 Other Factors

Increased levels of inflammatory markers such as epithelial neutrophil activating peptide-78 (ENA-78) and IL-1b have been found in the seminal fluid of men with a varicocele and infertility. ENA-78 is shown to negatively affect sperm motility, while administration of an IL-1b antagonist alleviated damage to germ cells and seminiferous tubules in rats with induced oxidative testicular damage. Animal studies link varicocele with overexpression of proinflammatory cytokines, which can increase the permeability of the blood–testis immunological barrier. Molecular evidence of the disrupted blood–testis barrier and a higher rate of anti-sperm antibodies have been demonstrated in subfertile men with a varicocele, proposing a role of inflammation and altered immune response in varicocele-induced infertility [7]. Furthermore, spermatozoa of men with a varicocele have been shown to have a decreased expression of androgen receptors and display lower rates of capacitation, which leads to decreased fertilization ability. Finally, an influx of adrenal metabolites with retrograde venous flow has been also implicated in the adverse effect of varicoceles on testicular function [5].

15.4.7 Genetic Predisposition

Men with varicoceles have been shown to have a decreased expression of the Heat-Shock Protein gene (HSPs) and Metallothionein-1 M (MT1 M) gene, known to protect against heat stress and oxidative damage. This may result in an increased sensitivity to the insult of testicular hyperthermia and oxidative stress on spermatogenesis in a subgroup of men. Such intrinsic susceptibility provides a possible explanation for genetic predisposition to infertility in men with varicoceles. Genetic polymorphisms have been implicated as a susceptibility factor for infertility and a possible cause for a less favorable response to varicocele repair. The association between genetic aberrations and varicoceles is intriguing; however, the data is scant and the findings are pending further replication [5].

15.5 Classification and Diagnosis

The most widely used classification of varicoceles is the modification of a clinical classification proposed by Dubin and Amelar, endorsed by the World Health Organization (WHO) [8]. According to the WHO classification system, varicoceles are classified as following:

Grade 0 *or subclinical*: varicocele diagnosed only with imaging techniques and not palpable or visible on physical examination;

Grade 1: varicocele palpable in the upright position with Valsalva maneuver;

Grade 2: varicocele palpable in the upright position without the Valsalva maneuver;

Grade 3: varicocele visible through the scrotal skin in the upright position.

Physical examination represents the cornerstone for detection of a clinically significant varicocele. The majority of men with varicoceles are asymptomatic, but some may present with testicular or groin pain that worsens after prolonged standing or exertion. A common finding on physical examination is painless scrotal swelling. The examination is performed in a warm and relaxed environment, both in the standing and supine positions with and without a Valsalva maneuver. In the context of a varicocele, the examination should include palpation of pampiniform plexus, and assessment of testicular size and consistency. Unfortunately, physical examination is subjective and is limited by intra-observer and inter-observer bias. Factors that limit detection and grading of varicoceles include scrotum tightening due to patient distress or cold temperature, obesity, hydrocele, prior scrotal surgeries and lack of sufficient clinical experience. Physical examination has a diagnostic sensitivity of 71% and a specificity of 69% [9].

Imaging modalities that have been described include ultrasound, computerized tomography (CT), magnetic resonance imaging (MRI), thermography, scintigraphy and venography.

Scrotal ultrasound with Doppler examination is the most widely used modality for detecting varicoceles and testicular pathology. When compared to venography, ultrasound-Doppler has a sensitivity of 97% and a specificity of 94%. Ultrasound of the scrotum is performed in the supine position with a high-frequency linear array transducer 7.5–14 MHz. The study can be then extended with the patient upright and/or with a Valsalva maneuver. The main sonographic criteria of varicocele include multiple anechoic tubular structures in the superior and lateral aspects of the testis with intermittent or continuous flow reversal with or without Valsalva. In general, it has been agreed that varicoceles of more than 2.5–3 mm diameter are clinically significant. However, the standardized diagnostic criteria regarding the extent of venous dilation or magnitude of reflux are lacking and there is limited correlation between the ultrasonographic findings and the clinical assessment of varicocele severity. The prognostic value of ultrasound findings for treatment outcomes is not well established. Ultrasonography remains the primary imaging modality for the evaluation of varicoceles as it is relatively inexpensive, non-invasive and readily available. The important limitations include the operator-dependent nature, limited field of view and poor tissue characterization [9,10]. The American Urological Association (AUA) and the American Society for Reproductive Medicine (ASRM) guidelines recommend scrotal ultrasound only as an adjunct to inconclusive physical examination [11].

CT imaging for the diagnosis of varicoceles is not superior to ultrasound and involves radiation exposure, higher costs and lower availability. Therefore, CT is not routinely used for detecting varicoceles and is mainly reserved for assessment of suspected retroperitoneal lesions [9].

MRI may be more advantageous than ultrasound as it is not operator-dependent and enables detailed visualization of retroperitoneal anatomy. In addition, MRI has the potential to accurately monitor testicular function and to determine the associated testicular damage, such as testicular fibrosis. Its diagnostic and prognostic utility is yet to be established and the exact role in the diagnostic algorithm remains undetermined [9].

Venography is primarily used as an adjunct to therapeutic intervention with embolization and has a value in identifying collateral circulation in patients with failed surgical ligation and is not a primary diagnostic tool. Other methods such as thermography and scintigraphy are not used in routine clinical practice [9].

15.6 Indications for Treatment

According to the ASRM recommendations, varicoceles should be treated when all of the following conditions are met: (i) palpable varicocele; (ii) abnormal semen parameters; (iii) the couple has documented infertility; and (iv) the female partner with normal or potentially reversible fertility [11]. Additional indications for treatment are reversing testicular atrophy in adolescent males, treating testicular pain from varicocele and improving hypogonadism in men with varicocele [11,12]. The factors to consider when making a decision regarding the surgical treatment include the degree of varicocele-related physical discomfort in affected men, potential cost-effectiveness of varicocele repair versus fertility treatments and determinants of female reproductive potential. Improvement in semen parameters usually takes up to 6 months post repair. Varicocelectomy may not be suitable for couples with advanced maternal age or diminished ovarian reserve to avoid wasting precious fertile time.

15.7 Methods of Varicocele Repair

The aim of varicocele treatment is to protect the testis from harmful heat and adrenal metabolites by interrupting the venous reflux to the testis. The techniques of varicocele repair include microsurgical approach, percutaneous embolization, laparoscopy and open surgery. Limited data demonstrates improved semen parameters with each repair method and largely comparable reproductive outcomes [11, 13].

15.7.1 Microsurgical Approach

A microsurgical varicocelectomy is a procedure performed under a high-power operating microscope. The technique involves a 3–4 cm transverse incision made in either inguinal or sub-inguinal regions in the groin followed by identification of the spermatic vessels for microsurgical repair. There are two most common microsurgical techniques, depending on the level of incision: microsurgical sub-inguinal varicocelectomy (MSV) and microsurgical inguinal varicocelectomy (MIV). MIV involves opening of external oblique aponeurosis, which may cause more postoperative pain compared to MSV. MIV has the advantage of encountering fewer larger-diameter internal spermatic vessels, including the arteries at this proximal level prior to their branching at the sub-inguinal level. In both techniques, all veins within the spermatic cord are ligated either with ties or clips. Vas deferens and its vessels are not disrupted. Every effort is made to save arteries and lymphatics. Use of intraoperative micro-Doppler ultrasound or spraying the exposed vessels with papaverine can aid in finding arteries quickly, but their use is rarely required in MIV [13,14].

Both microsurgical approaches have lower complication profile than the other methods. A meta-analysis that evaluated an efficacy and safety of different varicocele repair techniques demonstrated that the most common surgical complications such as hydrocele and arterial injury are observed in fewer than 1% of cases and the recurrence rate averages at 1% [15]. The authors demonstrated that microsurgery results in a 42% rate of spontaneous pregnancy, versus 33% achieved with embolization, 30% with laparoscopy and 36–38% with open surgery [15]. Given the high success rate and minimal morbidity, microsurgical varicocelectomy takes its place as the gold standard in contemporary urology [13–15].

15.7.2 Percutaneous Embolization

Embolization is a minimally invasive approach performed under intravenous sedation or local anesthesia. In general, embolization is associated with quicker recovery and remains a suitable alternative to the open surgical management of varicoceles. Venous access is routinely made at the right common femoral vein for left-sided varicoceles or the internal jugular vein for right-sided or bilateral varicoceles. Once venography identifies the varicocele, it is embolized with occlusive agents such as coils, vascular plugs or liquid embolic agents [13].

Several complications are unique to embolization. Successful embolization requires adequate access to the spermatic vein and ability to maneuver the catheter within the vein. On-table failure due to technical difficulties occurs in approximately 13% of patients but can be as high as 30% [15]. The complication rates of embolization vary between the studies and rely on the experience of the interventional radiologist performing the procedures [11]. Importantly, percutaneous embolization does not lead to hydrocele formation as it does not affect the lymphatic drainage. The recurrence rate following embolization is much higher than after microsurgical repair and varies broadly between the studies (3–13%) [13,15]. There are also concerns about gonadal radiation exposure, especially in prolonged embolization procedures. The reported improvement in fertility outcomes after emboliza-tion are not superior to the surgical methods [13,15]. As such, embolization is commonly reserved for patients wishing to avoid surgery or those with recurrence after varicocele surgery [11,13].

15.7.3 Other Methods

15.7.3.1 Laparoscopic Varicocelectomy

Even though urologists are proficient in laparoscopy, there is no advantage in performing laparoscopic varicocelectomy. When compared to microsurgical varicocelectomy, the laparoscopic approach is associated with 3% postoperative hydrocele and 4% recurrence rate [15]. Main disadvantages of **laparoscopic varicocectomy** include: (i) failure to address the cremasteric veins, which are only accessible at the inguinal and sub-inguinal level; and (ii) the possibility of intra-abdominal organ injury. As microsurgery became increasingly available, laparoscopic varicocelectomy is not generally offered, unless the patient requires trans-peritoneal laparoscopic procedure for other indications [11,13].

15.7.3.2 Open Surgery

Traditional techniques such as the open inguinal (Ivanissavich) and the retroperitoneal approach (Palomo) without an operating microscope are no longer routinely offered due to the high complications and recurrence rates. Open surgery has been associated with 7–8% hydrocele formation and 3–15% recurrence [15]. In current practice, the open approach by either method is largely replaced by microsurgical varicocelectomy among trained urolo-gists [11,13].

15.7.4 Postoperative Follow up

Following varicocele repair, a patient should undergo clinical evaluation for recurrence or persistence. Overall, clinical varicocele is eliminated in 90–99% following the repair. ASRM recommends a three-monthly semen analysis during the first year post surgery or until pregnancy is achieved [11]. ART treatments should be considered in couples with persistent infertility, despite successfully repaired varicocele.

15.8 Benefits of Varicocelectomy

15.8.1 Reproductive Outcomes

Multiple studies showed that varicocele repair resulted in improved sperm parameters, lower DNA fragmentation and overall enhanced sperm quality [13]. One meta-analysis demon-strated that after varicocelectomy sperm concentration increased by a mean of 12 million sperm/ml, motility increased by 11% and there was a positive effect on sperm morphology [16]. A retrospective analysis of 400 men demonstrated an increase in total motile sperm count by more than 2.5 following varicocelectomy with more prominent effect in men with the lowest TMC [28]. Another meta-analysis demonstrated that 43.9% (range 20.8–55.0%) of men with non-obstructive azoospermia had return of sperm in ejaculate 4.5–11 months post varicocelectomy [17]. The chance of finding sperm in postoperative ejaculate did not significantly differ between men with different severity of varicocele, although this observation was made in a group of 76 men. It has been suggested that varicocelectomy may allow some couples to achieve spontaneous pregnancy or to undergo less invasive fertility treatments [7,18].

The ultimate goal of a couple seeking fertility assistance is to bring home a healthy baby. Therefore, the efficacy of varicocele correction should be evaluated based on the ability to improve the most relevant reproductive endpoints, such as pregnancy and live birth rates. A meta-analysis of five observational and randomized controlled trials (RCTs) in 568 men with clinical varicoceles demonstrated that varicocelectomy improved the odds of spontaneous pregnancy with odds ratio (OR) = 2.87, p = 0.07 and the number needed to treat at 5.7 [19]. Two earlier systematic reviews that included eight RCTs in 385 men, did not find benefit of varicocele repair over expectant management [20,21]. These reviews, however, included studies in men with subclinical varicoceles or normal semen parameters. When the analysis was limited to oligo/azoospermic men with a clinical varicocele, the recalculated data from these meta-analyses showed significantly higher pregnancy rates after varicocelectomy than in men who did not undergo surgical treatment (36.4% vs 20% respectively, p = 0.009) [19].

The studies on the benefit of varicocelectomy for assisted conception demonstrate contradicting results. Recent meta-analysis of seven retrospective studies in 1,241 men concluded that varicocelectomy before ART significantly improve pregnancy rate (OR = 1.760, p = 0.011) and live birth rate (OR = 1.761, p = 0.024) in men with severely impaired semen parameters and clinical varicocele [22]. The authors also demonstrated an increased rate of surgical sperm retrieval in men with azoospermia after varicocelectomy (OR = 2.509, p = 0.0001). Additional systematic review analyzed 18 studies (11 retrospective and 7 prospective) involving 468 men with non-obstructive azoospermia and clinical varicoceles [17]. The surgical sperm retrieval rate was significantly higher after varicocele repair, either by the surgical method or by embolization compared to untreated controls (OR = 2.65, p < 0.001). Clinical pregnancy and live birth rates following use of testicular sperm were higher after varicocelectomy, but the difference did not reach statistical significance (OR = 2.07, p = 0.08 and OR = 2.19, p = 0.05, respectively). In azoospermic men, who had a return of sperm in ejaculate after varicocelectomy, spontaneous pregnancy rate was 13.6% and pregnancy rate with ART was 18.9% [17].

The effect of varicocelectomy on the outcomes of intra uterine insemination (IUI) has been explored in several studies with conflicting results [7]. The reported pregnancy rates after IUI in men with a corrected varicocele range from 7.7% to 50%, undermining the ability to estimate the true effect [23].

One RCT involving 136 couples with a history of recurrent miscarriage and clinical varicocele demonstrated that varicocelectomy resulted in significantly higher pregnancy rate (44.1% vs 19.1%, p = 0.003) and decreased miscarriage rate (13.3% vs 69.2%, p = 0.001) compared to the couples with untreated varicocele [23]. Conversely, large retrospective study in 248 men with oligospermia and varicocele reported similar miscarriage rate after ART cycles in men who underwent varicocelectomy and in those who had expectant management (23.9% vs 21.7%, respectively).

15.8.2 Hypogonadism

While some studies linked varicocelectomy with increased serum testosterone levels, this effect has not been confirmed by other studies. Varicocelectomy has been proposed to reverse symptomatic hypogonadism and to improve men's overall health, known to be directly correlated with the testosterone levels. A meta-analysis of nine studies including a total of 814 men showed a mean increase in serum testosterone of 97.48 ng/dL (3.4 nmol/ L) compared to the preoperative levels [1]. Several of these studies included men with normal preoperative serum testosterone levels and did not address hypogonadism as a primary outcome measure, which could have undermined the effectiveness of varicocelectomy. Whether an increase in serum testosterone of 100 ng/dL translates into the improvement of clinically significant symptoms remains to be seen.

15.8.3 Subclinical Varicocele

Management of subclinical varicoceles further adds to the controversy surrounding varicocelectomy. While current evidence supports repair of clinically apparent varicocele, correction of subclinical varicocele appears to have little benefit on fertility and hence is not routinely offered [11]. The 2016 systematic review of seven RCTs in 548 infertile men with subclinical varicocele and otherwise unexplained infertility demonstrated that varicocelectomy improved progressive sperm motility but did not influence the pregnancy rates [24]. The 2018 meta-analysis that comprised 13 studies (2 RCTs and 11 retrospective) in a total of 1,357 men with subclinical varicocele failed to show a positive effect of varicocelectomy on sperm parameters or spontaneous pregnancy rates [25]. A meta-analysis of four RCTs in 637 men with mixed clinical-subclinical disease showed significant improvement in progressive sperm motility, morphology and spontaneous pregnancy rates following repair of left clinical and right subclinical varicocele [26]. Based on the available evidence, treatment of subclinical varicocele should be guarded and individualized.

15.9 Varicocele in Adolescents

Adolescents with a varicocele should be offered varicocele repair if they present with ipsilateral testicular atrophy or abnormal semen parameters. Varicocele repair in adolescents has been shown to improve testicular testosterone production, which allows for testicular catch-up growth and improvement in semen parameters [3]. Experts agree that in the absence of testicular size reduction, discomfort or abnormality in semen parameters, annual follow-up with physical examination and semen analysis is appropriate. The effect of varicoceles diagnosed during adolescence or young adulthood on future paternity is less clear. According to one longitudinal study in 661 adolescent boys with a varicocele treated with embolization or observation, paternity rates were not different between the groups, reported as 78% and 85%, respectively [27]. Another observational study in over 400 adolescents demonstrated 3.6 times greater chance of paternity after microsurgical varicocele repair compared to the observation group [28]. This reiterates the desperate need for well-designed future studies. At this stage, there is no conclusive evidence to justify the repair of adolescent varicoceles for improving future fertility as a sole indication.

15.10 Challenges and Uncertainties

The growing body of evidence suggests that in the absence of other causes of infertility, repair of varicocele can help to achieve natural conception, eliminate the need for ART or enable less complex fertility treatments. When ART is still recommended, pre-treatment correction of clinical varicocele results in increased likelihood of finding sperm in men with azoospermia and improved reproductive outcomes in men with severely impaired semen parameters. Although the benefit of varicocelectomy has been solidified in several meta-analyses, these findings should be interpreted with caution.

First, the meta-analyses on different aspects of varicocele yield low to moderate quality evidence due to heterogeneity and risk of bias in the included studies. The methodological flaws of individual studies include poorly defined inclusion criteria of the study participants, unclear definition of oligospermia, varying treatment end-points, small-size, unclear time-line from repair to pregnancy and short follow-up. Most of these studies are retrospective and often do not examine the factors that may have confounded fertility outcomes of the couple. This includes duration of infertility, concurrent infertility diagnosis of the female partner, female age and previous reproductive experience.

Second, the methodology of the published meta-analyses themselves has been subjected to numerous critiques on data collection and synthesis [7]. This can add to error in producing and interpreting evidence.

Finally, the validity of research findings may be influenced by a highly variable nature of semen characteristics, frequently used as the surrogate end-points in studies on varicocele. Semen parameters may improve over time without any intervention or may be influenced by various lifestyle factors, which are rarely reported. The "normal fertility cut-offs" from the WHO 2010 manual do not always correlate with pregnancy rates and there is no defined cut-off for TMC, the most clinically relevant parameter of semen analysis. Overall, this urges the need for well-designed sufficiently powered studies with using a standardized methodology and clinically meaningful outcomes.

The number of areas in varicocele management remains underexplored. In a context of ART, it is unclear if varicocelectomy improves reproductive outcomes in couples of advanced paternal or maternal age, or in those with mild oligospermia who undergo ART for other indications. There is also insufficient knowledge regarding the most optimal surgery-to-ART time interval and long-term efficacy of varicocele repair on fertility. Several studies reported the mean of 6–7 months between varicocelectomy and ART cycles and the mean of 2.5–3 years to successful pregnancy [7]. These observations need to be prospectively confirmed in different patient cohorts. Importantly, the supposed financial benefits of varicocele repair rely on sound assumptions of preventing the need for ART or reducing the number of treatment cycles. However, the cost-effectiveness of varicocelect-omy in achieving live birth has not been formally assessed.

15.11 Conclusive Remarks

There is a strong physiological rationale for managing of varicoceles in the context of male infertility. Men should be assessed for the presence of a varicocele at early stages of a couple's fertility journey to enable concurrent timely care for both partners.

Despite the limitations in current evidence, couples should be made aware of increased likelihood of achieving pregnancy after varociclelctomy, even when ART is recommended. This holds true even with marginal improvement in semen parameters, since varicocele repair also improves semen quality. It is also anticipated that the couple would require a lower number of ART cycles with a potential to reduce the financial burden and stress associated with complex ART treatments. The decision to undergo varicocele repair is often complex, particularly when there is the readily available alternative of immediate ART. This requires the consideration of multiple factors, including semen characteristics, desired number of children, accessibility to ART, costs, timing, age and presence of other fertility factors.

Currently, there is a paucity of high-quality data to support generalized treatment of varicocele in all infertile couples. There are no clear guidelines on how to select the right group of men that would benefit the most from the repair. It is also unclear when is the best time to initiate intervention in men with incidental varicocele who still do not have plans for parenthood, including those diagnosed in adolescence. Future studies should focus on specific well-characterized patient phenotypes, provide clear and standardized outcome measures, adjust for important confounders and allow sufficient follow-up interval. It is time for fertility specialists and urologists to make a concerted effort in directing varicocele research toward clinically meaningful patient-centered outcomes. This will help to guide and shape the clinical practice to serve our patients in a more effective way.

References

1. Clavijo, R., Carrasquillo, R. and Ramasamy, R. (2017) Varicoceles: prevalence and pathogenesis in adult men. *Fertil Steril* **108**:364–369.

2. Mohammadali Beigi, F., Mehrabi, S. and Javaherforooshzadeh, A. (2007) Varicocele in brothers of patients with varicocele. *Urol J* **4**(1):33–35.

3. Jacobson, D. and Johnson, E. K. (2017) Varicoceles in pediatric and adolescent population: treat to future fertility? *Fertil Steril* **108**:370–377.

4. Vanlangenhove, P. (2018) Contribution to the pathophysiology and treatment of varicoceles. *JBSR* **102**(1):1–14.

5. Hassanin, A. M., Ahmed, H. H. and Kaddah, A. N. (2018) A global view of the pathophysiology of varicocele. *Andrology* **6**(5):654–661.

6. Jung, A. and Schuppe, H. C. (2007) Influence of genital heat stress on semen quality in humans. *Andrologia* **39**:203–215.

7. Kohn, T. P., Kohn, J. R. and Pastuszak, A. W. (2017) Varicocelectomy before assisted reproductive technology: are outcomes improved? *Fertil Steril* **108**(3):385–391.

8. Rowe, P. J., Comhaire, F. H., Hargreave, T. B. and Mahmoud, A. M. (2000) World Health Organization. *WHO Manual for the Standardized Investigation, Diagnosis, and Management of the Infertile Male*, 1st edn. New York: Cambridge University Press,

9. Belay, R. E., Huang, G. O., Shen, J. K. and Ko, E. Y. (2016) Diagnosis of clinical and subclinical varicocele: how has it evolved? *Asian J Androl* **18**(2):182–185.

10. Lorenc, T., Krupniewski, L., Palczewski, P. and Gołębiowski, M. (2016) The value of ultrasonography in the diagnosis of varicocele. *J Ultrason* **16**(67):359–370.

11. Practice Committee of the American Society for Reproductive Medicine (2014) Society for Male Reproduction and Urology. Report on varicocele and infertility: a committee opinion. *Fertil Steril* **102**:1556–1560.

12. Hsiao, W., Rosoff, J., Pale, J., Powell, J. L. and Goldstein, M. (2013) Varicocelectomy is associated with increases in serum testosterone independent of clinical grade. *Urology* **81**(6):1213–1217.

13. Johnson, D. and Sandlow, J. (2017) Treatment of varicoceles: techniques and outcomes. *Fertil Steril* **108**(3):378–384.

14. Tatem, A. and Brannigan, R. (2017) The role of microsurgical varicocelectomy in treating male infertility. *Transl Androl Urol* **6**(4):722–729.

15. Cayan, S., Shavakhabov, S. and Kadioglu, A. (2009)Treatment of palpable varicocele in infertile men: a meta-analysis to define the best technique. *J Androl* **30**(1):33–40.

16. Baazeem, A., Belzile, E., Ciampi, A., Dohle, G., Jarvi, K., Salonia, A., et al. (2011) Varicocele and male factor infertility treatment: a new meta-analysis and review

of the role of varicocele repair. *Eur Urol* **60** (4):796–808.

17. Esteves, S. C., Miyaoka, R., Roque, M. and Agarwal, A. (2016) Outcome of varicocele repair in men with nonobstructive azoospermia: systematic review and meta-analysis. *Asian J Androl* **18** (2):246–253.

18. Samplaski, M. K., Lo, K. C., Grober, E. D., Zini, A. and Jarvi, K. A. (2017) Varicocelectomy to "upgrade" semen quality to allow couples to use less invasive forms of assisted reproductive technology. *Fertil Steril* **108**(4):609–612.

19. Marmar, J. L., Agarwal, A., Prabakaran, S., Agarwal, R., Short, R. A., Benoff, S., et al. (2007) Reassessing the value of varicocelectomy as a treatment for male subfertility with a new meta-analysis. *Fertil Steril* **88**:639–648.

20. Evers, J. L. and Collins, J. A. (2004) Surgery or embolisation for varicocele in subfertile men. *Cochrane Database Syst Rev* **3**: CD00479.

21. Kamischke, A. and Nieschlag, E. (2001) Varicocele treatment in the light of evidence-based andrology. *Hum Reprod Update* **7**:65–69.

22. Kirby, E. W., Wiener, L. E., Rajanahally, S., Crowell, K. and Coward, R. M. (2016) Undergoing varicocele repair prior to assisted reproduction improves pregnancy rate and live birth rate in azoospermic and oligospermic men with a varicocele:

23. Mansour Ghanaie, M., Asgari, S. A., Dadrass, N., Allahkhah, A., Iran-Pour, E. and Safarinejad, M. R. (2012) Effects of varicocele repair on spontaneous first trimester miscarriage: a randomized clinical trial. *Urol J* **9**(2):505–513.

24. Kim, H. J., Seo, J. T., Kim, K. J., Ahn, H., Jeong, J. Y., Kim, J. H., et al. (2016) Clinical significance of subclinical varicocelectomy in male infertility: systematic review and meta-analysis. *Andrologia* **48**(6):654–661.

25. Kohn, T. P., Ohlander, S. J., Jacob, J. S., Griffin, T. M., Lipshultz, L. I. and Pastuszak, A. W. (2018) The effect of subclinical varicocele on pregnancy rates and semen parameters: a systematic review and meta-analysis. *Curr Urol Rep* **19**(7): 53.

26. Niu, Y., Wang, D., Chen, Y., Pokhrel, G., Xu, H., Wang, T., et al. (2018) Comparison of clinical outcome of bilateral and unilateral varicocelectomy in infertile males with left clinical and right subclinical varicocele: A meta-analysis of randomised controlled trials. *Andrologia* **50**(9):e13078.

27. Bogaert, G., Orgye, C. and De Win, G. (2013) Pubertal screening and treatment for varicocele do not improve chance of paternity as adult. *J Urol* **189**:2298–2304.

28. Cayan, S., Bozlu, M. and Akbay, E. (2017) Update on the novel management and future paternity situation in adolescents with varicocele. *Turk J Urol* **43**:241–246.

a systematic review and meta-analysis. *Fertil Steril* **106**:1338–1343.

Donor Insemination: Past, Present and Future Perspectives

Christopher L. R. Barratt, Rachel Agnew, and Eleanor Heighton

Donor insemination (DI) has undergone radical changes in the last 25 years; for example, moving to exclusive use of cryopreserved semen, increasing treatment of patients who do not suffer from male factor infertility and changes in society's attitudes to the use of donor gametes, to name but a few. The main focus of this chapter is to briefly examine the past to gain some perspective of where we have been, present a discussion of what major changes have occurred and thoughts on where the future may lie.

In the 1980s, a dramatic event changed the way DI operated, namely the transmission of human T-cell lymphotropic virus type III (HTLV-III) (since termed HIV) to four of eight recipients of donor semen from a man who was HIV sero positive. This added further evidence that HIV was transmitted via semen but, for DI, it had a profound impact on the recruitment, selection and screening of donors [1]. It was also recognised that there was a delay in men sero-converting after they became infected. Effectively, not only did it mean the mandatory use of cryopreserved spermatozoa, but also that frozen donor semen needed to be quarantined prior to treatment. Although a number of authorities (e.g. CECOS – Centre d'Étude et de COnservation du Sperme) had operated a cryopreservation service prior to 1985, many other clinics used fresh semen for convenience and the perception of higher success rates. Unfortunately, the change to exclusive use of cryopreserved cells and quarantining samples was a gradual process with many reluctant to change their beliefs that cryopreservation dramatically reduced success rates as well as adding significant inconvenient steps and associated costs to the process. Remarkably, even 10 years after the recognition of the risk of HIV transmission, some clinics still used fresh semen. We do not know if this latency in uptake had an effect on the transmission of HIV, such as were there further unnecessary cases of HIV following insemination of non-quarantined semen? Technology took some time to catch up with clinical practice so that rapid testing of samples for HIV and other viruses would be robust and reliable; however, even with these available technologies, cryopreservation and quarantine remain the standard practice.

Further changes regarding the way DI services operated were catalysed by the introduction of intra-cytoplasmic sperm injection (ICSI), which enables the use of partners' sperm utilising in vitro fertilisation (IVF) technology, thus avoiding the need for donor sperm. Initial data in national registers showed a dramatic decrease in the use of DI as ICSI steadily replaced DI as a potential treatment. In fact, for some time it looked as though DI would become a redundant treatment and disappear altogether. On reflection, this doomsday scenario was premature. Data from the United Kingdom (UK), where ART is regulated by the Human Fertilisation and Embryology Authority (HFEA) shows that since 1992 (when data were recorded) there is a clear trend with a decline until about 2007 (3,901 cycles), but then an increase or at least stabilisation to current times (5,446 cycles, 2016) (Figure 16.1,

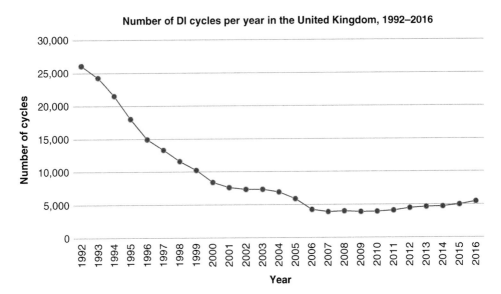

Figure 16.1 Number of DI cycles per year in the UK, 1992–2016.

Table 16.1). Moreover, the use of donor sperm in IVF/ICSI has increased steadily (1,288 cycles in 1992 compared to 3,041 in 2016, Table 16.1). A similar picture is seen in other countries, for example in Australia and New Zealand, where there has been a decline from 5,425 DI cycles in 1998 to 3,356 cycles in 2005, but this figure then stabilised to 3,198 in 2016. In parallel, there has been an increase in the number of ICSI cycles in the UK (137 in 1992 to 24,441 in 2016, Table 16.2, Figure 16.2), although the proportion of ICSI/IVF cycles has not changed since 2004 (~35%) (Figures 16.3 and 16.4).

Whilst it is not possible to accurately quantify the reasons for the decline in DI treatment, an overriding factor is the availability of ICSI. However, in the UK, as with a number of other countries (see below), there has been a significant number of changes in the regulatory framework, for example removal of anonymity of gamete donors which may have exacerbated the decline in the availability of donor sperm hence restricting the possibility of treatment. To counterbalance this there has been increased use of DI for non-male factor cases. As such, there appears to be a continual steady demand for DI (~100 per million population). For example, in 2016 in the UK, only 42% of the DI recipient cycles were for male partner infertility, 41% of patients had a female partner and 17% for no partner. DI is therefore a treatment which has evolved from almost exclusively treatment for male factor infertility to include almost equal numbers of social infertility (no male partner) cases.

A third key change in DI has been in the regulatory and operational landscape. Perhaps the most significant change was the removal of anonymity in a number of countries. Sweden was one of the first to effectively remove anonymity. On 18 March 1985, the Swedish Parliament enacted legislation providing the child with the right "when sufficiently mature" to receive identifying information about the semen provider. The reasons for the removal of anonymity include the principle that children have a right for information regarding their genetic parents. Following the example of Sweden, a number of countries have removed the

Table 16.1 Trends in donor insemination in the UK,1992–2016

Year	Number of DI treatment cycles[a]	% LBR	Number of IVF cycles with donor sperm[b]	% IVF cycles using donor sperm[b]
1992	26,081	5	1,288	9.0
1993	24,265	6	1,713	10.4
1994	21,490	8	1,670	8.9
1995	18,014	9	1,565	7.0
1996	14,927	10	1,401	5.6
1997	13,309	10	1,209	4.8
1998	11,581	10	1,114	4.2
1999	10,230	11	1,037	4.0
2000	8,414	11	979	3.8
2001	7,621	11	876	3.3
2002	7,332	11	916	3.4
2003	7,330	11	904	3.3
2004	6,917	11	940	3.2
2005	5,883	11	1,033	3.3
2006	4,254	11	916	2.7
2007	3,901	12	1,036	2.9
2008	3,999	12	1,269	3.3
2009	3,896	11	1,622	3.9
2010	3,948	13	1,993	4.6
2011	4,108	12	2,243	5.0
2012	4,478	13	2,371	5.4
2013	4,642	13	2,535	5.8
2014	4,696	14	2,695	6.2
2015	4,971	13	2,705	6.3
2016	5,446	12	3,041	7.3

[a] Excludes IVF with donor sperm
[b] Fresh cycles using own eggs
Abbreviations: DI, donor insemination; LBR, live birth rate; IVF, in vitro fertilisation

use of anonymous sperm donors, for example, the UK. Whilst there were initial concerns among infertility service providers that the change in policy would result in a significant decline in the availability of donors, at least in UK, the number of donors has stabilised so that the demand for treatment (~4,500 DI cycles per annum) can be satisfied. Interestingly, not all countries have adopted a regulatory framework whereby the children born from DI

Table 16.2 Treatment cycles per year for DI, IVF and ICSI in the UK, HFEA data, 2016

Year	DI	IVF	ICSI	Total
1992	26,081	18,208	137	44,426
1993	24,265	21,243	628	46,136
1994	21,490	23,539	1,345	46,374
1995	18,014	25,425	3,905	47,344
1996	14,927	27,241	6,236	48,404
1997	13,309	25,481	8,552	47,342
1998	11,581	25,155	10,512	47,248
1999	10,230	24,128	10,752	45,110
2000	8,414	24,154	11,284	43,852
2001	7,621	24,344	11,938	43,903
2002	7,332	25,185	12,331	44,848
2003	7,330	24,941	12,552	44,823
2004	6,917	26,272	13,853	47,042
2005	5,883	27,013	14,991	47,887
2006	4,254	27,584	17,079	48,917
2007	3,901	28,542	18,419	50,862
2008	3,999	30,402	20,394	54,795
2009	3,896	31,650	22,991	58,537
2010	3,948	33,883	24,144	61,975
2011	4,108	34,997	25,582	64,687
2012	4,478	34,922	25,314	64,714
2013	4,642	36,658	25,190	66,490
2014	4,696	38,158	25,383	68,237
2015	4,971	40,392	24,983	70,346
2016	5,446	43,649	24,441	73,536

Abbreviations: DI, donor insemination; IVF *in vitro* fertilisation; ICSI, intracytoplasmic sperm injection; HFEA, Human Fertilisation and Embryology Authority

can find out the identity of their biological father and there is wide variation, even within the European Union (EU).

The change in anonymity status has been in place in several countries for some time, hence we have more research, albeit variable, in its conclusions, to indicate the magnitude of these changes. Clearly, despite existence of regulation/legislation, at least initially, not all couples had told their children about the mode of conception let alone their ability to identify their biological father [2]. The inevitable conclusion is that

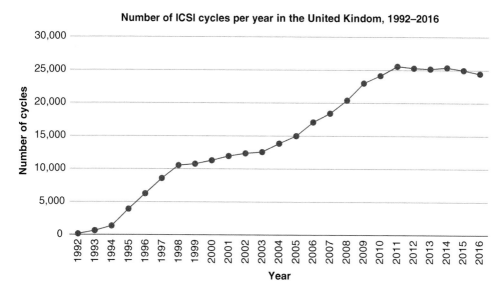

Figure 16.2 Number of ICSI cycles per year in the UK, 1992–2016.

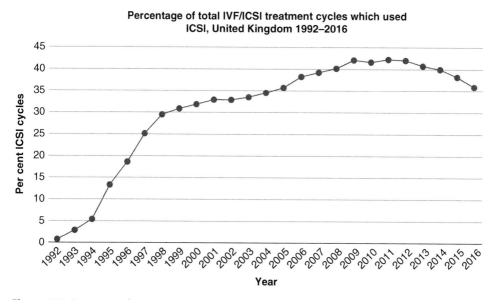

Figure 16.3 Percentage of total IVF/ICSI treatment cycles which used ICSI, in the UK 1992–2016.

considerable support needs to be in place for recipient couples. A 20-year follow-up study in Sweden provided encouraging data in that the majority of couples were relatively open about their treatment and their likelihood of disclosure to the offspring. Moreover, data from a single CECOS centre where sperm donation is anonymous showed that an overwhelming majority of parents of DI-conceived children had

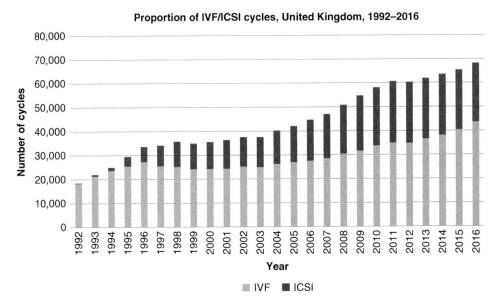

Figure 16.4 Proportion of IVF/ICSI cycles in the UK, 1992–2016.

disclosed the use of donor gametes to their children [3]. Furthermore, a nationwide study of CECOS centres came to similar conclusions [4]. In contrast, an Australian study found that only one in three couples had told their offspring about their origins [5]. However, further research is necessary to determine exactly how this information is presented to the offspring, at what stage, in what format and what support structures both formal and informal are necessary to facilitate the information sharing process [2,6].

Whatever the intellectual arguments for/against anonymity, we must be cognisant of the real-world situation. Critically, in this age that genetic testing is widely available to individuals such as "23and me" (www.23andme.com/en-gb/), it is inconceivable that we can maintain a system where children are prevented from discovering the identity of their biological father. McGovern and Schlaff present this eloquently in their article "Sperm donor anonymity: a concept rendered obsolete by modern technology" [7]. It may be a difficult transition for some countries/states to move to a system whereby the children are able, by regulation or legislation, to identify the biological father but we can learn from other examples such as Sweden and be proactive in this important arena.

16.1 Outcomes from Donor Insemination

In general, the data suggests that there are minimal significant concerns over the health of offspring of donor conceived children [8,9]. For example, a recent large retrospective study of HFEA data (n = 95,787 cycles) on IVF/ICSI with donor sperm compared to partner sperm showed no increased risk in adverse perinatal outcomes following use of donor sperm [10]. Moreover, a retrospective analysis of data from the Centre for Disease Control

United States of America on offspring produced from donor sperm with IVF/ICSI compared to partner sperm, provided similar reassuring conclusions [11].

16.2 Challenges of Future

Whilst some things have changed dramatically, a number unfortunately have not. Among those include the following.

16.2.1 Overall Success Rates

A plethora of studies continually show the influence of the female factors on success in DI. This is not surprising as the male component is effectively stabilised. Female age is of course a sentinel factor. For example, HFEA data showed a 15% live birth rate (LBR) per treatment cycle in women under 35, but only 5% in those 40–42 years of age (2016 data on 5,446 cycles, Table 16.1).

As with natural *in vivo* conception, critical factors apart from age, such as pelvic pathology and ovulation status, are also important and need to be taken into account when providing prognostic information to patients. However, it appears remarkable that the overall success rates of DI have remained relatively low and, in stark contrast to general IVF/ICSI, DI success rates have not significantly improved in the last 20 plus years. For example, in the UK, there has been no notable increase in the success rates of DI (overall live births/treatment cycle) since 1996 (~10% LBR/cycle in 1996 compared to 12% in 2016)). Similar trends are observed elsewhere. For example, in Australia and New Zealand, the current live delivery per cycle is 13% (2016 data). The average success rates in the EU were 11% delivery per cycle (EIM data 2017). This just does not make sense. David and colleagues were achieving a comparable standard of success – in the 1970s using cryopreserved semen [12]. Bearing in mind the technological advances in assisted conception, which have undoubtedly facilitated the increase in success of IVF/ICSI, it is very surprising that success in DI remains so low. DI is a very simple treatment and as long as the female has no significant pathology and sperm is inseminated at the correct time (just prior to ovulation), greater success rates should be achieved. This is clearly an area for future research and focus.

16.2.2 Questions over Methods

However, again, despite decades of research, we are still uncertain about critical areas of treatment regimes for DI, for example, the correct timing of inseminations or number of inseminations to perform. A classic example is the conclusions of the recent Cochrane review: "We concluded that the current evidence was too limited to choose between IUI or ICI, in natural cycles or with ovarian stimulation, in donor sperm treatment" [13]. There were remarkably few randomised controlled studies (RCTs) to use in the analysis and much of the data presented is on low numbers, so the overall quality of the data was deemed "very low." It is difficult to determine exactly why more comparative studies have not been performed. This is of course a continual failure in the field of infertility treatment where few large RCTs are conducted. Clearly we need more robust studies and the recent Capri consensus outlines ways in which this may be achieved [14]. However, there are some new trials appearing. For example, Rodriguez-Purata performed a randomised controlled trial examining the effect of inseminated volume of semen against DI success rates. No difference in success rates was observed between volumes of 0.2 versus 0.5 ml [15]. More of these types of studies are required.

16.2.3 Optimal Cryopreservation Regimens of Human Spermatozoa Remain to be Established

Initial advances in sperm storage and cryopreservation techniques resulted in the first human pregnancy from cryopreserved semen – reported in 1953. This was truly transformational and allowed the universal shipment and storage of semen, and facilitated the development of DI as a treatment for male infertility, and promised a new area of scientific endeavour. However, since this time there has been comparatively little progress on the cryobiology of human spermatozoa [16,17]. This is difficult to explain but perhaps because it "sort of works" and there are millions of cells, there has been little clinical imperative to improve success rates. It is likely that the low success rates of DI are in part due to the lack of optimised protocols for sperm cryopreservation, which do not allow maximal expression of fertilising capacity of the cells.

16.3 DI as a Potential Research Tool in Andrology

DI remains a powerful but underutilised research tool. A number of studies have compared various semen parameters as related to success. Generally, this shows a statistical relationship between the number/concentration of motile cells and success rates. However, what is particularly interesting is the observed differences in donor fecundity. Thyer and colleagues examined approximately 800 cycles of IUI DI with cryopreserved sperm and analysed the fecundability of 20 donors [18]. Remarkably, despite meeting minimal semen criteria for recruitment and all having minimal criteria after thawing, there was a substantial difference in fecundability ranging from 0.05 to 0.23 (after 40 cycles). This is not new information and has been observed by others, for example, Barratt and colleagues who compared fecundity levels of 33 donors in a minimum of 15 cycles [19]. As in the Thyer's study, there was no difference in semen characteristics and each passed the minimal criteria. However, in this study patients were inseminated with a minimum number of motile cells yet there were still large differences in donor fecundability ranging from 0.05 to 0.39. This has an important context as we know that men with relatively normal semen parameters have wide ranging fertilising ability [20]. As such, DI provides an ideal tool to assess the performance of new (and old) sperm function tests to assess their clinical value. Current methods to assess sperm fertilising ability are relatively poor and new ones are urgently required [21]. Surprisingly, this approach has received little attention [22], but as the search for elusive sperm function assays continues it would be an ideal complementary tool as part of a comprehensive testing system.

16.4 Summary

DI is a relatively straightforward treatment that now encompasses couples and single women where there is no male factor. Despite the increasing success rate of IVF/ICSI over the last 10 years, the success rates of DI have not improved. This is clearly a challenge for the future. Moreover, changes in the nature of access to genetic information will make secrecy a thing of the past for DI. This will be another key challenge and will require a plethora of support mechanisms in place for patients, clinics and offspring.

16.5 Acknowledgements

Work in CLRB laboratory is supported by MRC, Tenovus Scotland, Chief Scientist Office/NHS research Scotland and the Bill and Melinda Gates Foundation.

16.6 Authors' Roles

CLRB wrote the main and initial part of the manuscript. RA and EH analysed the data and prepared the figures and edited the manuscript. All authors contributed to the writing and approval of the final article.

16.7 Conflicts of Interest

CLRB was the Editor-in-Chief of Molecular Human Reproduction (2013–1018), has received lecturing fees from Merck and Ferring and is on the Scientific Advisory Panel for Ohana BioSciences. CLRB was chair of the World Health Organization Expert Synthesis Group on Diagnosis of Male infertility (2012–2016) and is an editor of RBMO.

References

1. Stewart, G. J., Tyler, J. P., Cunningham, A. L., Barr, J. A., Driscoll, G. L., Gold, J., et al. (1985) Transmission of human T-cell lymphotropic virus type III (HTLV-III) by artificial insemination by donor. *Lancet* 14:581–585.

2. Indekeu, A., Dierickx, K., Schotsmans, P., Daniels, K. R., Rober, P. and D'Hooghe, T. (2013) Factors contributing to parental decision-making in disclosing donor conception: a systematic review. *Hum Reprod Update* 19:714–733.

3. Lassalzede, T., Paci, M., Rouzier, J., Carez, S., Gnisci, A., Saias-Magnan, J., et al. (2017) Sperm donor conception and disclosure to children: a 10-year retrospective follow-up study of parental attitudes in one French center for the study and preservation of eggs and sperm (CECOS). *Fertil Steril* 108:247–253.

4. Kalampalikis, N., Doumergue, M. and Zadeh, S. (2018) French Federation of CECOS. Sperm donor regulation and disclosure intentions: results from a nationwide multi-centre study in France. *Reprod Biomed Soc Online* 10(5):38–45.

5. Kovacs, G., Wise, S. and Finch, S. (2013) Functioning of families involving primary school-age children conceived using anonymous donor sperm. *Hum Reprod* 28:375–384.

6. Zadeh, S. (2016) Disclosure of donor conception in the era of non-anonymity: safeguarding and promoting the interests of donor-conceived individuals? *Hum Reprod* 31:2416–2420.

7. McGovern, P. G. and Schlaff, W. D. (2018) Sperm donor anonymity: a concept rendered obsolete by modern technology. *Fertil Steril* 109:230–231.

8. Thepot, F., Mayaux, M. J., Czyglick, F., Wack, T., Selva, J. and Jalbert, P. (1996) Incidence of birth defects after artificial insemination with frozen donor spermatozoa: a collaborative study of the French CECOS Federation on 11,535 pregnancies. *Hum Reprod* 11:2319–2323.

9. Lansac, J. and Royere, D. (2001) Follow-up studies of children born after frozen sperm donation. *Hum Reprod Update* 7:33–37.

10. Kamath, M. S., Antonisamy, B., Selliah, H. Y., La Marca, A. and Sunkara, S. K. (2018) Perinatal outcomes following IVF with use of donor versus partner sperm. *Reprod Biomed Online* 36:705–710.

11. Gerkowicz, S. A., Crawford, S. B., Hipp, H. S., Boulet, S. L. and Kissin, D. M. (2018) Assisted reproductive technology with donor sperm: national trends and perinatal outcomes. *Am J Obstet Gynecol* 421.e1–421.e10.

12. David, G., Czyglik, F., Mayaux, M. J., Martin-Boyce, A. and Schwartz, D. (1980) Artificial insemination with frozen sperm: protocol, method of analysis and results for 1,188 women. *Br J Obstet Gynaecol* 87:1022–1028.

13. Kop, P. A., Mochtar, M. H., O'Brien, P. A., Van der Veen, F. and van Wely, M. (2018) Intrauterine insemination versus

intracervical insemination in donor sperm treatment. *Cochrane Database Syst Rev* **1**: CD000317.

14. ESHRE Capri Workshop Group (2018) Protect us from poor-quality medical research. *Hum Reprod* **33**:770–776.

15. Rodriguez-Purata, J., Latre, L., Ballester, M., González-Llagostera, C., Rodríguez, I., Gonzalez-Foruria, I., et al. (2018) Clinical success of IUI cycles with donor sperm is not affected by total inseminated volume: a RCT. *Hum Reprod Open* **2**:hoy002.

16. Hezavehei, M., Sharafi, M., Kouchesfahani, H. M., Henkel, R., Agarwal, A., Esmaeili, V., et al. (2018) Sperm cryopreservation: a review on current molecular cryobiology and advanced approaches. *Reprod Biomed Online* **37**:327–339.

17. Benson, J. D., Woods, E. J., Walters, E. M. and Critser, J. K. (2012) The cryobiology of spermatozoa. *Theriogenology* **78**:1682–1699.

18. Thyer, A. C., Patton, P. E., Burry, K. A., Mixon, B. A. and Wolf, D. P. (1999) Fecundability trends among sperm donors as a measure of donor performance. *Fertil Steril* **71**:891–895.

19. Barratt, C. L., Clements, S. and Kessopoulou, E. (1998) Semen characteristics and fertility tests required for storage of spermatozoa. *Hum Reprod* **13** (Suppl 2):1–7.

20. Barratt, C. L. R., Björndahl, L., De Jonge, C. J., Lamb, D. J., Osorio Martini, F., McLachlan, R., et al. (2017) The diagnosis of male infertility: an analysis of the evidence to support the development of global WHO guidance-challenges and future research opportunities. *Hum Reprod Update* **23**:660–680.

21. Schinfeld, J., Sharara, F., Morris, R., Palermo, G. D., Rosenwaks, Z., Seaman, E., et al. (2018) Cap-Score™ prospectively predicts probability of pregnancy. *Mol Reprod Dev* **85**:654–664.

22. Bonache, S., Mata, A., Ramos, M. D., Bassas, L. and Larriba, S. (2012) Sperm gene expression profile is related to pregnancy rate after insemination and is predictive of low fecundity in normozoospermic men. *Hum Reprod* **27**:1556–1567.

DNA Damage in Spermatozoa

Russell P. Hayden, Ahmad Aboukhshaba,
and Peter N. Schlegel

17.1 Introduction

DNA damage is a common feature of all spermatozoa. The relative magnitude and clinical meaningfulness of sperm genomic integrity varies from cell to cell, with each man producing a population of spermatozoa that will carry a unique distribution of DNA damage. Additionally, this distribution will vary with time, sperm source, and the lifestyle/exposures that occur during the period of spermatogenesis. Given the ubiquity of genomic lesions that occur in the male germ line, it is apparent that the embryo is capable of robust DNA repair with high fidelity. However, the embryo's ability to compensate for defects in the paternal genome does have limitations, which is apparent in data correlating male subfertility with progressively higher levels of DNA fragmentation. These observations are apparent in natural conception rates and time to pregnancy studies, a trend that has also translated to outcomes of assisted reproductive technologies (ART). Despite these data, reproductive medicine has been slow to adopt sperm DNA testing due to the lack of assay standardization, controversy regarding normal thresholds, and a body of literature that suffers from significant design/cohort heterogeneity with equally heterogeneous results. In the following review, the pathophysiology of sperm DNA damage will be discussed along with a description of the sequalae that can be expected. Finally, the data associating DNA fragmentation in sperm with reproductive outcomes will be outlined, including therapeutic options currently available for men faced with significant levels of sperm DNA damage.

17.2 Genomic Integrity

17.2.1 Categorization of Genetic Damage

The unique process of spermatogenesis exposes the male germ line to a specific set of genetic insults that are not typically encountered by somatic cells. Relevant hallmarks of spermatogenesis include the life-long maintenance of a stem-cell population, differentiation, meiosis with genetic recombination, successful production of a haploid cell line, and ultimate maturation into functional spermatozoa. The success of spermatogenesis is also dependent upon appropriate support and surveillance by surrounding Sertoli cells, the creation of a suitable paracrine and endocrine milieu, and the careful regulation of testis temperature. Impaired function at any of these levels can result in male subfertility. In terms of genomic integrity, aberrant function of the aforementioned processes can directly or indirectly affect the viability of the sperm product. Regardless of the cause, the majority of genetic damage can be categorized into three non-mutually exclusive endpoints: chromosomal abnormalities, errors in DNA packaging, and DNA fragmentation.

Chromosomal abnormalities include errors of chromosome number, deletions, and transversions. The majority of these types of genetic faults are associated with errors in meiosis. Overall, the testis is efficient in recognizing cells that have suffered an error of meiosis, and typically eliminates them prior to maturation into functional sperm. In men with proven fertility, the rate of aneuploidy is low in ejaculated specimens, with rates ranging below 1% [1]. The proportion of sperm with abnormal ploidy is elevated in both men with impaired semen parameters and in men who contribute to recurrent pregnancy loss with otherwise reassuring semen analyses [2]. The assay used to detect sperm aneuploidy has conventionally been fluorescent *in situ* hybridization with probes designed against specific chromosomes of interest (typically the sex chromosomes with the addition of 13, 18, and 21 [1]).

The second category of genetic damage encompasses errors in DNA packaging. Unlike somatic cells that carry their genetic material around histones, the majority of sperm DNA is compacted with protamines. The tertiary structure of protamines is approximately half the size of histones, but compacts the genome to approximately one-sixth the size observed in somatic cells [3]. Beyond size considerations, the function of protamination also engenders the genome with a significant level of protection from attack by reactive oxygen species (ROS) [4]. To achieve the level of compaction characterized by protamination, the DNA backbone becomes progressively supercoiled during rewinding around these protein structures. To limit torsional stress, topoisomerases cause temporary physiologic nicks in the DNA [5]. These DNA breaks allow for relief of torsional stress and are normally repaired without consequence. However, defective repair of these DNA nicks can lead to persistent DNA double-strand breaks in mature sperm, one possible mechanism of DNA fragmentation [6]. Although there are no widely utilized assays to measure protamination clinically, defective chromatin compaction has been linked to subfertility in both animal models and humans [7.8].

The third category of DNA damage is typically termed "DNA fragmentation," since it is measured by direct or indirect assays of DNA strand breaks (Table 17.1). However, the range of DNA damage that may ultimately result in fragmentation is broad. Table 17.2 provides a brief list of the types of DNA damage that may occur in spermatozoa. Although grouping these distinct processes under the DNA fragmentation header is imprecise, no widely used tests exist to assay each specific type of genetic insult in clinical practice. In lieu of mechanism-specific damage measurement, the clinician must therefore rely upon the global assessment of DNA fragmentation to provide an impression of genomic integrity.

Unlike errors of meiosis, some level of DNA fragmentation is thought to exist in every sperm, with the relative degree of genetic damage varying from cell to cell [9,10]. As a result, depending upon the type and severity of genomic damage, viable embryos will undergo a round of DNA repair prior to the first cleavage [6]. Although the embryo is well equipped to address this type of damage, viability will ultimately hinge upon the quality and quantity of DNA damage. A variety of risk factors have been linked to DNA fragmentation (Figure 17.1). Despite the myriad of causes, many investigators have effectively argued that oxidative stress forms a common mechanistic pathway [6,11,12]. Given the ubiquitous nature of DNA fragmentation in all males, the remainder of this chapter will concentrate on the pathophysiology, clinical consequences, and treatment of this type of genetic damage.

17.2.2 Pathophysiology of DNA Fragmentation

DNA fragmentation has been linked to an array of male infertility risk factors, including widely disparate conditions such as age, varicocele, cigarette smoking, and infection/

Table 17.1 Description of commonly used assays for assessment of DNA fragmentation.

Assay	Fragmentation assessment	Chemistry	Application
COMET	Direct	DNA with single and double strand breaks will migrate during gel electrophoresis, producing a tail stemming from the sperm nucleus	Capable of assessing DNA damage of individual cells. Requires a fresh semen sample. Time and labor intensive. Lacks well established protocols.
TUNEL	Direct	Exposed single and double strand DNA nicks are labeled with fluorescent dUTP with a template independent deoxynucleotidyl transferase	Commercially available kits. Can be conducted on fresh or frozen specimens. Also lacks established protocols and standardized thresholds.
SCSA	Indirect	Acridine orange fluoresces at differing wavelengths for intact vs denatured DNA. DNA with fragmentation will denature more readily and produce more signal	Frozen specimens are mailed to a commercial lab. Requires samples with large numbers of spermatozoa. Benefits from established clinical thresholds.
SCD	Indirect	Single cells are embedded in agarose gel, lysed, and the DNA is denatured. Undamaged DNA will produce a "halo" around the nucleus	Inexpensive commercial assays can be purchased that do not require fluorescent imaging. Noisy/unclear cells may be misinterpreted.

TUNEL: Terminal deoxynucleotidyl transferase-mediated dUTP nick end labeling. SCSA: Sperm chromatin structure assay. SCD (also known as "halo"): Sperm chromatin dispersion assay.

Table 17.2 Types of DNA damage possible in the sperm nucleus.

Types of DNA damage
Base adducts
Abasic sites
Guanosine oxidation
Pyrimidine dimerization
Thymidine glycol
Base modifications
Crosslinks
Mismatches

These types of genetic lesions are not directly measured by DNA fragmentation assays.

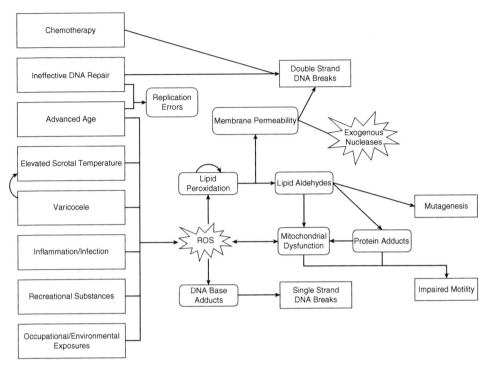

Figure 17.1 Risk factors associated with sperm DNA fragmentation.

inflammation. The pervasive endpoint of genomic instability would suggest a common mechanistic pathway for the conditions outlined in Figure 17.1. Seminal work by De Iuliis and colleagues explored the correlation of oxidative damage with a specific base adduct, 8-hydroxy-2′-deoxyguanosine (8OHdG), to the level of DNA fragmentation [4]. 8OHdG is a type of DNA modification that occurs following a direct oxidative insult of the DNA molecule itself, and has traditionally served as a robust biomarker of oxidative stress. The abundance of 8OHdG residues correlated so well with the amount of DNA fragmentation that some investigators "have been forced to conclude that most DNA damage in spermatozoa is oxidatively induced" [4,6]. It is worth mentioning that in correlated studies most of the risk factors listed in Figure 17.1 were also tied to an excessive oxidative state [13].

The role of ROS in male fertility is complex, with evidence showing that a mild oxidative state is necessary for appropriate sperm function. Early studies demonstrated improvement of fertilizing capability of human spermatozoa subjected to low levels of oxidative stress [14]. It is now appreciated that ROS are required for effective capacitation of sperm in multiple species, including humans [13,15]. The presence of ROS increases intracellular cAMP, inhibits tyrosine phosphatases, and promotes the oxidation of sterols in the spermatozoon head, all of which are necessary for effective capacitation [11]. The process may be initiated by either endogenous or exogenous ROS. H_2O_2 appears to be a key element, as the addition of catalase can prevent hyperactivation, membrane fusion, and the acrosome reaction [15]. The balance between ROS and antioxidants is critical however, as too much oxidative stress will result in DNA damage and possibly initiate apoptosis. To this end, it has been observed that morphologically normal sperm with hyperactive motility can harbor significant genomic damage, yet they can still perform well in terms of the ability to fertilize [16]. It is conceivable that sperm primed for capacitation, which may have already accrued pathologic levels of DNA fragmentation, will outperform sperm with less DNA damage as a function of ROS exposure.

As oxidative stress increases, the apparent continuum shifts away from the physiologic state described above and switches toward a form of apoptosis. Nearly all sperm are ultimately destined to either undergo apoptosis or senescence, as only a few will actually participate in fertilization. The unique process of sperm cell death is significant, as these cells must be consumed by phagocytic leukocytes in both the male and female reproductive tract without triggering an inflammatory response. The silent removal of these cells is ensured by the display of apoptotic markers on dead sperm, the most important being phosphatidylserine [12]. Although this is a common feature of apoptosis in general, the process of apoptosis in spermatozoa deviates substantially from somatic cells.

Apoptosis is an active process that relies upon intact transcription, translation, the expression of FAS (exogenous pathway), and the co-compartmentalization of the nucleus and mitochondria (endogenous pathway). A characteristic feature of somatic apoptosis is the laddering of nuclear DNA on gel electrophoresis, which is a consequence of endonuclease fragmentation of the genome. However, apoptotic sperm do not exhibit this laddering pattern [12]. Additionally, sperm do not respond to the conventional chemical triggers of apoptosis [12]. To understand these fundamental differences and how they are important clinically, one must recognize the exceptional barriers to efficient apoptosis that exist in sperm.

Initially, the developing germ line is capable of traditional apoptosis. The number of maturing gametes is controlled by surrounding Sertoli cells, which express FAS-ligand and triggers the exogenous apoptosis pathway [9–12]. This population control ensures that Sertoli cells have enough resources to provide proper support. However, as spermatocytes advance toward spermatozoa, they progressively lose the ability for transcription and translation. Additionally, the replacement of histones with protamines during spermiogenesis impacts on how endonucleases react with DNA, since the primary endonuclease Caspase-Activated-DNase (CAD) usually acts upon the linker segment between histones [12]. As spermatids elongate, the cytosol and mitochondria become compartmentalized into the midpiece, effectively sequestering them from the nucleus located in the sperm head. As a result, much of the dormant CAD in the cytosol can no longer access the nuclear material.

Beyond ineffective endonuclease activity, the unique structure of the sperm carries additional implications for canonical apoptosis. The mitochondria are a keystone to the endogenous pathway of apoptosis, and similar to the discussion regarding CAD, in sperm they are also functionally sequestered from the nucleus. The mitochondria are potent producers of ROS, which will typically be activated by the absence of "survival" signals presented to the spermatozoon via the PI3 K-AKT pathway [12]. The mitochondria will also initiate the endogenous pathway if they sense significant cellular damage, mainly in the presence of lipid aldehydes or exogenously produced ROS. Regardless of the initial precipitator, once the mitochondria switch to an apoptotic mode a progressive cycle begins that leads to cellular death.

Mitochondria initially increase their production of ROS, which begin to react with cellular components necessary for sperm function. These reactive molecules tend to attack polyunsaturated fatty acids, which are particularly abundant in spermatozoa. A lipid peroxidation cascade begins that culminates in the formation of toxic lipid aldehydes [16]. Both free unsaturated fatty acids and the presence of lipid aldehydes provoke the mitochondria to release more ROS. The positive feedback loop that ensues generates a surge of oxidative damage. One of the first elements to be affected is motility, which is thought to be secondary to depletion of ATP. Another possible mechanism is the production of protein adducts within the axoneme machinery via mitochondrial derived ROS and reactive lipid aldehydes. It has been shown experimentally that the mere addition of lipid aldehydes, at physiologic concentration, will impair sperm motility [12]. Simultaneously, accumulating oxidative damage within the cell membrane impairs the ability of the sperm to fuse with an oocyte.

The positive feedback loop that results in the surge of endogenous oxidative stress is likely adaptive since spermatozoa cannot undergo full apoptosis. To remove themselves from the pool of viable spermatozoa, the cell must incapacitate both its fertilizing capability (plasma membrane and motility) and dismantle its genetic payload. Since sperm cannot dispose of its DNA with endonucleases, the only element in the system that can reach the genetic material is the ROS that are produced. The toxic metabolites, such as lipid aldehydes, in addition to direct oxidative damage of DNA, produce a variety of genetic defects, as presented in Table 17.2. With time, DNA fragmentation becomes a final common endpoint as profound damage ensues and the spermatozoon progress toward death. Unfortunately, a period will exist in which the sperm has begun the process of apoptosis, but remains capable of fertilization. This state has been loosely termed "abortive apoptosis," whether it originates during maturation in the seminiferous tubules or in transit through the male or female genital tracts [5].

It is important for the fertility specialist to understand the process of sperm apoptosis and its link to genetic integrity. First, some amount of oxidative stress is needed to prime sperm for capacitation and fertilization. However, it is unclear when this balance may shift and moderation has been surpassed, potentially resulting in significantly damaged sperm outperforming unprimed cells with preserved genomes. Although motility is one of the first functions to diminish in the process, again the state of abortive apoptosis is misleading. Men with apparently "normal" semen parameters, motility being the most relevant variable, may be generating spermatozoa with moderate levels of DNA damage that is sufficient to affect reproductive outcomes. Finally, in terms of advanced reproductive technology, the selection of morphologically normal and motile sperm for ICSI is helpful, but not a guarantee, for selecting a cell that has minimal DNA damage. As a result, this latter concept may provide the basis for why ICSI seems to outperform IVF for men with significant levels of DNA fragmentation [17].

17.3 Clinical Sequelae of Sperm DNA Damage

The connection between sperm DNA damage and reproductive outcomes has been marked by inconsistent findings in the primary literature. The proclivity of evidence points to a negative association between increasing DNA damage of sperm and reproductive outcome measures. However, the human data is fraught with non-uniform cohorts, the use of differing DNA fragmentation tests, variable assay cutoffs, and superficial endpoints (i.e. clinical pregnancy rate vs live births). As a result, the heterogeneity of these studies is considerable, which should raise caution when interpreting meta-analyses. It is also worth mentioning that including couples with a female factor can drastically attenuate the signal between DNA damage in the male gamete and reproductive success [17]. Consequently, the current guideline from the American Society for Reproductive Medicine does not recommend "the routine use of sperm DNA integrity tests in the evaluation and treatment of the infertile couple" [18].

Experiments in animal models, in which variables can be readily controlled, clearly demonstrate an association between increasing DNA fragmentation and poor reproductive outcomes. In one of the more illuminating studies, Fernandez-Gonzalez and colleagues induced DNA damage in mouse spermatozoa and tracked the long-term health outcomes of offspring conceived with ICSI [19]. The use of low DNA-integrity sperm resulted in poor embryo development and generated smaller litter sizes compared to controls. At 12 months of age, offspring from compromised sperm exhibited objective differences in behavior. More concerning, animals generated from ICSI of damaged sperm exhibited shorter life spans, an increased propensity for mesenchymal tumors, and accelerated aging. These data corroborate evidence in primates connecting poor reproductive outcomes with DNA damage [20].

In humans, the strongest data regarding the effects of sperm DNA damage is seen in natural conception and intrauterine insemination (IUI). Evenson and colleagues reviewed the literature for natural conception rates using the SCSA assay [21]. In their analysis, they examined thresholds for the DNA fragmentation index (DFI, the total percentage of abnormal sperm) of both 30% and 40%. Men with a DFI below 30% were 6.5 (CI 1.7–24.9) times more likely to contribute to a pregnancy than men with a DFI above 30%. Using the alternative cutoff of 40% for DFI increased the odds ratio for natural conception to 7.5 (CI 2.5–22.6) when comparing men below and above the 40% DFI level. Bungum and colleagues conducted one of the largest series examining IUI results, which spanned 387 cycles [22]. They found that an SCSA above 30% resulted in decreased clinical pregnancy rates (OR 0.1, CI 0.02–0.42) and delivery rates (OR 0.07, CI 0.01–0.48). Within their cohort, 19% of cycles with SCSA of less than 30% achieved a live birth, as opposed to 1.5% for men with levels above the 30% threshold.

As mentioned earlier, the data linking sperm DNA fragmentation to the success of standard IVF and ICSI has been inconsistent, mainly due to heterogeneity of study design. Unfortunately, results can be skewed by small changes in study design, the most prominent example being the inclusion of female factors. In the meta-analysis by Osman and colleagues, the authors conducted a sensitivity analysis to assess the influence of different subgroups within their pooled cohort [23]. The risk ratio for failure of standard IVF was 1.27 (CI 1.05–1.52) comparing men with low and high levels of DNA fragmentation. However, when controlling for female factors, the risk ratio increased to 2.76 (CI 1.59–4.8).

In one of the most exhaustive reviews to date, Simon and colleagues attempted to control for assay type, ART technique and, for the outcome of clinical pregnancy, female factors [9,10]. They highlight a relationship between sperm DNA integrity and fertilization for the specific case of microdrop IVF, which was not as strong for ICSI or mixed IVF-ICSI cohorts. Regarding embryo quality, assay type appeared to be the most influential. The relationship between DNA fragmentation and poor embryo development was best supported by studies utilizing the COMET assay. To assess the outcome of clinical pregnancy, they controlled for assay type in addition to female factor. Their pooled analysis of 70 studies spanning 17,744 treatment cycles favored an impact of DNA fragmentation on ART outcomes, demonstrating an overall odds ratio of 1.15 (CI 1.08–1.23). For IVF, ICSI, and mixed IVF-ICSI subgroups, the odds ratios were 1.15 (CI 1.05–1.27), 0.89 (CI 0.8–0.99), and 2.0 (CI 1.66–2.41), respectively. Direct DNA fragmentation assays (TUNEL, comet) had a pooled odds ratio of 2.4 (CI 2.03–2.84), whereas indirect assays (SCSA, SCD) yielded an odds ratio of 0.99 (CI 0.92–1.06).

The review by Simon and colleagues supports the use of standard IVF or ICSI over IUI when the male partner has significant amounts of sperm DNA damage [9,10]. The data suggests that ICSI is the least sensitive to DNA fragmentation of the male gamete. However, it should not be assumed that the ICSI procedure prevents the consequences of using spermatozoa with poor genomic integrity. Simon and colleagues also published a second analysis, which utilized stricter inclusion/exclusion criteria of candidates studied to improve data heterogeneity [9,10]. This analysis demonstrated an odds ratio of 1.31 (CI 1.08–1.59) for clinical pregnancy rate when comparing ICSI cycles with high and low DFI sperm. Although their findings were more statistically significant compared to their first analysis, ICSI still outperformed standard IVF. The observed differences in clinical outcomes may be due to a selection bias inherent to the ICSI technique. When an embryologist selects a sperm for injection, cells with the best motility and morphologic characteristics are chosen. As mentioned in Section 17.2.2 discussing pathophysiology, these selection criteria will improve the probability of selecting sperm with relatively low DNA fragmentation. However, even morphologically normal sperm with intact motility tend to have higher amounts of genomic damage in subfertile males [17]. In this scenario, the ramifications of successful fertilization may not be realized in the early embryonic period. In a meta-analysis by Zhao and colleagues, pregnancy and miscarriage rates were assessed based upon ART techniques [24]. Similar to the aforementioned studies, Zhao and colleagues demonstrated a significant inverse association between sperm DNA damage and pregnancy rate after standard IVF, but not with ICSI. However, they found the reverse relationship regarding pregnancy loss, where cycles initiated with ICSI carried an increased odds ratio of 2.68 (CI 1.4–5.14). It has been postulated that significant DNA damage of the male genome results in a "late paternal effect," which can result in miscarriage. This effect differs from impairments of fertilization and early embryonic development observed prior to embryo transfer [17]. Thus, caution should be observed when using ICSI for men with high DFI rates, as the hypothetical delayed paternal effect may increase the risk of pregnancy loss and ultimately subvert the primary goal of treatment.

17.4 Treatment

Therapeutic options are evolving for couples facing elevated sperm DNA damage. With the lack of modifiable risk factors, enough data now exists to justify the use of standard IVF or ICSI earlier in a treatment plan. Since the risks and benefits of utilizing ART for the case of significant sperm DNA damage was reviewed in Section 17.3, the following discussion will focus on alternative therapies designed to modify known risk factors. Of note, the emerging role of antioxidants for the treatment of men with elevated DFI is specifically addressed in an accompanying chapter.

17.4.1 Lifestyle

A multitude of lifestyle factors have been linked with male subfertility, semen parameters, and sperm DNA integrity (Figure 17.1) [25]. A detailed discussion of the various lifestyle choices and xenobiotic exposures relevant to male fertility is beyond the scope of this chapter. The reader is directed to another book in the CUP series "How to Improve Preconception Health to Maximize IVF Success" by Kovacs and Norman. However, tobacco smoke warrants a discussion as it is common, modifiable, and carries notable consequences for the genetic integrity of spermatozoa. Tobacco smoke itself contains high levels of ROS, diminishes the availability of systemic antioxidants, and correlates with the level of seminal oxidative stress [25]. As a result, DNA integrity of smokers declines significantly. One study of 160 fertile men found a near doubling (5.8% vs 10.8%, $p < 0.05$) of DNA fragmentation of nonsmokers compared to smokers [26].

Not only are smokers exposed to greater oxidative stress, but they also have a diminished ability to repair base adducts that form as a consequence. Tobacco smoke serves as one of the principle routes for ingestion of cadmium [6]. Base adducts are repaired through the base excision repair pathway, which begins in the sperm with removal of the damaged base by the enzyme OGG1. Completion of this type of DNA repair mechanism only ensues after fertilization. Oocytes carry the next critical enzyme, APE1, which is not otherwise present in spermatozoa. Conversely, OGG1 is not expressed within oocytes, and so sperm must contribute this enzyme to the embryo. Cadmium inhibits the activity of OGG1, thereby inhibiting the base excision repair pathway that an embryo must rely upon [6]. Disruption of the base excision repair process is one possible explanation for why pre-conception paternal smoking, and not maternal smoking status, increases the risk of childhood cancer in resulting offspring [6].

17.4.2   Varicocele

The association between a palpable dilation of the pampiniform plexus and male subfertility is longstanding. Only recently, however, have investigators begun to link varicoceles to oxidative stress, DNA damage, and poor chromatin packaging [27]. In an early meta-analysis by Agarwal and colleagues, the presence of varicocele mediated infertility was strongly correlated with increased seminal ROS and a concomitant decrease in total antioxidant capacity [28]. These observations carried forward in studies assessing DNA damage in men with subfertility and a coexisting varicocele, a relationship that appears to correlate with clinical grade. In a pooled analysis that encompassed 12 studies, Wang and colleagues found that men with a varicocele had a 9.8% (CI 9.2–10.5) higher level of DNA fragmentation [29]. Their review also assessed the benefit of varicocele repair, which resulted in a 3.4% (CI 2.7–4.1) decrease in fragmentation rates.

It is apparent that varicocelectomy modestly improves genomic integrity, although it should be acknowledged that post-procedure these men continue to have higher rates of DNA damage as compared to controls [27]. The clinical value of varicocele repair for the indication of sperm DNA fragmentation is therefore limited, especially considering the substantial advantages afforded by IVF and ICSI. A role for varicocele repair does exist for couples who desire natural conception, as varicocelectomy will provide one means to optimize the male's reproductive potential.

17.4.3   Post-Testicular Factors

The use of testicular sperm in lieu of ejaculated samples is an emerging and controversial option for men with elevated DFI. The rationale for this treatment is based upon the belief that sperm will accrue genomic damage as a result of oxidative stress in the seminiferous tubules and epididymis. The principle exogenous sources of ROS in the male genital tract include nonviable spermatozoa that are in the process of apoptosis, an epididymal epithelium under stress and, if present in the epididymis, leukocytes responding to inflammation/infection. Two recent meta-analyses have addressed the utilization of testicular sperm in this setting. In the first, Esteves and colleagues pooled the data for men who were either oligozoospermic or normozoospermic with a history of recurrent ICSI failure [30]. All men included in the analysis had elevated DFI. Their results revealed a lower DNA fragmentation rate in testicular sperm than for ejaculated sperm, 8.9% versus 33.4% ($p < 0.0001$). Testicular-derived sperm yielded higher clinical pregnancy rates (OR 2.42, CI 1.57–3.73), live birth rates (OR 2.58, CI 1.5–4.35), and a lower occurrence of pregnancy loss (OR 0.28, CI 0.11–0.68) [30]. There was significant heterogeneity among the studies, which included differing assay types for DNA damage and inconsistent reporting of potential confounders (e.g. female factors).

Abhyankar and colleagues conducted a similar meta-analysis but restricted their review to studies that encompassed cryptozoospermic men [31]. Given the technical difficulty of performing genetic integrity testing on rare ejaculated sperm, the studies included by Abhyankar did not restrict patient selection based upon pre-operative DNA fragmentation testing. In this analysis of men with unknown sperm DNA damage, no clinical meaningful improvement was found using testicular sperm over ejaculated [31]. The discrepancy between Abhyankar and Esteves may be due to patient selection, whereas Esteves only included men with known elevated DFI, and therefore would be predicted to benefit from the use of testicular sperm [30,31]. Overall, the data grouped in these two meta-analyses were derived from observational studies with significant limitations. Given the procedural risks of obtaining testicular sperm, in addition to the theoretical risk of higher sperm aneuploidy, further work is needed to clarify the benefits of testicular sperm, which patient criteria will serve as indications, and if there is any additional risk to the offspring [1].

17.5 Conclusions

The demands required for delivery of the male genome to the oocyte has produced a cell type with a unique set of characteristics. The consequences of spermatozoon physiology results in a truncated and altered form of apoptosis, an ROS-dependent process for capacitation, and a form of DNA compaction that deviates from all other somatic cell lines. The interplay of sperm production, storage, and function produces inevitable DNA damage that is present in all spermatozoa. Current evidence points to oxidative stress as the principle mediator of DNA fragmentation in the male germ line. The embryo compensates for this defect with a robust mechanism of DNA repair. However, the embryo cannot overcome dramatic levels of paternal DNA damage. Elevated sperm DNA fragmentation results in a longer time to pregnancy among natural pregnancy planners, impaired IUI outcomes, and decreased pregnancy rates for standard IVF. ICSI appears to overcome many of the negative consequences associated with sperm DNA damage, possibly due to a favorable selection bias when sperm are chosen for injection. Unfortunately, it is apparent that ICSI is still affected by an impaired male genome as evidenced by an increased rate of pregnancy loss. Additionally, the downstream health outcomes for offspring produced by ICSI in men with elevated sperm DNA fragmentation have yet to be established.

Despite the body of evidence supporting the role of sperm DNA fragmentation in human reproduction, the field has been slow to adopt the technology due to lacking assay standardization, unclear normal thresholds, and inconsistent study results. To improve the clinical utility of sperm DNA testing, standardized assays must be created that also provide a dynamic range capable of matching the distribution of DNA damage that will exist in a population of spermatozoa. Only once these critical hurtles have been addressed will sperm DNA testing become a practical and necessary adjunct to the traditional semen analysis.

Acknowledgments

Salary support provided by Frederick J. and Theresa Dow Wallace Fund of the New York Community Trust, Mr. Robert S. Dow Foundation, and the Irena and Howard Laks Foundation.

References

1. Ramasamy, R., Besada, S. and Lamb, D. J. (2014) Fluorescent *in situ* hybridization of human sperm: diagnostics, indications, and therapeutic implications. *Fertil Steril* **102**:1534–1539.

2. Ramasamy, R., Scovell, J. M., Kovac, J. R., Cook, P. J., Lamb, D. J. and Lipshultz, L. I. (2015) Fluorescence *in situ* hybridization detects increased sperm aneuploidy in men with recurrent pregnancy loss. *Fertil Steril* **103**:906–909.e901.

3. Gonzalez-Marin, C., Gosalvez, J. and Roy, R. (2012) Types, causes, detection and repair of DNA fragmentation in animal and human sperm cells. *Int J Mol Sci* **13**:14026–14052.

4. De Iuliis, G. N., Thomson, L. K., Mitchell, L. A., Finnie, J. M., Koppers, A. J., Hedges, A., et al. (2009) DNA damage in human spermatozoa is highly correlated with the efficiency of chromatin remodeling and the formation of 8-hydroxy-2'-deoxyguanosine, a marker of oxidative stress. *Biol Reprod* **81**:517–524.

5. Gunes, S., Al-Sadaan, M. and Agarwal, A. (2015) Spermatogenesis, DNA damage and DNA repair mechanisms in male infertility. *Reprod Biomed Online* **31**:309–319.

6. Aitken, R. J., Smith, T. B., Jobling, M. S., Baker, M. A. and De Iuliis, G. N. (2014) Oxidative stress and male reproductive health. *Asian J Androl* **16**:31–38.

7. Bell, E. L., Nagamori, I., Williams, E. O., Del Rosario, A. M., Bryson, B. D. and Watson, N., et al. (2014) SirT1 is required in the male germ cell for differentiation and fecundity in mice. *Development (Cambridge, UK)* **141**:3495–3504.

8. Zhang, X., San Gabriel, M. and Zini, A. (2006) Sperm nuclear histone to protamine ratio in fertile and infertile men: evidence of heterogeneous subpopulations of spermatozoa in the ejaculate. *J Androl* **27**:414–420.

9. Simon, L., Emery, B. R. and Carrell, D. T. (2017a) Review: diagnosis and impact of sperm DNA alterations in assisted reproduction. *Best Pract Res Clin Obstet Gyn* **44**:38–56.

10. Simon, L., Zini, A., Dyachenko, A., Ciampi, A. and Carrell, D. T. (2017b) A systematic review and meta-analysis to determine the effect of sperm DNA damage on *in vitro* fertilization and intracytoplasmic sperm injection outcome. *Asian J Androl* **19**:80–90.

11. Aitken, R. J. and Baker, M. A. (2013) Causes and consequences of apoptosis in spermatozoa; contributions to infertility and impacts on development. *Int J Devel Biol* **57**:265–272.

12. Aitken, R. J., Baker, M. A. and Nixon, B. (2015) Are sperm capacitation and apoptosis the opposite ends of a continuum driven by oxidative stress? *Asian J Androl* **17**:633–639.

13. Bui, A. D., Sharma, R., Henkel, R. and Agarwal, A. (2018) Reactive oxygen species impact on sperm DNA and its role in male infertility. *Andrologia* **2018**:e13012.

14. Aitken, R. J., Gordon, E., Harkiss, D., Twigg, J. P., Milne, P., Jennings, Z., et al. (1998) Relative impact of oxidative stress on the functional competence and genomic integrity of human spermatozoa. *Biol Reprod* **59**:1037–1046.

15. Aitken, R. J., Gibb, Z., Baker, M. A., Drevet, J. and Gharagozloo, P. (2016) Causes and consequences of oxidative stress in spermatozoa. *Reprod Fertil Devel* **28**:1–10.

16. Koppers, A. J., Garg, M. L. and Aitken, R. J. (2010) Stimulation of mitochondrial reactive oxygen species production by unesterified, unsaturated fatty acids in defective human spermatozoa. *Free Rad Biol Med* **48**:112–119.

17. Bach, P. V. and Schlegel, P. N. (2016) Sperm DNA damage and its role in IVF and ICSI. *Basic Clin Androl* **26**:15.

18. ASRM (2013) The clinical utility of sperm DNA integrity testing: a guideline. *Fertil Steril* **99**:673–677.

19. Fernandez-Gonzalez, R., Moreira, P. N., Perez-Crespo, M., Sanchez-Martin, M., Ramirez, M. A. and Pericuesta, E., et al. (2008) Long-term effects of mouse intracytoplasmic sperm injection with DNA-fragmented sperm on health and behavior of adult offspring. *Biol Reprod* **78**:761–772.

20. Burruel, V., Klooster, K. L., Chitwood, J., Ross, P. J. and Meyers, S. A. (2013) Oxidative damage to rhesus macaque spermatozoa results in mitotic arrest and transcript abundance changes in early embryos. *Biol Reprod* **89**:72.

21. Evenson, D. P. and Wixon, R. (2008) Data analysis of two *in vivo* fertility studies using Sperm Chromatin Structure Assay-derived DNA fragmentation index vs. pregnancy outcome. *Fertil Steril* **90**:1229–1231.

22. Bungum, M., Humaidan, P., Axmon, A., Spano, M., Bungum, L., Erenpreiss, J., et al. (2007) Sperm DNA integrity assessment in prediction of assisted reproduction technology outcome. *Hum Reprod (Oxford, UK)* **22**: 174–179.

23. Osman, A., Alsomait, H., Seshadri, S., El-Toukhy, T. and Khalaf, Y. (2015) The effect of sperm DNA fragmentation on live birth rate after IVF or ICSI: a systematic review and meta-analysis. *Reprod Biomed Online* **30**:120–127.

24. Zhao, J., Zhang, Q., Wang, Y. and Li, Y. (2014) Whether sperm deoxyribonucleic acid fragmentation has an effect on pregnancy and miscarriage after *in vitro* fertilization/intracytoplasmic sperm injection: a systematic review and meta-analysis. *Fertil Steril* **102**:998–1005. e1008.

25. Wright, C., Milne, S. and Leeson, H. (2014) Sperm DNA damage caused by oxidative stress: modifiable clinical, lifestyle and nutritional factors in male infertility. *Reprod Biomed Online* **28**:684–703.

26. Taha, E. A., Ez-Aldin, A. M., Sayed, S. K., Ghandour, N. M. and Mostafa, T. (2012) Effect of smoking on sperm vitality, DNA integrity, seminal oxidative stress, zinc in fertile men. *Urology* **80**:822–825.

27. Roque, M. and Esteves, S. C. (2018) Effect of varicocele repair on sperm DNA fragmentation: a review. *Int Urol Nephrol* **50**:583–603.

28. Agarwal, A., Prabakaran, S. and Allamaneni, S. S. (2006) Relationship between oxidative stress, varicocele and infertility: a meta-analysis. *Reprod Biomed Online* **12**:630–633.

29. Wang, Y. J., Zhang, R. Q., Lin, Y. J., Zhang, R. G. and Zhang, W. L. (2012) Relationship between varicocele and sperm DNA damage and the effect of varicocele repair: a meta-analysis. *Reprod Biomed Online* **25**:307–314.

30. Esteves, S. C., Roque, M., Bradley, C. K. and Garrido, N. (2017) Reproductive outcomes of testicular versus ejaculated sperm for intracytoplasmic sperm injection among men with high levels of DNA fragmentation in semen: systematic review and meta-analysis. *Fertil Steril* **108**:456–467.e451.

31. Abhyankar, N., Kathrins, M. and Niederberger, C. (2016) Use of testicular versus ejaculated sperm for intracytoplasmic sperm injection among men with cryptozoospermia: a meta-analysis. *Fertil Steril;***105**: 1469–1475. e1461.

Chapter 18

Prevention of Male Infertility: From Childhood to Adulthood

Alberto Ferlin

18.1 Introduction and General Remarks on the Importance of Andrological Prevention

Sexual and reproductive health is a fundamental part of a person's health and wellbeing and it is defined by the World Health Organization (WHO) as a state of complete physical, mental and social wellbeing in all matters relating to the reproductive system. Importantly, it implies also that people should be able to have a satisfying and safe sex life and they should maintain sexual and reproductive health during their entire life. Reproductive health has emerged as an important healthcare need involving many clinical and public health issues, including sexually transmitted infections (STIs), declining fertility and rising rates of testicular cancer [1–4]. Importantly, it is now recognized that many causes and risk factors for testicular dysfunction and infertility indeed act early during life [5]. Many andrological pathologies that we see in adults actually arise at a younger age, due to the strong susceptibility and vulnerability of the male gonad to external insults, starting from gestation age and during all growth phases.

Three main phases of a man's life are particularly susceptible for subsequent normal testis development and function (Table 18.1, Figure 18.1): the intrauterine phase, the neonatal phase comprising the so-called "minipuberty" in the first months of life, and puberty. However, even during infancy, when the testes are apparently "sleeping," damaging causes with permanent effects on testicular function can occur. This is, for example, the case of the iatrogenic, devastating effect of chemotherapy in this period of the life. Risk factors acting via the mother during pregnancy might compromise definitively testicular function later in life, by disrupting foetal germ cell proliferation and differentiation, Sertoli

Table 18.1 Critical vulnerability phases of male gonadal development and subsequent function

Phase	Major external (non-congenital) risk factors of subsequent testicular function
Intrauterine	Environmental toxic agents, endocrine disruptors, maternal factors (diabetes, smoking, alcohol)
Neonatal	Lack of minipuberty
Childhood	Overweight/obesity, lifestyle behaviour (diet, physical exercise), chemo/radiotherapy, varicocele, testicular trauma/torsion/orchitis
Puberty	Overweight/obesity, lifestyle behaviour (diet, physical exercise, smoking, alcohol, drug abuse, steroid abuse), sexual behaviour, STIs, chemo/radiotherapy, varicocele, testicular trauma/torsion/orchitis

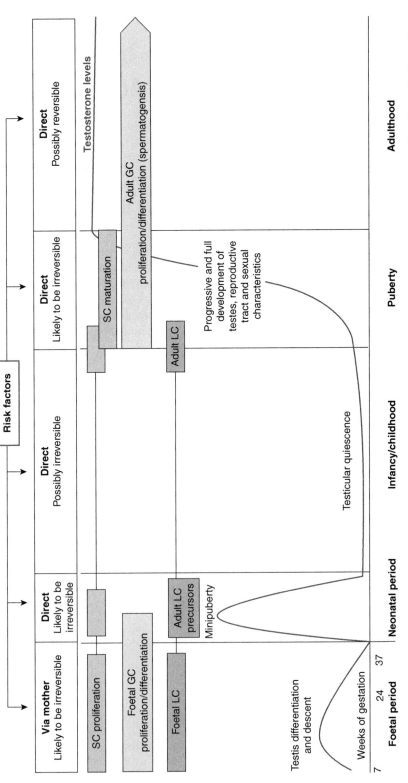

Figure 18.1 Effect of risk factors for testicular development and function from the foetal period to adulthood. SC: Sertoli cells; GC: germ cells; LC: Leydig cells. Modified from (6).

Table 18.2 Risk factors for infertility (and general testicular function) that might have negative effects from gestation to puberty

Environmental toxic agents, endocrine disruptors during pregnancy

Maternal factors (diabetes, smoking, alcohol)

Cryptorchidism

Known genetic factors (e.g. karyotype anomalies, cystic fibrosis, thalassemia)

Iatrogenic causes (pelvic and inguinal surgery, chemotherapy, radiotherapy, medications)

Systemic diseases and/or endocrine diseases (e.g. diabetes mellitus, renal diseases, hepatic disease)

Overweight/obesity

Testicular trauma

Testicular torsion

Orchitis

Varicocele

Cigarette smoking

Alcohol and substances of abuse

Steroid abuse

Sexually transmitted infections

Environmental exposition

cell proliferation and establishing of the Leydig cell population (Figure 18.1). Similarly, risk factors acting directly on minipuberty might compromise germ, Sertoli and Leydig cell differentiation and proliferation. Iatrogenic, environmental and lifestyle risk factors during childhood might interfere above all with the germ cell compartment and those acting during puberty might disrupt Sertoli cell maturation, the establishment of adult Leydig cell population and spermatogenesis (Figure 18.1) [5,6].

Apart from the intrauterine phase, childhood and adolescence therefore represent key times and windows of vulnerability in which andrological prevention and early risk factor detection could take place, including: (i) correct management of pathologies of the reproductive tract (e.g. cryptorchidism, varicocele); (ii) early detection of causes and risk factors of subsequent infertility (e.g. testicular hypotrophy, Klinefelter syndrome, obesity); and (iii) identification and information on health risk behaviours and lifestyles that might compromise future fertility and testicular function (e.g. alcohol, tobacco use, drug abuse and unprotected sex) (Table 18.2) [7].

Adolescence in particular is considered a vulnerable time for the development and maturation of the genitourinary tract [8]. Risk factors and lifestyles adopted in adolescence may negatively affect adult health as well as that of future generations, through epigenetics. Prevention is the most efficacious way of improving sexual and reproductive health, as further confirmed by the high prevalence of undiagnosed (and hence untreated) andrological disorders. Indeed, the US Center for Disease Control and Prevention (CDC) Healthy 2020 Objectives identified several targets relevant to adolescents, focusing on weight, substance use and abuse, smoking and sexual and reproductive health [9]. According to

Table 18.3 Estimates of risk for subsequent infertility for the major risk factors when present in pre-pubertal and adolescent age

Risk factor	Probability of infertility
Cryptorchidism (corrected)	30–40%
Testicular hypotrophy (<12 ml at the end of puberty)	60–80%
Klinefelter syndrome	90–100%
Chemo-radiotherapy	70–80%
Orchitis/testicular torsion/testicular trauma	20–30%
Varicocele	30–40%
Sexually transmitted diseases	20–30%
Overweight/obesity	30–40%
Smoking, alcohol, drug abuse	20–30%
Steroid abuse	50–60%

the WHO's 2004 Global Burden of Disease study, the main risk factors for incident disability adjusted life year (DALYs) in 10–24-year-olds are alcohol (7% of DALYs), unprotected sex (4%), lack of contraception (2%) and illicit drug use (2%) [10].

Prevention of future infertility should therefore pass through information and modification of bad lifestyles during childhood and adolescence, although definite risks are not easily defined (Table 18.3). For example, contrasting data exist regarding smoking and male fertility, the association between marijuana use and non-seminoma testicular germ cell tumours needs to be confirmed, and late effects on fertility of alcohol consumption are not clear. Indeed, some lifestyles are clearly associated with reproductive fitness and wellness [5,13]. This is the example of steroid abuse, as recently stated by the Endocrine Society [14]. About 2% of American high school students reported having used anabolic agents abuse in the previous months [14], and the detrimental effect of them on the endocrine function of the testis and spermatogenesis is well documented. The WHO estimates that adolescent alcohol abuse is increasingly widespread [10]. Binge drinking is common in this age group and is associated with reduced testosterone levels [15]. *In vivo* and *in vitro* studies showed that excessive alcohol intake suppresses the hypothalamic-pituitary-gonadal axis [16]. Importantly, in adolescents, even moderate alcohol consumption impairs pubertal development and testicular endocrine function far beyond the period of consumption [17]. Recent data also suggest that substance abuse, particularly alcohol, during adolescence is associated with impaired testicular volumetric development.

Another area of concern is related to the possible consequences on reproductive fitness and wellness of sexually transmitted infections (STIs) and diseases (STDs) during adolescence [18]. STIs represent one of the most important risk factors able to impair sexual and reproductive health, but the exact effect later in life is not well known, although predictable. Professionals in reproductive medicine should disseminate the information and be committed to appropriate studies on STIs and STDs. As reported by the WHO, about 357 million treatable STDs are detected worldwide each year, and in most countries the prevalence of STDs has increased in recent years. The prevention of STDs is at the centre of health policy guidelines worldwide, in order to halt the spread of infection.

Among STIs, human papillomavirus (HPV) is one of the most prevalent and has become a major source of morbidity and mortality worldwide. Unfortunately, the research focus has been exclusively on women for too long, but men are also affected. Indeed, the prevalence and consequences of HPV infection in males are not negligible and men might be carriers of continuous HPV transmission among sexually active couples. Furthermore, HPV infections usually clear without intervention in most cases, but can cause long-term consequences and, most importantly, might compromise the couple's fertility [19]. However, most studies of HPV have analysed diagnosis, treatment and prevention in women. Moreover, strategies in sexual and reproductive health programmes in many countries have focused on epidemiological control in women, but they have tended to overlook the role of this infection in men, despite its high prevalence. The same is true for HPV vaccination [20]. In fact, men may constitute a reservoir for inadvertently transmitting infection to women, due to its asymptomatic nature in most cases, thus contributing to the persistence of infection and cancer.

Finally, we should bear in mind that health risk behaviours could worsen the reproductive potential in boys with andrological disorders (undescended testes, varicocele, genetic disorders). Therefore, great effort should be done to promote primary and secondary prevention in this period of life. Preventive interventions could improve the chance of healthy development [21]. Greater attention to the importance of andrological health in adolescence is needed and strategies that place the adolescent years at centre stage could offer valuable opportunities to improve fertility later in life.

We will now examine specific strategies for early detection, management and follow-up of some classic causes of infertility that can occur early in life to minimize their negative consequences on the reproductive system: undescended testes, varicocele, Klinefelter syndrome, obesity, sexually transmitted infections and diseases, health risk behaviours and abuse of substances (Table 18.4).

18.2 Prevention and Management of Defects of Testicular Descent and Their Consequences on Testicular Function

Cryptorchidism affects 3–5% of term infants and 9–30% of preterm infants. Spontaneous testicular descent in the first months of life occurs in about 50% of term infants, with a 1.5% prevalence at age one year, whereas it is more frequent in preterm infants with a 7% prevalence at age one year. The incidence of undescended testes is increasing, possibly due to *in utero* exposure to oestrogenic or anti-androgenic endocrine disruptors [22]. Long-term sequelae of cryptorchidism include infertility, hypogonadism and testicular cancer [22], therefore appropriate follow-up programmes should be offered to these subjects.

The prevention of cryptorchidism and other defects of testicular descent is limited to removal, when possible, of known risk factors, such as low birth weight, small for gestational age (SGA), and maternal factors such as gestational diabetes, smoking, alcohol, caffeine, and exposure to endocrine disruptors (e.g. phthalates, pesticides, herbicides, PDEs) [5]. Other possible areas of prevention could be the transmission of genetic factors involved in testicular descent and development (mutations in genes responsible for HH, INSL3, RXFP2, AR, or mutations and chromosomal alterations causing complex genetic syndromes) [22,23].

At birth, testes position should be carefully evaluated by palpation at scrotal, suprascrotal and inguinal level, together with annotation of other genital disorders, in particular hypospadias. If chromosomal and complex genetic syndrome might be suspected, specific

Table 18.4 Andrological stages for management of the most important risk factors for infertility from birth to puberty

	Birth	0–6 months	6–12 months	1–9 years	10–15 years	16–18 years
TESTICULAR DESCENT AND POSITION DEFECTS	Examine position of testes, observe any associated malformations of the urogenital tract and other organs and systems. Genetic analysis in the suspect of Klinefelter syndrome (karyotype). HH (multiple genes) and/or DSD (multiple genes)	Verify spontaneous testes descent. If hypogonadism suspected measure FSH, LH, AMH, inhibin B, testosterone	Orchidopexy if hypogonadism. Suspected measure AMH and inhibin B and perform hCG stimulation test	Annual examination and testicular ultrasound	If hypogonadism suspected measure FSH, LH, testosterone, oestradiol, inhibin B, AMH. Teach testicular self-examination	Semen analysis and eventual cryopreservation
HYPOGONADISM	Check for ambiguous genitalia, micropenis and/or cryptorchidism. If a genetic syndrome is suspected, perform karyotype and specific gene analysis	In the presence of genital abnormalities, measure FSH, LH, testosterone, AMH, inhibin B	If hypogonadism suspected, measure AMH and inhibin B and perform hCG stimulation test. If a genetic syndrome is suspected, perform karyotype and specific gene analysis		Look for absence/delay/arrest of pubertal development, abnormal development of testes and secondary sexual characteristics, eunuchoid body proportions, childlike voice, retarded bone development, asthenia, increased fatty mass, metabolic syndrome. In these cases, measure FSH, LH, testosterone. If a genetic form is suspected, perform karyotype and specific gene analysis	Semen analysis and eventual cryopreservation
KLINEFELTER SYNDROME	Assess micropenis, hypospadias, cryptorchidism. Karyotype if indicated		Check for language problems, attention disorder, difficulty in articulating and managing emotions, judgement and decision-making difficulties, reduced muscle tone and fine motor skills, tremors, difficulty in running, high stature with long lower limbs. Karyotype if indicated. Speech therapy		Monitor timing of start of puberty and pubertal and testicular development. Check for eunuchoid proportions, gynecomastia, testicular atrophy. Karyotype if indicated. Measure FSH, LH, testosterone, oestradiol, SHBG, inhibin B, AMH. Correct diet and physical exercise. Check weight, height, BMI, waist circumference, testicular volume and pubertal stage every 3 months. Assess blood glucose, lipid profile, thyroid function, calcium, phosphorus and vitamin D annually. Prevention of thromboembolic events, early diagnosis of breast cancer and mediastinal germ cell tumours; calcium and vitamin	

	D supplementation; DXA every 2 years. Educate adolescents in infertility risk behaviours (smoking, alcohol, drugs, STD). Answer patients' questions on wellbeing, physical exercise, energy/ sexuality	Semen analysis and eventual cryopreservation and/or TESE
VARICOCELE, HYDROCELE AND TESTICULAR SWELLING	Check for any congenital hydrocele. Wait until age 2 years for possible spontaneous reabsorption, thereafter surgery Physical examination of genitals at each paediatric visit for early diagnosis of any lumps Physical examination of testes while standing and lying down and during Valsalva's manoeuvre; assessment of any lumps and measurement of testicular volume using Prader orchidometer; testicular colour Doppler ultrasound to establish varicocele grade and any testicular asymmetry. For right varicocele, perform ultrasound for early diagnosis of any retroperitoneal mass	
	US-documented testicular asymmetry ≥20% for ≥1 year	Semen analysis and eventual cryopreservation
	Symptomatic patient with progression of asymmetry: surgery	Semen analysis: if pathological, semen cryopreservation and surgery. If normal, annual scrotal US and semen analysis
	Testicular symmetry or US-documented testicular asymmetry <20% for ≥1 year: annual check up to Tanner stage V, then perform semen analysis	Semen analysis. If pathological, semen cryopreservation and surgery. If normal, annual scrotal US and semen analysis
	Subclinical varicocele: annual check up to Tanner stage V, then perform semen analysis	
OVERWEIGHT AND OBESITY	Identify overweight and obese subjects and intervene Periodic measurement of weight, height, BMI, waist circumference, blood pressure, blood glucose, insulin, lipid profile and thyroid function; assess any complications associated with overweight/obesity and monitor timing of start of puberty and pubertal and testicular development (testicular US, FSH, LH, testosterone, oestradiol, SHBG, prolactin, testosterone precursors and hand/wrist X ray to determine bone age) Education in healthy lifestyle (diet, physical exercise)	

Table 18.4 (cont.)

	Birth	0–6 months	6–12 months	1–9 years	10–15 years	16–18 years
SEXUALLY TRANSMITTED INFECTIONS, RISK BEHAVIOURS AND SUBSTANCE USE					Discourage risk behaviours. Sexual education. Discourage smoking, alcohol and drug use. HPV vaccination. Investigate sexual relations, erection, ejaculation. Specific tests if STD suspected. Semen analysis and genital US	Educate in infertility risk behaviours (smoking, alcohol, drugs, STD). Semen analysis

genetic tests should be performed. Testicular position should be regularly checked in the first years of life, both to recognize spontaneous postnatal descent of testes (generally within the first 6 months of age) and to identify acquired cryptorchidism.

Early orchidopexy (1–2 years of age), although reduces the risk for infertility, hypogonadism and testicular cancer, does not completely abolish it, but it represents the ideal treatment [24].

Minipuberty, the period between birth and 6 months, represents an extraordinary window for the diagnosis of endocrine disturbances. In this period, in selected cases with suspicion of very early onset or congenital hypogonadism, hormonal assessment with determination of FSH, LH, testosterone, AMH and inhibin B could be performed. Thereafter, and until the onset of puberty, the only endocrine assessment that could be performed for early detection of hypogonadism secondary to cryptorchidism is limited to AMH and inhibin B determination and hCG stimulation test.

Ex-cryptorchid subjects should be carefully and regularly followed up during pubertal development to identify possible disorders in pubertal and testicular development involving both the spermatogenic and hormonal compartments. Testicular volumes, Tanner stages, growth curves, hormonal determinations (FSH, LH, testosterone), as well as scrotal ultrasound (US), should be monitored. Semen analysis should be considered in ex-cryptorchid subjects, ideally when Tanner V is reached, and eventual semen cryopreservation should be offered whenever abnormal findings are present and progression of testicular damage is conceivable.

In any case, andrological follow-up with physical examination, semen analysis, scrotal ultrasound and hormonal (FSH, LH, testosterone) determination should be annually offered to ex-cryptorchid patients. Furthermore, patients and parents should be informed and educated on testicular self-examination.

18.3 Prevention of Consequences on Testicular Function caused by Varicocele

Varicocele is not infrequent in prepubertal boys, but unfortunately it is frequently not recognized or it is misdiagnosed. Indeed, varicocele could be a risk factor for future fertility and testicular function. The prevalence of varicocele is about 3% in boys at Tanner stage 1 (<10 years), it increases to 3–7% in boys at Tanner stages II–IV (11–14 years), and to 15% in boys at Tanner stage V (>15 years) [25,26].

Debate still exists to identify clear prognostic factors influencing testicular development and long-term consequences of prepubertal varicocele, as not all cases should be treated [27]. On the other hand, evidence suggests that, if treatment is indicated, early varicocelectomy has better long-term effects than postponing treatment later [27].

During regular paediatric visits, physical examination of testes while standing and lying down and during Valsalva's manoeuvre should be performed. If varicocele is suspected, measurement of testicular volume using a Prader orchidometer and, better still, by testicular colour Doppler US is a key factor to identify those subjects who best will benefit from treatment. Colour Doppler US is necessary to establish varicocele grade and better identify any testicular asymmetry, which represents a fundamental parameter in selecting subjects who are candidates for varicocelectomy.

Based on current evidence, varicocelectomy is suggested when the US-documented testicular asymmetry is over 20% and lasting for more than one year or in symptomatic patient with progression of asymmetry. Varicocelectomy in these patients is particularly recommended when semen analysis shows alterations, whereas repeated semen analyses in the normal range could indicate strict follow-up by scrotal US and semen test. On the contrary, when both testes have similar volumes or the US-documented testicular asymmetry is less than 20% for more than one year, it is suggested to annually check up to Tanner stage V, then performing semen analysis in order to decide whether varicocelectomy is necessary. Subclinical varicocele might be followed up annually up to Tanner stage V, then performing semen analysis. In any case, it is suggested that semen analysis is performed at 16–18 years (Tanner V): if pathological, semen cryopreservation and surgery are indicated, whereas a normal finding could suggest just to follow up the patient with annual scrotal US and semen analysis.

18.4 Management of Klinefelter Syndrome and Prevention of Its Consequences on Testicular Function

Klinefelter syndrome (KS) is the most common sex chromosome disorder, with a prevalence in 1:600 new born males. It is characterized by an excessive number of X chromosomes, with the most frequent karyotype observed represented by 47, XXY [28,29]. Although the clinical picture is extremely variable, KS is the most frequent chromosomal disorder found in infertile males. Only about 10% of adult KS have few sperm in the ejaculate, the remaining 90% being azoospermic. In these latter cases however, sperm can be retrieved by testicular sperm extraction (TESE) in 40–50% [30]. KS subjects are at increased risk for metabolic alterations (glucose and lipid metabolism), obesity, osteoporosis, and CVD, due to a combination of low testosterone and genetic factors linked to the extra X chromosome [29]. The timing of start of puberty is generally regular in these subjects, but then an arrest of progression with testicular atrophy is observed [28]. It is therefore fundamental to correctly manage KS subjects when diagnosis is made prenatally (actually 5–10% of cases), and to pay attention to symptoms and signs suggestive of KS from birth onwards in order to make an early diagnosis, bearing in mind that there are no clinical hallmarks typical for this syndrome and the phenotype is extremely variable [31].

At birth, micropenis, hypospadias and cryptorchidism are the only signs that could be associated with KS (20–30% of cases), whereas during infancy the symptoms that could prompt to suspect KS are linked to neuropsychological problems that are present in variable frequency and sometimes associated with high stature with long lower limbs, language and learning problems, attention disorder, difficulty in articulating and managing emotions, judgement and decision-making difficulties, reduced muscle tone and fine motor skills, tremors, difficulty in running, etc. [28,29].

Most frequently, KS is diagnosed during pubertal development, because at mid-puberty an arrest of testicular development might be observed together with eunuchoid proportions, gynecomastia and increased levels of gonadotropins with testosterone levels in the mid-low range [28,29]. When KS is diagnosed, the clinical work up should include the general measures highlighted in Table 18.4 and fertility management should consider semen analysis with eventual cryopreservation or TESE in azoospermic men [30,31]. The timing of fertility evaluation is dependent on different variables, including psychological and familial aspects. Testosterone treatment could then be necessary to complete pubertal development and prevent clinical sequelae caused by hypogonadism.

18.5 Management of Overweight/Obesity in Children and Prevention of Its Consequences on Testicular Function

It is well known that overweight and obesity represent an important risk factor for infertility and endocrine testicular function. Childhood obesity is continuously increasing in incidence and the effect of increased fat mass on pubertal and testicular development is serious [32]. It is therefore necessary to pay attention to children with overweight/obesity and correctly intervene (mainly by life style modifications) to prevent the transition from an obese child to an obese adult [33]. Periodic measurement of anthropometric and metabolic data is recommended, as well as the monitoring of timing of start of puberty and pubertal and testicular development. Early (at the end of puberty) semen analysis is recommended for early detection of possible fertility problems, together with endocrine assessment of reproductive hormones. Transition to adult endocrinologist/andrologist is suggested in order to have a regular follow-up of these patients by semen analysis, scrotal ultrasound and endocrine assessment.

18.6 Information and Prevention of Sexually Transmitted Infections and Their Consequences on Reproductive Health

As reported by the WHO, STIs and STDs show an increasing incidence, especially in the under-25 age group: 1 adolescent in 20 contracts a treatable STI every year and almost half of the 19 million cases of STI diagnosed every year in the United States affect adults aged 19–24 years.

A number of risk behaviours (practices and factors encouraging the spread of STIs) can be mentioned and should constitute the core for information programmes from Health Agencies [34]: unprotected sex, multiple sexual partners, relations with a partner who has multiple sexual partners, poor awareness of STIs, difficulty in accessing mechanical (barrier) contraceptives, younger age of first sexual relations, poor intimate hygiene, use of inadequately cleaned facilities (public toilets, gyms, swimming pools, etc.), sharing of towels used for intimate hygiene, tendency to self-diagnose and self-treat, drug use, smoking and alcohol.

Other than primary prevention, early detection and treatment of STIs and STDs are crucial to minimize the negative effects on the reproductive system. Therefore, adolescents should be regularly seen and interrogated regarding the mentioned sexual behaviours to identify at-risk subjects. Physical examination and laboratory analyses (microbiological and viral test on urine, semen, urethral or anal swab, Stamey test) should be done to have a correct diagnosis. Furthermore, subjects with STI/STD diagnosis should undergo semen analysis and reproductive tract ultrasound for early detection of reduced fertility potential. In cases of irreversible damage of the testes/reproductive tract with obstructive and/or non-obstructive azo-oligozoospermia, semen cryopreservation and/or TESE seem reasonable.

Finally, an important part of prevention could come from the correct application of a vaccination programme for HPV in those countries where it is offered to male adolescents in addition to females [20].

18.7 Conclusion

Prevention screening and early diagnosis programmes in the andrological and reproductive sciences are not developed as for other areas of medicine, although differences

Table 18.5 Proposed timetable, interventions and personnel involved for the correct identification and management of andrological diseases and risk factors for infertility

Age	Interventions	Involved personnel	Main pathologies/risk factors
Birth	• Testes position and genital appearance, distinguishing the different forms of anomalies of testis descent and position, evaluating associated malformations for possible DSD • Congenital penile anomalies, including micropenis and hypospadias • Register gestational age, weight at birth, SGA • Register possible maternal factors (diabetes, endocrine disruptors, drugs) • Consider genetic analysis in the suspect of Klinefelter syndrome (karyotype), HH (multiple genes) and/or DSD (multiple genes) • Counselling to parents	• Paediatrician/paediatric endocrinologist • Surgeon/paediatric urologist • Geneticist • Parents	• Cryptorchidism • DSD • Congenital penis malformation/hypospadias • Congenital hypogonadism • Klinefelter syndrome
0–6 months	• Window period to diagnose congenital hypogonadism (FSH, LH, testosterone, AMH, inhibin B) • Verify spontaneous testes descent in cases of cryptorchidism at birth and note eventually acquired cryptorchidism	• Paediatrician/paediatric endocrinologist • Geneticist • Parents	• Congenital hypogonadism
6–12 months	• Verify spontaneous testes descent in cases of cryptorchidism at birth and note eventually acquired cryptorchidism • Consider FSH, LH, testosterone, AMH, hCG-test and surgical exploration in cases of non-palpable testicles • Consider karyotype, mutation analysis for AR, NR5A1 and HH genes or other selected genetic analysis based on clinical suspicion • Programme orchidopexy within 1–2 years of age • Counselling to parents	• Paediatrician/paediatric endocrinologist • Surgeon/paediatric urologist • Geneticist • Family care paediatrician • Parents	• Cryptorchidism • Congenital hypogonadism

Age	Professionals involved	Actions	Conditions
1–2 years	• Family care paediatrician • Parents	• Verify eventual acquired cryptorchidism	• Acquired cryptorchidism
3–5 years	• Paediatric neuropsychiatrist/Speech therapist • Family care paediatrician • Parents	• Pay attention to neuropsychological disturbances for Klinefelter syndrome and eventually perform karyotype analysis • Pay attention to boys with overweight/obesity and intervention • Verify eventual acquired cryptorchidism • Counselling to parents	• Overweight/obesity • Klinefelter syndrome
6–9 years (pre-puberty)	• Family care paediatrician • Parents	• Testes examination in clinostats, orthostatism and during Valsalva manoeuvre • Scrotal ECD in the suspect of varicocele • Pay attention to boys with overweight/obesity and intervention • Growth curves • Identify precocious puberty • Consider AMH and inhibin B (ev. hCG test) whether iatrogenic causes of testicular damage or endocrine diseases are present • Pay attention to symptoms of possible gender dysphoria • Counselling to parents	• Varicocele • Precocious puberty • Overweight/obesity • Gender dysphoria • Iatrogenic causes of testicular damage or endocrine disorders
10–15 years (puberty)	• Paediatrician/paediatric endocrinologist • Family care paediatrician • Surgeon/paediatric urologist • Geneticist	• Timing of onset and development of puberty and testicular growth, with eventual specific analyses • Scrotal ultrasound and colour doppler if suspect varicocele • Consider follow-up vs varicocelectomy and eventual semen analysis	• Varicocele • Pubertal disorders • Gynecomastia • Congenital and acquired hypogonadism • STDs and at risk behaviours

Table 18.5 (cont.)

Age	Interventions	Involved personnel	Main pathologies/risk factors
	• Pay attention to gynecomastia, measure anthropometry and other signs during pubertal development suggesting hypogonadism and/or Klinefelter syndrome	• Patients and parents	• Overweight/obesity
			• Lifestyle potentially damaging
	• Growth curves		• Sexual dysfunction
	• Consider karyotype analysis and genetic analysis for HH in suspicious cases		• Gender dysphoria
			• Klinefelter syndrome
	• Consider endocrine assessment in the suspect of hypogonadism and/or Klinefelter syndrome (LH, FSH, testosterone, oestradiol, inhibin B, AMH and eventually others)		• Iatrogenic causes of testicular damage or endocrine disorders
	• Pay attention to boys with overweight/obesity and intervention		
	• Diagnosis and treatment of precocious and delayed puberty		
	• Pay attention to sexual habit and at risk sex relations (sexual intercourses, masturbation, erection, ejaculation)		
	• Pay attention and information on lifestyle		
	• Pay attention and information on STDs		
	• Pay attention to symptoms of possible gender dysphoria		
	• Information and educating on testis self-examination		
	• Counselling to patients and parents		
16–18 years (late adolescence)	• As previous stage	• Paediatrician/paediatric endocrinologist	• Varicocele
	• Transition to adult endocrinologist/andrologist for evaluation of gonadal function (semen analysis and	• Family care paediatrician	• Pubertal disorders
			• Gynecomastia

eventual semen cryopreservation and specific analyses; scrotal ultrasound and colour doppler; FSH, LH, testosterone; genetic analyses; etc.)

- Surgeon/paediatric urologist
- Geneticist
- Endocrinologist/andrologist
- Psycosexologist
- Patients and parents

- Congenital and acquired hypogonadism
- STD and at risk behaviours
- Overweight/obesity
- Lifestyle potentially damaging
- Sexual dysfunction
- Gender dysphoria
- Klinefelter syndrome
- Iatrogenic causes of testicular damage or endocrine disorders
- Follow up of ex-cryptorchid patients and other pathologies with testicular dysfunction

exist among countries. In many countries, fewer than 5% of young adults (<20 years) has ever undergone an andrological visit and in many cases children and boys become adults without adequate information and counselling regarding risk factors for reproductive and sexual health. On the contrary, females are much more inclined for prevention and early diagnosis and adolescent girls have gynaecological evaluation in much higher percentages. Since a great number of risk factors for future male fertility might already be present in young ages, the possibility for early diagnosis and prevention of negative sequelae is unfortunately low if systematic health and information programmes are lacking. Indeed, interventions focused on childhood, prepubertal boys, as well as during pubertal development, could have a profound effect on sexual and reproductive health later in life. To do this, multiple level interventions are necessary, from politic awareness and national healthcare programmes, to more consciousness of the different health professionals, to information/formation of parents, children and adolescents. Table 18.5 provides an example of a timetable programme for andrological prevention and early detection of diseases and risk factors.

The decline in fertility rates and birth rates in many countries have obviously many causes, in most cases not directly related to medical conditions (i.e. economic, social, politic). Similarly, the continuous increase in assisted reproduction techniques has different justification. However, an intensified prevention (primary, secondary prevention) and correct management and follow-up of andrological disorders and risk factors detected early at young ages could actually improve the reproductive fitness in adulthood.

References

1. Khabbaz, R. F., Moseley, R. R., Steiner, R. J., Levitt, A. M. and Bell, B. P. (2014) Challenges of infectious diseases in the USA. *Lancet* **384**:53–63.

2. Slater, C. and Robinson, A. J. (2014) Sexual health in adolescents. *Clin Dermatol* **32**:189–195.

3. Stephen, E. H., Chandra, A. and King, R. B. (2016) Supply of and demand for assisted reproductive technologies in the United States: clinic- and population-based data, 1995–2010. *Fertil Steril* **105**:451–458.

4. Nigam, M., Aschebrook-Kilfoy, B., Shikanov, S. and Eggener, S. (2015) Increasing incidence of testicular cancer in the United States and Europe between 1992 and 2009. *World J Urol* **33**:623–631.

5. Skakkebaek, N. E., Rajpert-De Meyts, E., Buck Louis, G. M., Toppari, J, Andersson, A. M., Eisenberg, M. L., et al. (2016) Male reproductive disorders and fertility trends: influences of environment and genetic susceptibility. *Physiol Rev* **96**:55–97.

6. Sharpe, R. M. (2010) Environmental/lifestyle effects on spermatogenesis. *Philos Trans R Soc Lond B Biol Sci* **365**:1697–1712.

7. Sawyer, S. M., Afifi, R. A., Bearinger, L. H., et al. (2012) Adolescence: a foundation for future health. *Lancet* **379**:1630–1640.

8. Abreu, A. P. and Kaiser, U. B. (2016) Pubertal development and regulation. *Lancet Diabetes Endocrinol* **4**:254–264.

9. US Department of Health and Human Services (2013) *2020 Topics and Objectives.* www.healthypeople.gov/2020/topics-objectives/topic/Adolescent-Health?topicid=2.

10. Gore, F. M., Bloem, P. J., Patton, G. C., et al. (2011) Global burden of disease in young people aged 10–24 years: a systematic analysis. *Lancet* **377**:2093–2102.

11. Henriksen, T. B., Hjollund, N. H., Jensen, T. K., et al. (2004) Alcohol consumption at the time of conception and spontaneous abortion. *Am J Epidemiol* **160**:661–667.

12. Curtis, K. M., Savitz, D. A. and Arbuckle, T. E. (1997) Effects of cigarette

smoking, caffeine consumption, and alcohol intake on fecundability. *Am J Epidemiol* **146**:32–41.

13. Tournaye, H., Krausz, C. and Oates, R. D. (2017) Concepts in diagnosis and therapy for male reproductive impairment. *Lancet Diabetes Endocrinol* **5**:554–564.

14. Pope, H. G., Jr., Wood, R. I., Rogol, A., Nyberg, F., Bowers, L. and Bhasin, S. (2014) Adverse health consequences of performance-enhancing drugs: an Endocrine Society scientific statement. *Endocr Rev* **35**:341–375.

15. Frias, J., Torres, J. M., Rodriguez, R., Ruiz, E. and Ortega, E. (2000) Effects of acute alcohol intoxication on growth axis in human adolescents of both sexes. *Life Sciences* **67**:2691–2697.

16. Rachdaoui, N. and Sarkar, D. K. (2013) Effects of alcohol on the endocrine system. *Endocrinol Metab Clin N Am* **42**:593–615.

17. Diamond, F., Ringenberg, L., Macdonald, D., et al. (1986) Effects of drug and alcohol-abuse upon pituitary testicular function in adolescent males. *J Adol Health* **7**:28–33.

18. Weinstock, H., Berman, S. and Cates, W., Jr. (2004) Sexually transmitted diseases among American youth: incidence and prevalence estimates, 2000. *Perspect Sex Reprod Health* **36**:6e10.

19. Foresta, C., Noventa, M., De TonI, L., Gizzo, S. and Garolla, A. (2015) HPV-DNA sperm infection and infertility: from a systematic literature review to a possible clinical management proposal. *Andrology* **3**:163–173.

20. Harder, T., Wichmann, O., Klug, S. J., van der Sande, M. A. B. and Wiese-Posselt, M. (2018) Efficacy, effectiveness and safety of vaccination against human papillomavirus in males: a systematic review. *BMC Med* **16**:110.

21. Catalano, R. F., Fagan, A. A., Gavin, L. E., et al. (2012) Worldwide application of prevention science in adolescent health. *Lancet* **379**:1653–1664.

22. Foresta, C., Zuccarello, D., Garolla, A. and Ferlin, A. (2008) Role of hormones, genes, and environment in human cryptorchidism. *Endocr Rev* **29**:560–580.

23. Ferlin, A., Zuccarello, D., Zuccarello, B., Chirico, M. R., Zanon, G. F. and Foresta, C. (2008) Genetic alterations associated with cryptorchidism. *JAMA* **300**:2271–2276.

24. Radmayr, C., Dogan, H. S., Hoebeke, P., Kocvara, R., Nijman, R., Silay, S., et al. (2016) Management of undescended testes: European Association of Urology/European Society for Paediatric Urology Guidelines. *J Pediatr Urol* **12**:335–343.

25. Oster, J. (1971) Varicocele in children and adolescents: an investigation of the incidence among Danish school children. *Scand J Urol Nephrol* **5**:27–32.

26. Zampieri, N. and Cervellione, R. M. (2008) Varicocele in adolescent: a 6-years longitudinal and follow-up observational study. *J Urol* **180**:1653–1656.

27. Silay, M. S., Hoen, L., Quadackaers J., Undre S., Bogaert G., Dogan, H. S., et al. (2019) Treatment of varicocele in children and adolescents: a systematic review and meta-analysis from the European Association of Urology/European Society for Paediatric Urology Guidelines Panel. *Eur Urol* **75**:448–461.

28. Gravholt, C. H., Chang, S., Wallentin, M., Fedder, J., Moore, P. and Skakkebæk, A. (2018) Klinefelter Syndrome: integrating genetics, neuropsychology, and endocrinology. *Endocr Rev* **39**:389–423.

29. Bonomi, M., Rochira, V., Pasquali, D., Balercia, G., Jannini, E. A. and Ferlin, A. (2017) Klinefelter ItaliaN Group (KING). Klinefelter syndrome (KS): genetics, clinical phenotype and hypogonadism. *J Endocrinol Invest* **40**:123–134.

30. Corona, G., Pizzocaro, A., Lanfranco, F., Garolla, A., Pelliccione, F., Vignozzi, L., et al. (2017) Klinefelter ItaliaN Group (KING). Sperm recovery and ICSI outcomes in Klinefelter syndrome: a systematic review and meta-analysis. *Hum Reprod Update* **23**:265–275.

31. Nieschlag, E., Ferlin, A., Gravholt, C. H., Gromoll, J., Köhler, B., Lejeune, H., et al. (2016) The Klinefelter syndrome: current

management and research challenges. *Andrology* **4**:545–549.

32. Ogden, C. L., Carroll, M. D., Kit, D. K. and Flegal, K. M. (2012) Prevalence of obesity and trends in body mass index among US children and adolescents, 1999–2010. *JAMA* **307**:483–490.

33. Berenson, G. S., Srinivasan, S. R., Bao, W., Newman, W. P., 3rd, Tracy, R. E. and Wattigney, W. A. (1998) Association between multiple cardiovascular risk factors and atherosclerosis in children and young adults. The Bogalusa Heart Study. *N Engl J Med* **338**:1650–1656.

34. Centers for Disease Control and Prevention (2012) Youth risk behavior surveillanced United States, 2011. *MMWR Surveill Summ* **61**.

Index